TRANSACTIONS

OF THE

AMERICAN PHILOSOPHICAL SOCIETY

HELD AT PHILADELPHIA
FOR PROMOTING USEFUL KNOWLEDGE

NEW SERIES—VOLUME 44, PART 2
1954

FORGOTTEN LEADERS IN MODERN MEDICINE

Valentin, Gruby, Remak, Auerbach

BRUNO KISCH, M.D.

Professor of Philosophy and History of Science,
Yeshiva University, New York

THE AMERICAN PHILOSOPHICAL SOCIETY
INDEPENDENCE SQUARE
PHILADELPHIA 6

JUNE, 1954

Dedicated to

Ruth Kisch-Arndt

never-failing friend,

great artist,

indefatigable leader in the

propagation of fine music

1928 1953

Library of Congress Catalogue
Card Number: 54-7498

PREFACE

The various *Who's Whos* in medicine and in science contain thousands of names and biographical sketches. The bearer of each of these names may be justly proud to have contributed his share to modern medicine, and to have played a more or less prominent role in the contemporary medical world. But probably not many of them are really aware of the fact that, very shortly after their death, their names will be forgotten. For several years they may still be quoted in certain scientific papers. They may appear occasionally in footnotes of pertinent publications, but finally they will only help to fill the files of our big libraries with cards referring to their books and articles which are no longer read. New generations of teachers and scholars will write new scores of books and articles, and new scores of pupils will buy and read only the latest works on a subject, preferring those written by their own teachers, while the kind, prosperous, and flattering vanity fair of *Who's Who* will go on without harming anybody.

Medicine is only one sector of human life; there are other sectors, such as law, science, philosophy, politics, literature, each of which has its own efficient and comforting *Who's Who*. No one can remember the innumerable and ephemeral celebrities, and certainly no longer than the passing moment when one may have personal contact with them. It is understandable, therefore, that, when a celebrity is no more a living member of the profession, he is forgotten, and rightfully so, except by his family and his friends, who may fondly remember his kindness, helpfulness, and personal charm for a lifetime, quite apart from his scientific importance.

Outstanding among those listed in the *Who's Who* are, for instance, those medical men or scientists who contributed to our knowledge an important and original idea or discovery of lasting value. If the average name in a *Who's Who* deserves from posterity only the type of salute reserved for the unknown soldier, killed in the course of military service, the outstanding men deserve a salute befitting the unknown *officer* in science. Today this is accomplished only inadequately by the various *Who Was Who* collections in literature.

Here begins the justified and valuable work of writing history, especially history of science and medicine. At least the student of medicine, if not every educated man, should know something more than he generally does about those scholars to whom we owe the advancement of our knowledge in medicine and the progress in our struggle to rule the world around us in accordance with the Biblical commandment (Gen. 1: 28) and to help suffering mankind in a kindly, brotherly, and efficient manner. We should know more about the life of those who have changed our points of view and have helped greatly to foster our progress. We should learn about the paths of their progress and the ways of their success, about their obstacles, shortcomings, failures. Finally, we should also learn how their endeavor, if it was for the purpose of expanding our knowledge and not to enhance their personal success only, was never in vain but always contributed to a final success.

When a battle is fought, each soldier's conduct is of importance and a gifted field officer, with vision, courage, and ability to make correct decisions, is often of greater significance for the outcome of the fray than a commanding general.

It is proper that people, after a war is won, worship the leading generals. It is also right and justified that people learn from popular books and motion pictures about the romance of the scientific life of the great heroes in medicine, such as Pasteur, Magendie, Ehrlich. The interested layman and by all means the professional colleague and the scientist should also know about those who made important contributions to science and medicine without being leading generals. In military history, the details of the facts may remain forever forgotten or buried in military archives. In science and medicine, posterity is able to judge the value of past contributions from published papers and on the basis of modern views and knowledge. And this is so, though the achievements of a modest worker may have remained hidden for long years because facts were concealed and his findings were later rediscovered independently by those who came after him. Here lies the important task of an ***honest and unbiased*** historian and here the outstanding value of his research.

The four scholars selected for biographical sketches in this volume are all outstanding pioneers of modern medicine. Their activity begins in the first half of the nineteenth century, that wonderfully great period when experimental and critical science conquered the field of medicine, wrestling it triumphantly from the clutches of the so-called philosophy of nature (*Naturphilosophie*), which especially in Germany was dominant at that time. Today these four are barely known even by name to the profession; certainly no one knows anything about the circumstances of their life. The average physician is not even acquainted with Dr. Gruby, although several biographical sketches have been written about this colorful personality in the last twenty-five years.

The medical heroes to whom this volume is devoted have one more characteristic in common; they all were Jews and, as such, in spite of the enlightening movement of the eighteenth and nineteenth centuries, were prevented by discrimination from employing their talents as fully as they might have done otherwise. Had they accepted baptism, as was suggested to each of them in one way or another, they would have been given great opportunities, but true to themselves and to their religion, they rejected offers made on such a humiliating condition.

The present volume of biographies has by no means an apologetic intention, nor is its aim to show how much these men would have been able to accomplish and to contribute to medicine under more favorable conditions. The purpose is to record, in humble admiration, what they contributed in spite of all obstacles. It is intended to give a portrait of four heroes in medicine who, inspired by an unquenchable thirst for knowledge and an eagerness to help in the development of a better framework for medical science than that which existed in their time, remained to the last days of their lives faithful servants in the realm of research. Each of these idealists was well aware that he would be justly rewarded only by the fruits of his studies. They are the noble prototypes of scientists for science's sake, true philosophers. To prevent their names from vanishing from the annals of medicine and the memory of mankind is the purpose and the aim of this book, entitled *Forgotten Leaders in Modern Medicine.*

The author wishes to acknowledge the helpful cooperation of the various libraries and institutions that supplied him valuable material for this work. Outstanding among these are: the library of the New York Academy of Medicine, New York; the Historical Library of Yale University School of Medicine, New Haven, Connecticut; the library of the Surgeon General, Washington, D. C.; the libraries of Columbia University, New York; the Welch Medical Library of Johns Hopkins University, Baltimore, Maryland; the unique library of the Marine Biological Laboratories in Woods Hole, Massachusetts; the library of Mount Sinai Hospital in New York City; the Archives of the Medical Faculty of the University of Berlin, Germany, where Miss Annemarie Dieterici, secretary of the Faculty, was especially helpful; the University of Wraclaw, Poland, which was good enough to supply the photograph of Leopold Auerbach, nowhere else available; the library of the Royal Swedish Academy of Sciences in Stockholm, where, thanks to the head librarian, Dr. A. Holmberg, five letters and part of a manuscript of Valentin, directed to Professor Retzius, were put at my disposal. Letters and other material of the greatest value concerning G. G. Valentin's life were found in the Archives of the Burger-Bibliothek, Bern, Switzerland, where the kind and very valuable cooperation of Director Hans A. Haeberli and Professor Dr. E. Hintzsche were highly appreciated. Valuable new material concerning David Gruby was supplied by the Vienna Universitäts Bibliothek through the kind offices of Direktionssecretär Dr. Hugo Alker.

FORGOTTEN LEADERS IN MODERN MEDICINE

Bruno Kisch

Vixere Fortes Ante Agamemnona
Multi, Sed Omnes Illacrimabiles
Urgentur, Ignotique Longa
Nocte: Carent Quia Vate Sacro.
Horace, Carminum Lib. IV.
Ode Ad Lollium.*

CONTENTS

* Many heroes lived before Agamemnon. Unwept and unknown are they, covered by endless night, because they did not find a devoted poet.

I. GABRIEL GUSTAV VALENTIN

1810–1883

INTRODUCTION

The development of modern medicine began at the same time as the general revolutionary development that took place in the world in the second half of the eighteenth and the first half of the nineteenth century. This development had different aspects in Europe and in America, but it was marked all over the world by the tendency of singular personalities and entire populations to rid themselves, in every single sector of human life, of the bondage of tradition in so far as this tradition tried to block new, independent, desired developments. Since the time of the Renaissance, the trend has been to gain for the individual the freedom to search for better and more profound knowledge of the material world and to pursue new ways of making life easier, happier, and freer from damage inflicted by other people, by nature itself, and by the unhealthy conditions of the human body.

In the political field such a movement got under way all over Europe at the end of the eighteenth century. In the scientific field it had already begun with Paracelsus in the sixteenth century, but the use of methods of exact research did not usher in a new era in medicine until the eighteenth century. In Italy, G. B. Morgagni (1682–1771) and F. Fontana (1720–1805) were outstanding. They tried to overcome traditional superstition in science and in medicine by exact observation of the facts. In spite of the pioneer work of such men, the romantic attitude of the school of the philosophy of nature (*Naturphilosophie*) was just blooming in Germany in the early part of the nineteenth century. This school attempted to adapt the facts of natural history and medicine to metaphysical systems. Scholars like Goethe, Oken, Hegel, and Schelling, and their followers endeavored to solve problems of science by applying their philosophical systems and poetical intuition to them and by adapting the facts to their own preformed concepts. However, the dominant spirit in the great American and French Revolutions, the spirit of a realistic approach to political situations as well as to all problems of life, could no longer be suppressed in the following centuries. A personage like the leading French physiologist, François Magendie (1783–1855), a contemporary of the congenial F. X. Bichat (1771–1802), was really an outgrowth of the time and the spirit of the French Revolution, of the spirit of admiration for reason, and the disposition to put the facts and their intelligent evaluation above traditional imagination and misinterpretation.

The ideals of Francis Bacon began to penetrate the medical world. Magendie was the true, worthy follower of Morgagni's and Fontana's approach to natural science, creating, together with some of the best clinicians of Paris, a school of modern medicine to preach new aspects in medicine. In England, Charles Bell (1774–1842) and the younger William Bowman (1816–1892) were leaders in the new development. In Germany the great progress in modern medicine started with the work of Johannes Müller (1801–1858), full Professor of Anatomy, Physiology and Pathology in Berlin. Through his position as well as through his outstanding work in anatomy, through his *Handbook of Physiology* and his achievements in comparative zoology, he was the leading representative of Germany's modern physiology. Purkinje (1787–1869) in Breslau was another of these early leaders toward a new way, to objective medicine, and so was his pupil Valentin (1810–1883) in Switzerland. In Vienna it was the pathologist Rokitansky (1804–1878) and the clinician Skoda (1805–

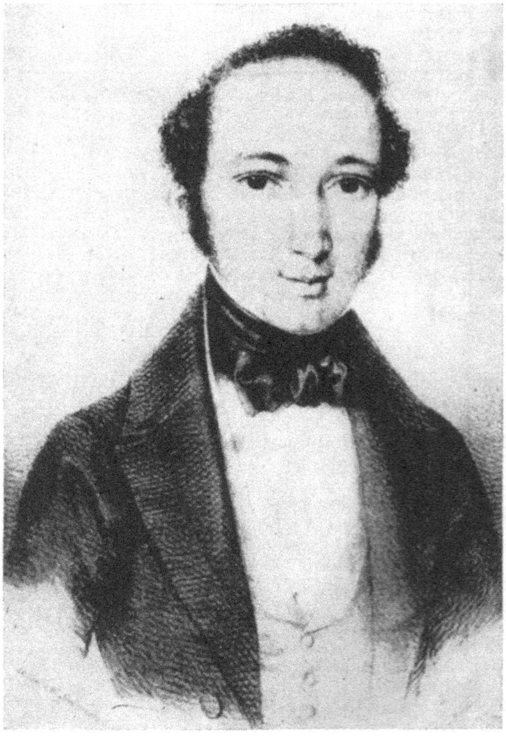

FIG. 1. Valentin's portrait. A lithograph by F. Koska made in the Lithographic Institute of W. Steinmetz in Breslau. The picture was published together with a short biography of Valentin in K. Klein's *Jahrbuch des Nützlichen und Unterhaltenden für Israeliten* **4**: 87, Breslau, J. Urban Kern, 1844–1845.

1881) who, each in his field, were instrumental in building the new framework of medicine as a science.

Around these central figures—Purkinje, Müller, Valentin, and Rokitansky—soon formed schools of gifted young doctors eager to follow the new course of objectivism against the old talkative, philosophical approach to medical problems. Different methods and different instruments, some inherited from former generations—like the microscope—but now developed to undreamed of importance, and some devised by this generation of physicians—like those for the investigation of bioelectricity (DuBois)—were the weapons that soon decided the contest between the new realistic spirit and the old Romanticism.

It was probably the most exciting and most inspiring time in all the history of medicine, the first half of the last century, when almost every day brought fresh fundamental discoveries, many of which became the foundation of new branches of modern medical science. The competition in the large laboratories, like those of Johannes Müller and Purkinje, must have been feverish, as was the competition among the various famous laboratories of France, Germany, Austria, and England. Physically, these laboratories in the first half of the nineteenth century were most modest in appearance but the spirit that prevailed there conquered the world of science.

In the first half of the nineteenth century Paris was still the center of medical knowledge in Europe because of its outstanding scholars and clinicians and because of the activities of its Academy of Sciences. The most prominent scientists and medical men of Germany were happy to be permitted to present the results of their work at the meetings of the Paris Academy. It was the dream of every physician graduated from a German university to spend at least a few months after graduation in Paris, if his means permitted such luxury, in order to learn at the source about the new trends in medicine. Time and again in the first half of the last century German physicians competed for the great awards the Paris Academy of Sciences offered for the best solution to medical problems, and some scholars from Germany, like Valentin and Pappenheim, both pupils of Purkinje, succeeded in capturing the Grand Prix, the highest award of the Academy in a particular field.

The middle of the nineteenth century saw leadership in medicine and science taken over by Germany. Among the many prominent persons to whom we are indebted for widening the horizons of our medical knowledge, the pupils of the great leaders, Johannes Müller and Purkinje, and those of Carl Ludwig played an outstanding role.

Some of these pioneers in physiology and experimental medicine are no less famous in our day than they were at the time when they lived and worked. Among them are François Magendie, Claude Bernard, Johannes Müller, and Hermann Helmholtz. Others, famous in their own time, are today generally known to the members of the medical profession only because a certain fact or organ is connected with their names, for example, Purkinje (Purkinje's fibers in the heart) and E. Hering and L. Traube (Hering-Traube's waves of blood pressure).

It is most surprising, however, that a few of these formerly well-known protagonists in the development of modern experimental medicine should be completely forgotten in our day. This neglect is by no means justified. It may therefore be worth while to revive the memory at least of some of the contributors to our present knowledge who were famous in their time, revered leaders in medicine because of their discoveries as well as their fascinating personalities, their extraordinary insight into problems, and their influence on the younger generation.

Such a man was Gabriel Gustav Valentin.[1]

There is no comprehensive biography of Valentin, and the present endeavor cannot be regarded as exhaustive; it is still only an outline. The available data were collected partly from Valentin's own work and original letters, and partly from references to his personality and his lot in life made by himself and by his personal friends and contemporaries. The information here gathered together was obtained from various sources mainly from the following:

1. Valentin's own publications. A good bibliography up to 1845 is given in Callisen's *Encyclopedia of Medical Authors* (9).[2] Especially noteworthy is his short autobiography contained in his doctoral thesis in 1832 (40).

2. Probably the first biography of Valentin was published in 1845 in the fourth volume of a Jewish Almanac in Breslau (32). My attention was called to this long-forgotten source by Rabbi A. Kober in New York. It is of interest because the author (Neumann), a teacher at the Wilhelm-School in Breslau, was well acquainted with the local details and because the biography is accompanied by a lithograph portrait of young Valentin. The artist was F. Koska of the Lithographic Institute of W. Steinmetz in Breslau. (See fig. 1.)

3. A biographical sketch written by J. Hirschfeld in 1877, when Valentin was still alive (21). This sketch contains personal details that no one but Valentin himself or those nearest to him could have supplied.

---

[1] A preliminary outline of Valentin's biography was published by this author in the Memorial Volume for Victor Robinson, New York, Froben Press, 1948. Some statements made there have been corrected here on the basis of a better knowledge of the facts gained in personally studying the original material concerning Valentin's life in the Archives of the Burger-Bibliothek in Bern.

[2] Numbers in parentheses indicate references at end of chapter, p. 191.

4. A short biographical sketch written in 1889 by J. Graetzer (15), one of Valentin's close friends from his university days.

5. Carl Vogt (64) in his autobiography gives an extremely vivid and interesting description of Valentin's activities in his first years in Bern. During that time Vogt, then a medical student, was an assistant and close collaborator of Valentin.

6. Some data appear in the eulogies of Professor Forster (75) and Professor Grützner (75), the latter being Valentin's successor to the Chair of Physiology in Bern. Both these eulogies were published in 1883, shortly after Valentin's death.

In addition to these and some minor original sources, for instance, a sketch of Valentin's personality in the Berlin journal, *Der Freihafen* (1839), and the autobiography of Ludwig Bamberger (2), there is brief mention of Valentin's life and achievements in some encyclopedias and works on medical history, but these are easily recognizable as merely extracts from one or another of the aforementioned sources.

7. A remark in Gustav Retzius' volume of Johannes Müller's letters to his father made me aware that the entire correspondence of Anders Retzius (1796–1860), the famous anthropologist and anatomist of Stockholm, was preserved in the archives of the Stockholm Royal Academy of Sciences. With the assistance of the head librarian, Dr. A. Holmberg, five of Valentin's letters and part of a manuscript of his of the period from 1833 up to 1846 were found in the library. Photostats of this material were made available and were used in preparing Valentin's life story.

8. The most important and the most authentic source for this biography was the treasure of letters and documents from the possession of Valentin preserved in the Burger Bibliothek of Bern, Switzerland. A part of this material was photostated and will be cited as B.B.B. (Burger Bibliothek Bern) with the number as registered in the archives of this library as Mss.Hist.Helv. XXVIII.

9. Finally, in a second-hand bookshop in Bern four volumes of Valentin's principal publications, apparently his personal copies, were found. They are printed with an especially broad margin that is covered with interesting notes and remarks in Valentin's hand, also some of his notebooks, filled with mathematical calculations and several very interesting letters to Valentin by his friends Vierordt and M. Stern and by Valentin's son Adolf were there acquired.

10. Some interesting material has recently been published by Professor E. Hintzsche (18) in Bern, letters written to Valentin by his famous pupil and friend, Count Alfonso Corti.

With these sources at hand we shall be able to derive a fuller picture of Valentin's life and personality than was possible before.

When this book had already gone to press, a biography of Valentin was published by Erich Hintzsche.* A few facts of this biography, included in this chapter will be referred to as (Hintzsche, 1953).

VALENTIN'S PERSONALITY

All available sources establish that Valentin was prominent as a research worker and as a teacher as well in the fields of embryology, anatomy, physiology, zoology, and even botany. As unusual as such versatility may appear to us, it was not a singular phenomenon in the nineteenth century.

Valentin's books were translated into English, French, Dutch, Italian, and Danish. In his eulogy Professor Forster (75) said of him: "There is no question that he was the most prominent physiologist of his time." And though a eulogy delivered at a funeral usually tends toward benign over-exaggeration, some value must, nevertheless, be attributed to this judgment, for recently even Feller (12: 233), who does not speak very kindly about Valentin's personality, admitted that in 1862 Valentin was one of the most popular teachers of the entire University of Bern. When Valentin retired in 1881, the faculty, in awarding him a pension of 3,000 francs, stated that he had imparted to the Medical School of Bern its highest lustre (12: 331).

Very impressive is the statement of the famous biologist Jacob Moleschott (30) regarding Valentin's influence on the younger generation. In his autobiography Moleschott said: "Valentin's *Handbook of Physiology* opened up for us a new world." Still more fascinating for the young students in Bern than Valentin's handbook was his personality as a teacher. The zoologist and leading German revolutionary politician, Carl Vogt, in his autobiography describes how discouraging were the conditions as well as the teachers in the Bern Medical Faculty where he had just come in 1835 from the University of Giessen and from the inspiring laboratory of Justus Liebig. He then referred to the arrival of Valentin, who took over the professorship of physiology at that time (1836), in the following words: "A saviour in the time of need was G. Valentin, who was called from Breslau as Professor of Physiology and Comparative Anatomy" (64).

Valentin's *Handbook of Physiology* was a revelation not to the students alone; scholars and university professors were eager to study it. This we read in the letters that were exchanged between Griesinger and Robert Mayer, the discoverer of the law of conservation of energy (29: 215, 216, 220). Moleschott (30: 101) said: "I am obliged to him [Valentin] not only for the most intensive and manifold instruction, but also for the unending interest he showed in the development of my scientific career."

* Erich Hintzsche, Gabriel Gustav Valentin (1810–1883), *Berner Beiträge zur Geschichte der Medizin und Naturwissenschaften* 12, Bern, Paul Haupt, 1953.

Even the aged anatomist K. F. Burdach (6) spoke of young Valentin with the highest admiration and personal sympathy and was happy to have him as collaborator on his own *Handbook of Physiology* (7). Johannes Müller carried on a scientific correspondence with his young colleague (31: 174, B.B.B.). A lasting friendship existed between Valentin and his former pupil, Alfonso Corti, the discoverer of Corti's organ in the ear, who so greatly appreciated the inspiration and instruction received personally from Valentin that, in 1854, in one of the letters published by Hintzsche (18, 19), he wrote to Valentin: "You may have thousands of more gifted, but not a more sincere and eternally devoted servant and friend."

Such a statement reveals the somewhat exaggerated politeness of the Italian style which is especially evident in this letter in which Corti acknowledged the favor received of Valentin, who had been instrumental in his election to the Academia Leopoldino-Carolina. This letter gives a vivid picture of Corti's admiration for his former teacher, as does every one of Corti's letters published by Hintzsche (18).

Most of the outstanding scholars and personages who came in personal contact with Valentin felt the same way about him, and many remained his lifelong friends. The same affection speaks out of a letter from the Danish physiologist, Professor F. Eschricht (1798–1863), who informed Valentin of the impending visit of a young compatriot of his, Doctor Hannover, with the remark (20): "He will visit you with the purpose to learn. How fortunate and enviable is he!" When this young man, Adolf Hannover (1814–1894), later to become the most famous anatomist and pathologist in Copenhagen, finally arrived in Bern in 1840, he too was immediately captivated by the charm of Valentin's personality. "He was exactly as I imagined him to be" (3). During the short time Hannover was in Bern, he and Valentin spent the days together. "We worked together and we took walks together," wrote Hannover to his friend, Japetus Steenstrup (1813–1897), later zoologist of the University of Copenhagen (3). He would have loved to stay longer but Valentin was engaged to be married and had to leave for Breslau to visit his fiancée, his cousin, Miss Samosch. Various letters of Hannover are preserved (B.B.B.) from 1847 up to 1867, all in the same spirit of true affection, which lasted up to Valentin's death (3).

We also have an account of Valentin's character and his home in Bern, given by one of the leading German parliamentarians and politicians of the second half of the nineteenth century, Ludwig Bamberger (2). It was in 1848, when a flood of political refugees poured into Switzerland after the failure of the revolution in the nearby Grand Duchy of Baden, seeking shelter and safety. Bamberger, then twenty-six years of age, was among the crowd that was not too warmly received by the Swiss bourgeois. In Valentin's house, however, he and his friend, Oppenheim, always found a welcome, and there they really felt at home. Bamberger (2: 210) said of Valentin:

> He was a kind and courteous man, his wife an intelligent and inspiring, animated lady. Oppenheim and I were always welcome guests. We greatly appreciated the benevolent, kind spirit of their home in the midst of the dissolute activities of the refugees. Valentin was one of the luminaries of the new physiological school. . . . He retained an extreme reverence and attachment to his Judaism.

A valuable witness to Valentin's unselfish and lifelong enthusiasm for research is Louis Agassiz, the great scientist and friend of Valentin. In the introduction to his *Monographies d'échinodermes* (1: 9) and again in the preface to Valentin's contribution to these monographs (1: 1) he cannot find enough words to praise "my friend Valentin, an author by virtue of his works, rating high among the anatomists and physiologists of our epoch." Valentin, at the request of Agassiz, undertook to write a general anatomy of the echinodermata (marine animals, such as starfish and sea urchins) for the latter's monographs. In appreciation for this cooperation, Agassiz wrote (1: 10): "The scientific world knows what is to be expected from the scalpel and the pen of Mr. Valentin," and he added in admiration that it was necessary, in order "to do justice to his unselfishness, to emphasize here that Mr. Valentin went, at his own expense, on a research voyage along the coast of the Mediterranean for the special purpose of dedicating himself to the research necessary for the completion of this undertaking."

I have used all these quotations from various sources because they give us a different picture of Valentin's personality and character from what can be gained from Feller's *History of the University of Bern*.

If we now try to summarize the main features of Valentin's personality, not overlooking the criticism of those who, for one reason or another, were not his friends, we are first of all impressed by his eagerness to devote all his time to research and by his energy in working day and night in all fields of descriptive and experimental biology. We are also struck by his keen ability to notice facts that had gone unnoticed and to grasp their importance immediately, as demonstrated by his discovery of the ciliary movement in animals. We notice the tenacity of his mind in evaluating new discoveries and his often very sharp criticism of the work of other scholars, even when it was the work of a generally revered authority like Johannes Müller.

In his private life Valentin appears as a typical product of his time, somewhat romantic and sentimental. He was a member from early youth of the "Gesellschaft der Brüder," a humanitarian, philanthropic Jewish society founded in 1780 under the spiritual influence of Moses Mendelssohn and his group, which he joined on January 22, 1836 (B.B.B.). On September 28, 1836, Valentin was admitted to the first degree of free masonry in the St. Johannis Lodge "Zum Frankfurter Adler," in Frankfurt on the Main (B.B.B.); he also continued his membership in a lodge in Switzerland, as proven by a membership bill to T. C. F. Valentin from La R. Loge de l'espérance of October 13, 1841 (B.B.B.). When he informed the Prussian Minister of Education of his acceptance of a call to the chair on the faculty of Bern, touchingly he emphasized his reluctance to leave his old and sick mother alone in Germany, he being her only child.

As a child of the Romantic Age in Germany he longed for friendship and had faith in friendship, especially with outstanding persons whom he revered and admired, even when the latter felt only the sympathetic friendliness that one usually holds for an outstanding colleague; this Valentin had to find out the hard way in his correspondence with Johannes Müller (B.B.B.). Valentin himself was always ready to offer helpful service and real friendship to persons of his own age or younger. In many cases this friendship lasted a long time, sometimes even a lifetime, witness his relationship with Moleschott, Carl Vogt, Marchese Corti, Eschricht (20), A. Hannover (3), the mathematician, Professor M. Stern, and many others, some of whose letters, covering several decades and written in a spirit of friendliness and admiration, are preserved in Valentin's estate (B.B.B.).

Besides these striking and brilliant colors there were, in the picture of Valentin's personality, less pleasant tones, some of which provoked strong criticism. It would not be expected otherwise. In the strong bright light of the sun the shadows are darker than in the gray of the dawn.

It is apparent that Valentin was not indifferent to success and acclamation. Very few outstanding personalities are. He surely enjoyed personal and scientific success and watched over the reputation of his own work with a certain jealousy, always ready to challenge anyone who dared to doubt its validity. Most of his unfortunate literary controversies, for instance those with Johannes Müller and his pupil, Robert Remak, and some reproachful letters he wrote to the old physiologist, Burdach, and others, originated in this attitude, which occasionally led Valentin to somewhat biased and insufficiently grounded judgments. Today we would regard his avidness to receive credit for his work, his sometimes very sharp criticism of the work of other scholars, and his watchfulness over his own scientific reputation as the expression of an overcompensated inferiority complex. The same impression is created by Valentin's inclination to take mild objective criticism as a personal insult, as a sign of intrigue against his scientific reputation, or to regard an innocent delay in the publication of one of his papers as personal malevolence. This happened time and again. His suspicion in matters of this kind was as strong against young competitors, like Jacob Henle, as it was against distinguished authorities of generally acknowledged fame, and editors of journals such as Johannes Müller and Hecker.

To understand all these different facets of an undoubtedly great personality like that of Valentin, the historian and the biographer have to try to discover the most important factors that moulded the character of their hero, instead of merely recording what was good and what was bad in a notable life. Understanding them does not dim the brilliance of a character nor dull its importance, and the disagreeable sides of a personality do not become more sympathetic, but light and shadow become more meaningful and more human.

In the case of Valentin, an attempt to understand such a personality better is especially well justified, because his type of prominence and shortcomings is found in some of his other contemporaries, who came from backgrounds similar to his own, for instance, Robert Remak, Maurizio Schiff, and even Jacob Henle.

Valentin grew up in a time when German Romanticism still strongly affected the enlightened inhabitants of the Jewish Ghettos in all parts of Germany. "Art and Science" was the slogan. Religiosity, knowledge and education, friendship, moonbeam-poetry, and endless letter writing were on everyone's mind. Goethe was adored and modern natural science admired. Popularization of the results of scientific research became widespread, as probably never before. The Jewish milieu in which, in the first half of the nineteenth century, many leading figures in Germany's cultural life originated, had a lasting influence on both the good and the less desirable qualities of these late children of a remote point in the already vanishing Romantic Era in Germany.

At that time the Jews in Central Europe (Germany, Austria, Hungary, Poland, etc.) still lived in a material as well as a spiritual Ghetto, but it was already penetrated by the leading ideas of their non-Jewish environs. Except for the short, but important, Napoleonic era, in Europe in the early nineteenth century only a few humanistic idealists thought of the Jews as human beings with a right to a dignified existence, to education, active participation in public affairs, even the right to modest happiness. Not until 1812, at the time of its deepest humiliation and helplessness, did Prussia give her Jews a kind of partial citizenship.

The average Jewish boy living in these Ghettos had one goal concerning his future, and that was to help his parents as quickly as possible in the earning of his own and the entire family's livelihood. The struggle for daily bread was extremely hard in these Jewish communities within the communities of a country.

Of course, the days of fourteen-year-old Moses Mendelssohn were definitely over. Later a pioneer and leader in educating the German Ghetto-Jew to modern secular culture when he came from the little town of Dessau to Berlin, this young idealist had to hide carefully his greatest treasure, a German grammar; otherwise he would have been regarded and ostracized as an apostate of the Jewish faith. That was in 1743. Mendelssohn's lifework, his personal life, his generally recognized position in German literature and philosophy, his friendship with the great German poet Lessing, all this educated in a new spirit a generation of contemporary Jews and many generations to come. To speak and to write correct German, to contribute to the development and to the ideals of their non-Jewish neighbor's intellectual atmosphere, were in the early nineteenth century no longer regarded as signs of defection by the majority of the German Jews, though unfortunately they often led to real apostasy.

The Romanticism that bloomed in Germany at the end of the eighteenth and the beginning of the nineteenth century was strongly echoed in progressive Jewish circles. The religiosity, the mystic longing for a heavenly destination, the enthusiasm for the great poets, Schiller and especially Goethe, all this was warmly shared by progressive Jews and Jewesses. It is no coincidence that Jewish women were the principal figures in the Romantic circles of that center of Romanticism, Berlin. Around them developed some of the most famous "Berliner Salons" of the Biedermeier period. Moses Mendelssohn's daughter, Dorothea (1764–1834), was the wife of one of the leaders of German Romanticism, Friedrich von Schlegel. Henriette Herz (1764–1847) established in her Berlin home a social center where some of the leaders of Romanticism met, such as Jean Paul, the Schlegels, Schleiermacher, Wilhelm von Humboldt, and many others. Rahel Levin (1771–1833), friend of the Schlegels, Heine, Börne, Schleiermacher, and the wife of Varnhagen von Ense, was another such person. The Jews in every Ghetto of Germany were deeply impressed and affected by the reports about the Jews in Berlin and their way of living. In Breslau, under the influence of Mendelssohnian ideas, as early as 1780 a kind of Jewish lodge was organized, the "Gesellschaft der Brüder," with educational and romantic brotherly aims, which, as previously mentioned, Valentin joined when a very young man.

In spite of their spiritual development and eagerness to share in the great new humanistic aims of mankind, the legal status of the Jews in central Europe remained unchanged, and conditions became unbearable for those who were generally well educated. Many of them became baptized; those who were more steadfast in their faith suffered continuously.

Degrading enactments of the government and certain unwritten laws aggravated the constant humiliations of the Jewish part of the population. At the end of the eighteenth century Jews were still barred by law from most of the professions; in many countries they were not permitted to study; with some exceptions they could not even marry legally unless they emigrated from their home country or bought the marriage license, as in Bohemia and Prussia, for high sums from the government, and paid still higher amounts as bribes to petty government employees.

As in the case of non-Jews at that time, the most gifted boys in the Ghettos were destined by their parents for the ministry (rabbinate), and from earliest youth (among the Jews, as a rule, from the fifth year) were compelled to devote themselves to an extremely intensive study of all religious topics. This background and this kind of unhealthy double life had a great influence, both good and bad, on the character, especially in the formative years of the development of youth.

In the eighteenth and early nineteenth centuries, the ideas of enlightenment and the guiding example of Moses Mendelssohn having penetrated the walls of the Ghetto, most of the unusually talented youth there saw the possibility of a change in the Jewish situation. Many of them had an indomitable desire not to become rabbis, with no future other than life in the Ghettos; they wished to turn to secular studies, which promised a life of freedom, success, and prominence in the fatherland. Many of them secured admission to such a competitive career by accepting baptism, as the father of the anatomist, Jacob Henle, did for himself and his young children; all of them had this great eagerness and desire to become well known, to help in elevating the level of mankind, and in this way to demonstrate before the eyes of the world that the Jews are as qualified as the non-Jews to do great things for their country and people.

It was the time early in the nineteenth century, when each of the many existing Jewish journals eagerly reported every title, order, or rank of nobility conferred upon a Jew anywhere in the world, to prove to their readers and to the world that the Jews, if given the opportunity to do so, were able and willing to contribute their share to the cultural development and advancement of their respective countries. This educational factor unquestionably sharpened the eagerness of the Jewish scientist of this period to produce good work, to become an asset to the reputation of the Jews of his own country. Diligence, studiousness, assiduousness were fostered. Moreover, Jewish religious education insisted that the student be devoted to his work day and night and not permit himself to be distracted by any worldly pastime, to say nothing of wasting time, mind, and energy in frivolity. Their Jewish background intensified all the qualities we admire in the work of Valentin, Remak, and many others. Years of study, participation in profound discussions and in the logical hairsplitting that were part and parcel of talmudic investigations, made them eminently fitted also for critical evaluation of the publications of other scholars. Unfortunately, the less desirable aspects of Valentin's personality were also strengthened by this background. From his own experience and from that of adults, the

Jewish child was aware of the bias and unjustified prejudice that most non-Jews held against Jews. Being different often produces unwarranted hatred. Being different in appearance, religion, habitat, food, time of holidays, and so on produced in many non-Jews a hostile attitude toward their Jewish neighbors. They hated the Jews and tried to harm them or at least their reputation. This fostered a kind of allusion of persecution in the Jewish child, even on occasions when it was not justified. Often a criticism or a contrary opinion expressed was not simply accepted by a member of this group or rejected as such, but it was felt to be an expression of personal animosity, hostility, antisemitism, an attempt to deprive a Jew unjustly of his due credit. The reaction was one of militant aggression; it was not in keeping with the criticism, but far in excess of what was called for though it may have been a subconscious reaction only. Similarly, every statement in science, not in agreement with Valentin's previously stated opinion, had the same effect as criticism, as can be seen in the Valentin-Remak controversy and others of like nature.

This approach to Valentin's personality may be helpful in understanding his virtues and shortcomings better, but it should not lead us to believe that these shortcomings were typical of all Jewish scholars of the early nineteenth century, or were confined to them. For example, Adolf Hannover, David Gruby, Leopold Auerbach, Moritz Stern, and many others did not indulge in emotionalism. Physiological conditions may have been a factor also: Remak in his later years was diabetic; Valentin was probably hypertensive, as may be conjectured from his attacks of vertigo and the stroke he suffered. Such persons are often impatient and easily irritated. Finally, these qualities are completely human ones and were strongly pronounced in non-Jewish scholars of all times as well, as witness the various heated polemics of A. W. Volkmann, E. Pflüger, E. Du Bois Reymond and others.

An extremely interesting letter from Johannes Müller (B.B.B.) answering an attack by Valentin, who felt he had been insulted by Müller, shows how a wise man reacts to such outbreaks (p. 173). Müller firmly stated that Valentin, spoiled since youth by too much acclamation and admiration, simply had to learn to take criticism as well as to give it. Müller also showed him the psychological background of his oversensitivity. In spite of the aloofness of the Prussian Herr Geheimrat, he wrote with so much understanding for the light and shadow in Valentin's personality that his letter did not cause a break in the relations between the two scholars; indeed their friendly correspondence continued for many years (B.B.B.).

There has never been a scientist who was an angel, nor was Valentin one. Posterity should thankfully remember the contribution of a great man to the progress of mankind and place less emphasis on those qualities in him which were not admirable.

YOUTH

Gabriel Gustav Valentin was born on July 8, 1810, in the city of Breslau in Silesia (Germany), the only child of a Jewish goldsmith, Abraham Valentin. In his autobiography (1832) he says: "Natus ego sum a.d. vlll ld. Jul. MDCCCX (40)." His father died on November 20, 1830 (B.B.B.), his mother, Carolina (Kele) Bloch, had the satisfaction to see her son not only graduated as a medical doctor but also appointed Professor in Bern. According to a census of 1776 mentioning all Jews living in the town of Breslau (4), the only persons named Valentin at that time were Abraham Nida (Juda) Valentin, thirty-eight years of age, born in Zültz, his wife, Rosel Isaackin, thirty-five years old, born in Breslau, and two children. In 1776 their only son, Aaron, was twelve years old. Whether and how this family was related to G. G. Valentin cannot be ascertained.

There is in Bern (B.B.B.) a small booklet in red binding in which Valentin's father, Abraham, in a calligraphic hand wrote a kind of autobiographical sketch in German as well as in classic Hebrew. The literal translation of the short German entry reads:

> Birth register for Abraham Valentin. My birth took place the 28th of July, 1778 at Polish Lisha, and when Lisha burned down on June 2, 1790, my late father transferred his residence here to Breslau as his own, his parents', and his ancestors' birth place. Here he indeed enjoyed the protection of the elders and trustees (Aeltesten Vorstehern) of the honorable Jewish community who appointed him as Dajan [Assistant Rabbi]. The chief trustees (erste Vorsteher) were at that time my late uncle Mr. Aaron Neumegen and the late Mr. S. Kuh.
>
> On the evening of the 5th of March I went with my dear mother to the widow Lea Haendel to meet with Dem[oiselle] Carolina Bloch, an orphan without father or mother. On the 8th of the month, at the same place, our engagement was effectuated, and on the 16th of June 1808 the marriage took place between myself and the above-mentioned, who is now my dear wife.
>
> On July 8, 1810 the Lord blessed us. After a hard struggle Dr. Henschel took with a spoonlike instrument the child, our dear first-born son, who was consecrated on the 15th of this month in our religion and received the name Gabriel.

Unfortunately, here the manuscript comes to an end. The physician mentioned, Elias Henschel (1755–1839), was one of the outstanding Jewish physicians in the town of Breslau and one of the early proponents of vaccination. On the occasion of the fiftieth anniversary of his graduation as a physician, a medal was struck in his honor by the Jewish community of Breslau. A biographical sketch of Henschel was published in the Jewish journal *Sulamith*,[8] and in 1837 his biography was published in Breslau by one Dr. Davidson.

Abraham Valentin, Gabriel's father, was a jeweler or probably a goldsmith. In the inventory of his estate (B.B.B. Mss.Hist.Helv. XXVIII/62) he is designated as *Silberhaendler*, a dealer in silverware. The document that made Abraham Valentin a citizen of the town of

[8] 5 (2): 247, 1819.

Breslau is dated September 23, 1812, and signed by the Magistrat der Kgl. Preussischen Haupt- und Residenzstadt Breslau. The inventory mentioned contains all the sums that were left by Abraham Valentin, the amounts that came in from silverware out of the estate that was sold, and all the expenditures made for his widow and his son in the following years. According to this record Valentin's father was not wealthy; rather he was a bourgeois of small means.

The Hebrew portion of the entries in Abraham Valentin's booklet generally repeats the German part, but it gives some more interesting details. Here Valentin's father calls himself Abraham, son of the late Dajan Josúa Falk. He also gives the profession of his late father-in-law as goldsmith and his first name as Gabriel. Gabriel Valentin was, therefore, named in memory of his deceased grandfather.

In 1810, when Gabriel Valentin was born, living conditions for the Jews in Prussia were still very different from those of their non-Jewish fellow citizens, though the best German people at that time were enthusiastic about the new ideas of freedom, humanity, and enlightenment, which in the eighteenth century influenced the development of all Europe. However, this part of the population in Germany was then, as always, in the minority. In 1790, for instance, there was still opposition in all guilds to the admission of Jewish children as apprentices (17) and in 1818 the conversion of a non-Jewish person to Judaism was still forbidden in Prussia.[4] It was only two years after the birth of Valentin that the Prussian Government's Edict of 1812 was passed. This edict finally admitted Jews to citizenship for the first time, even though their ancestors had already lived within the confines of Prussia for centuries. After this decision of high political and economic importance, the Jewish community of Breslau developed very quickly, and the Jewish inhabitants of the town soon proved to be highly interested in all cultural, scientific, and educational problems, and helpful in their solution. Many of them also soon contributed an important share in the development of medicine and science in Germany.

Valentin attended first a private school, the Heilberg'sche Anstalt (32), and entered the Maria Magdalena Gymnasium in Breslau in 1821 (40), at the age of eleven. His first teacher there was the rector, Manso. In former years, Manso had written a book, *The Art of Love* (*Die Kunst zu lieben*), which was ridiculed by Goethe in his *Xenien*. In Valentin's time Manso was an old bachelor wearing a pigtail, white stockings, and shoes with buckles. He educated Valentin and the other pupils the strict way, occasionally even slapping their faces. He was later replaced by Kluge, a modern pedagogue (B.B.B.).

When Valentin was seventeen, his congratulatory poem in Greek distiches honoring this principal, Kluge,

[4] *Sulamith* 6: 65, 1820.

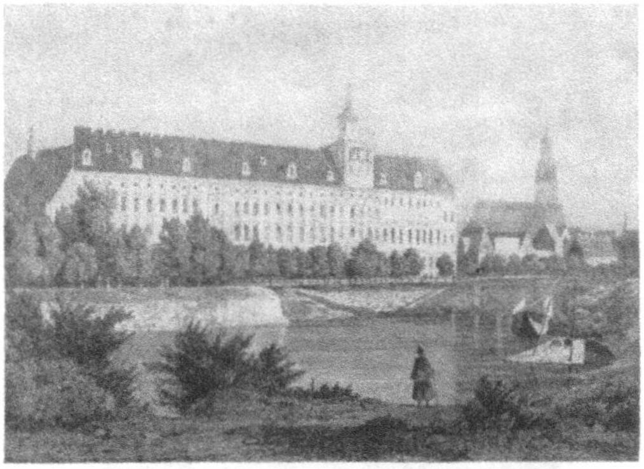

FIG. 2. The University of Breslau in the early nineteenth century. From the author's collection.

was published (32 and 75). These and many other valuable details of Valentin's early life are given in a short biographical sketch probably (Hintzsche, 1953) written by his son Adolf (B.B.B. XXVIII/68). Valentin graduated from the Gymnasium in 1828 (40). During the time of his attendance he was trained not only in various secular subjects taught in the school, but also in talmudic studies in accordance with the traditions of his family. Hirschfeld (21) mentions that Valentin's grandfather was a well known man in Jewish theological literature, probably referring to R. Josua Falk. According to Heppner (17), he was a descendant of the famous, and legendary, rabbi Loew of Prague.

In the fall of 1828 Valentin entered the medical faculty of the University of Breslau to study medicine and natural science. In spite of all the prejudice against the Jews in Germany at that time, no quota system existed to prevent gifted Jews from studying at a university.

A PUPIL AND FRIEND OF PURKINJE

One member of the medical faculty of Breslau at that time, without being a spellbinding speaker and teacher, exerted great influence on the entire following generation of students. Studies of problems of physiology and pathology took, under his leadership, an entirely new and experimental direction. That man was the Bohemian, Johann Evangelista Purkinje. He was famous as anatomist, microscopist, and physiologist, and also as founder (in 1824) of an experimental physiological laboratory for teaching and research purposes at a university in Germany.[5] This laboratory in Breslau, renowned for the work of Purkinje and his pupils, was by no means impressive in its physical appearance. It is quite probable that the lowliest assistant in New York's Rockefeller Research Laboratory would refuse

[5] Before that, in 1821, only Carl August Sigmund Schultz created in Freiburg an experimental physiologic laboratory, the first of its kind in Germany.

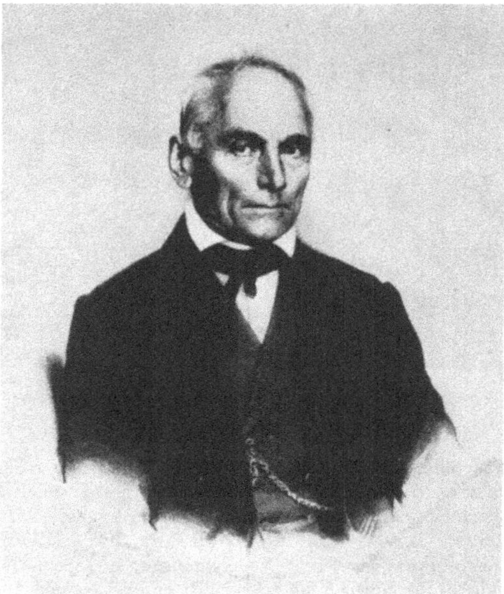

FIG. 3. J. Ev. Purkyně. Lithography by Rud. Hoffmann from a photograph (1856). From the author's collection.

to work in such a place. Later, the rooms of this laboratory were used as a *carcer,* a place of confinement for unruly students (15).

Purkinje himself was a strange and peculiar man, but he was recognized all over the world as one of the founders of modern physiology. Early in his career he was interested mainly in the physiology of the senses, and with his first publication, a booklet of 176 pages (1819), he attracted the interest of the poet and scientist Goethe, who received the young doctor very kindly when he visited him in Weimar in 1822, at which time they discussed problems of physiological optics. However, the statement appearing repeatedly in the literature, that Goethe was instrumental in Purkinje's being appointed as full professor in Breslau, is a mere legend.[6]

Purkinje was not only an independent thinker as a physiologist; he was also very much interested in social and political problems. Of Czech parentage, he felt deeply about the political and cultural re-awakening of the Czech nation. As a foreigner in a strange country, he suffered in Breslau not only from the jealous attitude of the anatomist, Otto, but also from homesickness for his native land. He became more and more a supporter and fighter for recognition of the nationalist aspirations of his people and grew less and less interested in the study of medicine. Finally, in 1850, he returned, a celebrated national hero, to Czechoslovakia and to Prague, there becoming, as professor at the University of Prague, the representative of his country in the field of physiology.

Prague honored him time and again, both as a great physiologist and as a great patriot. Medals were struck in his honor in the last years of his life in Prague. His bust stood in the Physiological Laboratory of the German University in Prague until the First World War when clumsy soldiers broke it. Such a man, himself an ardent nationalist, with all the necessary understanding for the suffering of a minority among an antagonistic majority, might have been expected to feel a profound sympathy for the difficulties of his Jewish collaborators, like Valentin and Pappenheim, and we know that there really existed a close collaboration and even friendship between him and those other national outsiders in the midst of a hostile, highly nationalistic German environment. How Purkinje personally approached the entire question of Jewish academic emancipation is worth while considering from the point of view of his personality as well as from that of his attitude towards Valentin and the other Jewish students. It is also useful in evaluating the attitude of the early leaders of the Renaissance of the Czech people toward their Jewish fellow citizens in Prague and Bohemia (26).

When, in 1847, a time of pre-revolutionary tension and political stress, the universities of Prussia were asked by the government to submit their opinion on the contemplated admission of Jews to teaching positions, the professors who held chairs on a Prussian faculty had to submit their individual opinions in a so-called separate vote. All these documents are preserved in an extremely instructive book by Dr. M. Kalisch (24). From Purkinje's lengthy report, which is probably the most interesting of them all, only the following need be mentioned. In the introduction Purkinje emphasized that he regarded the Jews as a separate race, distinguished as such by different, constant physical and psychological characteristics and by their Semitic language. After a detailed description of the situation existing between Jews and non-Jews in the various countries, he very strongly suggested intermarriage and complete assimilation of the Jews to their non-Jewish environment, but he always stressed that the Jew, on receiving all the rights of true citizenship, should not interfere with the preferred status and righteously developed egotism of the people among whom he lived. Purkinje recommended the religious reform movement among the Jews. He even mentioned, as a ridiculous idea, the very serious proposal of a contemporary, one Mardochäus Manuel Noah, to create a Jewish republic in North America.[7]

[6] See the excellent article by R. H. Kahn, Aus Goethe's Purkinje-Zeit, *Lotos* (Prag) **80**: 1, 1932.

[7] This Jewish merchant, Mardochai Manuel Noah (1785–1851), from New York (born in Philadelphia) acquired, on March 13, 1820, a large island on the Niagara River between Lake Erie and Lake Ontario with some thousand acres of land, for the purpose of settling the oppressed Jews from Europe (*Sulamith* **6**: 284, 1821). M. M. Noah, Major in the New

Purkinje insisted that the only possibility of a solution of the Jewish problem lay in a compromise between the population and the Jewish inhabitants on an agreeable basis. He concluded his statement as follows:

It is apparent from these meditations that it must be my sincerest wish that the Jews may take part in all our rights and freedoms, our means of culture and our fortune to reach their high humane destination, but all this without doing any injury to the children of the house. This should be achieved in such a way that by and by they give up their own racial and national peculiarities and amalgamate with us entirely as one people. As soon as they, by adequate institutions, gain our sympathy, our respect and our confidence to a higher degree than up to the present time and to a wider extent, and as soon as they become more assimilated to our way of viewing and feeling things, the time will come to give them access without any limitations to all the higher and highest offices in the state, among which I regard professorship at a university. At the moment I find it neither permissible nor proper to depart from the present constitution [i.e., not to admit any Jews to a teaching position].

It is of the greatest significance that Purkinje expressed such an opinion after his old Jewish collaborator and friend, Valentin, had already been full professor and one of the outstanding men in a Swiss university for more than a decade, and after his years of experience with this man and with Pappenheim, his pupil, who, like Valentin, once won a high award from the Academy of Sciences in Paris, and even after, in Prussia, King Frederic William IV had already admitted the Jew, Remak, to a teaching position in the Berlin University. This attitude and Purkinje's well-known personal peculiarities may explain why the friendly relationship between him and Valentin became impaired in the last year of Valentin's stay in Breslau, much to the regret of the latter (B.B.B.). (See also Hintzsche, 1953.)

Purkinje was, like Valentin, a Free Mason, and as such against oppression of individuals and nations. He was strictly opposed to any assimilation of the Czechs in Prague to their German environment. He was such a fanatic nationalist himself that when he left Breslau for Prague in 1850, he changed the spelling of his name from Purkinje to Purkyně. Yet this same nationalist zealot and fighter for justice for his own people would have deprived the Jewish minority in every country, including his own homeland, of equal rights of citizenship, unless they underwent complete assimilation, including their religion, and intermarried. There can hardly be any question that Purkinje's behavior must have influenced his leading compatriots in Prague, such as the historian Palacký, who was one of the central figures of the Czech Renaissance and with whom Purkinje corresponded years before he was recalled to his homeland (23).

In spite of his attitude on this question and probably partly because of his isolation in Breslau, his human feeling led him to close collaboration and even friendship with some of his Jewish pupils. By his personality and by his enthusiastic and even fanatic devotion to research, Purkinje in his younger years deeply influenced the young men who came to study medicine in Breslau. However, as a lecturer, at least in the German language, he was never very impressive.

Under Purkinje's leadership, Valentin was imbued with an unextinguishable, passionate love for research. His determination to devote his entire life to science was expressed by him in the preface to the first volume of his *Repertorium,* where he said that he regarded it as the main task of his life to acquire an exact knowledge of normal and pathological physiology, as the main basis of all medicine. Throughout his lifetime he remained the same indefatigable research worker. Even on his deathbed, when he was partially paralyzed, he continued to dictate the results and conclusions of his earlier experiments (75). From his days in Purkinje's laboratory to the end of his life, Valentin was a devoted servant of scientific medicine.

EARLY SCIENTIFIC ACHIEVEMENTS

On October 10, 1832, Valentin was graduated from the medical faculty of Breslau, having presented a thesis on the embryonic development of muscle tissue (40).

Of course, the young doctor had a great desire to continue in the scientific work he had just begun and to devote his entire life to science and research. At that time, however, a Jew could not hope to be appointed by the Prussian Minister as a teacher or even as an assistant at any institute of a Prussian University, and because his financial situation was precarious (32), Valentin had to decide to make his living as a practitioner.

In the account of his father's estate the expenses of Valentin's graduation as a doctor are given as more than 279 thaler (B.B.B.), and on July 25, 1833, there is an entry of expenses for a bell and a door plate. It was at that time, apparently, that he started his practice, in which he came to be highly esteemed by his patients, as shown by letters (B.B.B.), that have been preserved, but which, from the financial point of view, he did not conduct efficiently (32). Expenditures for cloth (velvet waistcoat, etc.) show that he was careful with his appearance in public. His greatest expenses for that time, mentioned in this account, were for books, for instance 31 thaler on October 9, 1833.

Valentin, in spite of being established as a general practitioner, was dissatisfied with merely practicing and was glad to be permitted to continue his research work

York militia and commander of its port, also for a time United States Ambassador in Tunis, founded on September 15, 1825, the day after the Jewish New Year, on this island a town called Ararat as a refuge for persecuted Jews (*Sulamith* 7: 72, 138, 1826). He did not succeed with his idea, for the time was not yet ripe, the facilities were not adequate, and the European Jews were not yet in a proper frame of mind for it. In 1838 he published a booklet at Hammerich in Altona in which he, as Dr. Boudinot (1816), Smith (1825), and Worsley (1828) before him, tried to prove that the American Indians are the descendants of the ten lost tribes of Israel.

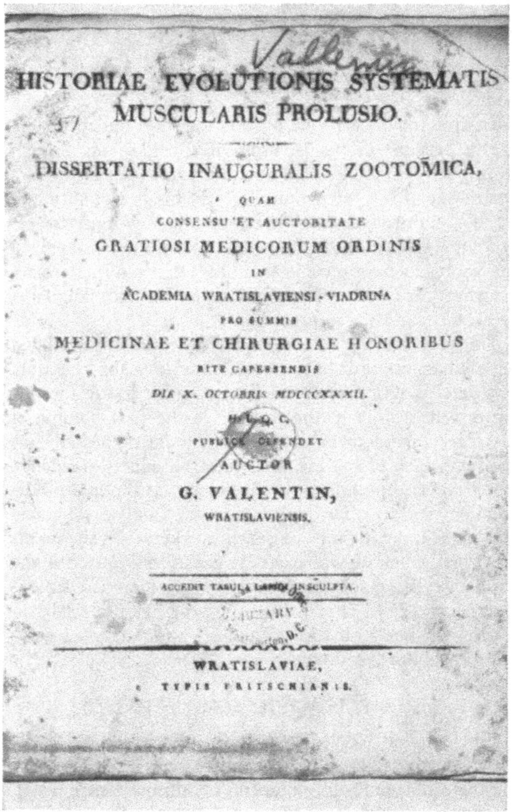

HISTORIAE EVOLUTIONIS SYSTEMATIS MUSCULARIS PROLUSIO.

DISSERTATIO INAUGURALIS ZOOTOMICA,
QUAM
CONSENSU ET AUCTORITATE
GRATIOSI MEDICORUM ORDINIS
IN
ACADEMIA WRATISLAVIENSI-VIADRINA
PRO SUMMIS
MEDICINAE ET CHIRURGIAE HONORIBUS
RITE CAPESSENDIS
DIE X. OCTOBRIS MDCCCXXXII.
H. L. Q. C.
PUBLICE DEFENDET
AUCTOR
G. VALENTIN,
WRATISLAVIENSIS.

ACCEDIT TABULA LAPIDI INSCULPTA.

WRATISLAVIAE,
TYPIS FRITSCHIANIS.

FIG. 4. Title page of Valentin's Doctoral Thesis (October 10, 1832). Courtesy of the Library of the Surgeon General, Washington, D. C.

in Purkinje's laboratory, for which he found time as his practice was small. In 1833–1835 he published, in Ammon's *Journal of Ophthalmology* and in Hecker's *Annalen,* his findings with respect to the anatomy of vessels and the ganglion intercaroticum [8] and on the foetal development of the eye of vertebrates, particularly the membrana capsulo pupilaris, which had just been discovered in the embryonic eye by the physiologist, Johannes Müller, and had been studied by his pupil, Jacob Henle, in his doctoral thesis, but which was still nonexistent in the opinion of the anatomist, Arnold (41). Valentin investigated the terminal ramifications of the nerves in the muscles,[9] rediscovering there the sarcolemma of muscle bundles (p. 71), and became the expert microscopist for which he later became famous. His most important contribution at this time was the discovery (together with Purkinje) of the ciliary epithelium in mammals and its function. This basic discovery was published in the first volume of *Müller's Archiv* in 1834 (34). The second volume of the same *Archiv* contained the continuation of these investigations. Johannes Müller reported it in the annual "Reports" in his *Archiv* [10] as one of the most outstanding and important developments in physiology. An exhaustive summary on the same subject was published in collaboration with Purkinje in 1835 in Breslau (35) and, finally, in the *Acta,* the proceedings of the Academia Leopoldino-Carolina.

Before the last mentioned publication came out, Valentin was made a member and secretary of the Academy in 1835. His predecessor in this position, up to 1830, was the physiologist, Johannes Müller, of Bonn, who resigned when its President Nees von Esenbeck accepted a call to the University of Breslau and when the seat of the Academy, on this occasion, was also transferred from Bonn to Breslau.

Valentin's early friendship with Purkinje and their scientific collaboration were very close. This is expressed in Valentin's reference to Purkinje in 1833 as his "dear teacher and friend" (41: 311). Young Valentin also enjoyed the privilege of becoming acquainted with his teacher's family and after many years in a letter to Retzius he gratefully remembered Purkinje's late wife as his highly revered friend. Together with Purkinje and Pappenheim he studied the histology of the mucous membrane of the stomach; simultaneously with Purkinje he discovered ciliary epithelium in the cavities of the central nervous system.[11] Purkinje inspired him to pursue histological studies of the central nervous system, which Valentin continued for many years.

It was Valentin's outstanding contribution to neurology and neurohistology to have recognized that the entire nervous system consists mainly of two constituents, ganglionic cells and nerve fibers, as we call these elements today; he also discovered the ganglionic cells in the retina.[12]

Valentin's fundamental publication in this field falls in the period when he was collaborating with Purkinje. On February 9, 1836, he submitted to the Carolo-Leopoldina Academy a paper on the course and the terminal parts of the nerves. This paper was published in 1836 in the *Proceedings* of the Academy.[13] Decades later the outstanding anatomist, Koelliker of Würzburg, called it "the epoch-making first good description of the elements of the nervous system." Fontana in 1779 (13: 357) had discovered the nerve fibers, and Ehrenberg (in 1833) the nerve cells, but only Valentin in his publication of 1836 showed that nerve cells and nerve fibers are the main constituents of each kind of nervous tissue. This was before the scientific and medical

[8] *Jour. Ophthal.* **26**: 398, 1833.
[9] Hecker's *Annalen* **2**: 1, 1835.
[10] *Archiv* 1835: 128.
[11] *Müller's Archiv* 1836: 289.
[12] *Repertorium,* 1837.
[13] **18** (1): 51–240, 1836.

Entdeckung continuirlicher
durch
Wimperhaare erzeugter Flimmerbewegungen,
als eines allgemeinen Phänomens in den Klassen der Amphibien, Vögel und Säugethiere.
Von Prof. Dr. *Purkinje* und Dr. *Valentin* in Breslau.

Die merkwürdige Eigenthümlichkeit gewisser thierischer Theile, continuirliche Strömungen in dem sie umgebenden, meist flüssigen Medium zu erregen, hat die Aufmerksamkeit sehr vieler Naturforscher mit Recht auf sich gezogen und anhaltende Beobachtungen veranlasst. Bei den Infusorien wurde diess Phänomen zuerst bekannt, da das leicht wahrzunehmende Räderorgan der Vorticellen zu diesem Zwecke dient. Späterhin wurden ähnliche Erscheinungen bei Muscheln von Erman, von Baer, Carus u. A. wahrgenommen. Die merkwürdige Drehung der Embryonen im Ei, welche bei diesen Geschöpfen leicht zu beobachten ist, hat man nicht ohne Glück auf dieses Phänomen reducirt. Auch viele andere wirbellose Thiere und deren Eier gaben zu ähnlichen Erfahrungen Gelegenheit. Bei den Wirbelthieren hat dagegen der treffliche Steinbuch zuerst etwas Aehnliches an den Kiemen der Batrachierlarven gefunden, wiewohl seine Beschreibung nicht ganz der Natur entspricht. Spätere Naturforscher, wie Carus, Hugi, E. H. Weber, Stiebel, Joh. Müller u. A., haben einzelne Zu-

FIG. 5. First publication of the discovery of the fibrillatory movement in vertebrates. *Müller's Archiv,* 1834.

world was enlightened by Schleiden and Schwann's cell theory. In his exact observations Valentin also gives in this paper a good description of the nucleolus, a structure within the nucleus of the cell, the latter known since Brown (1833). In this way he contributed, *quasi en passant,* a fundamental discovery important for all biology which he had published in 1836 in his *Repertorium* in describing the epithelium of the conjunctiva.

The only point he missed in his important investigations was the real connection between nerve cells and nerve fibers. His misconception of this problem led soon after to the deplorable controversy between Valentin and Remak, which was detrimental not only to these men, but to the progress of science as well. In spite of this, Valentin's paper on the structure of the nervous system was nevertheless a landmark in the history of neurophysiology and neuroanatomy.

MEDICAL MICROSCOPY IN THE EARLY NINETEENTH CENTURY

Valentin was renowned as and proud to be an outstanding authority in microscopy. In 1836 he discovered the nucleolus (45: 50); he was the first to recognize the general histologic structure of the central nervous system. His reputation as microscopist was great at a time—the middle of the nineteenth century—when, even in Berlin, some of the outstanding physicians, especially those of the older generation, did not yet realize the value of the microscope for clinical medicine, regarding it rather as a toy for children, just as the kaleidoscope was when it was invented in 1817 by Sir David Brewster, an English physicist. Professor J. J. Dieffenbach (1792–1847), one of the most outstanding German surgeons in Berlin, expressed this opinion on microscopy repeatedly to his revered colleague, Professor Stromeyer in Munich, in letters in the middle of the century. He shows a contempt for the microscopists in medicine in spite of the fact that he witnessed a lecture and demonstration by Valentin in Berlin in his own house. For instance, he wrote on December 1844 (10: 33):

> I do not like the present way of doing research in science. It makes the main factor microscopy, kaleidoscopy. I remember from my childhood, that the wing of a fly and the leg of a flee looked nice and large. But there remains so much to be seen in natural size with the eyes and to touch

DE
PHAENOMENO GENERALI ET FUNDAMENTALI
MOTUS VIBRATORII
CONTINUI
IN
MEMBRANIS CUM EXTERNIS TUM INTERNIS
ANIMALIUM PLURIMORUM
ET SUPERIORUM ET INFERIORUM ORDINUM
OBVII.
COMMENTATIO PHYSIOLOGICA.

SCRIPSERUNT
PROF. DR. JOH. EV. PURKINJE ET DR. G. VALENTIN,
WRATISLAVIENSES.

WRATISLAVIAE,
SUMPTIBUS AUG. SCHULZ ET SOCII.
AMSTELODAMI: APUD MUELLER ET COMP. LONDINI: APUD BLACK, YOUNG ET YOUNG.
PARISIIS: APUD HEIDELOFF ET CAMPE. ST. PETROPOLI: APUD W. GRAEFF.
MDCCCXXXV.

FIG. 6. Main publication of Purkinje and Valentin on the fibrillatory movements in vertebrates. Breslau, 1835.

with the fingers, and even about that we do not yet see clearly enough.

Again on May 13, 1846, this colleague of the leading microscopists, Johannes Müller and Ehrenberg, in the Faculty of Medicine in Berlin wrote (p. 39) to his friend:

I cannot become a friend of the new activities in science. They all stem from the attitude that all that we have seen with clear eyes has no further value, and is labelled as inadequate to the present-day status of science. This is the chant of those people who are only peeping through the microscope. Microscope-Kaleidoscope.

Valentin, of course, despite his youth was a leading figure in this new triumphant course that science took by using the microscope, not as a toy, but as one of the most valuable instruments in modern medicine. It is, therefore, psychologically understandable that this champion of the new science was not delighted by the appearance of a still younger champion among the group around Johannes Müller in Berlin, who proved new facts contradicting Valentin's observation.

Of course, it should not be assumed that Valentin opposed Remak's new discoveries only because of prejudice or vanity. His scientific idealism was too high for such a poor attitude. In 1837, when the differences of opinion had just started, he mentioned in a letter to Professor A. Retzius in Stockholm his hope that such differences might finally help to clarify the truth (see p. 164). He even frankly admitted his own mistake concerning the fine structure of certain layers of the brain, for Remak's contrary observations were correct beyond a doubt. In a footnote to page 98 of his *Anatomy of the Nervous System* (50) Valentin said: "On this point I entirely agree with Remak, when he corrects my previous mistake. . . ." Of course, no scientist is happy to be compelled to make such a statement publicly. In 1838 Valentin also admitted in a personal letter to Remak his confirmation of the existence of Remak's organic nerve fibers. It is quite understandable that with regard to all the other microscopic discoveries of Remak, Valentin was reluctant to concede one defeat after another. They were not so easily proven as the existence of Remak's fibers in the nervous system, and Valentin resisted yielding, as long as he was not convinced of his mistake, and resisted hailing a young rising star in the scientific firmament of Berlin.

VALENTIN'S RESEARCH IN EMBRYOLOGY

Valentin's favorite field of research, next to microscopy, was always embryology. Embryological studies led him to the above mentioned discovery of the ciliary movement in mammals, observed in the oviducts,[14] and to another discovery, on which he addressed the 1833 convention of German Natural Scientists and Physicians in Breslau, where, probably for the first time, he met Alexander von Humboldt. Here he reported on artificial production of freaks in chicken embryos, resulting in double monstrosities. Again Johannes Müller immediately realized the importance of the findings of the young doctor and characterized it as an outstanding observation in his *Archiv*.[15] Years later, Valentin again took this problem up, investigating fish embryos in collaboration with Marchese Corti when the latter worked with him in Bern (25).

The early years of Valentin's scientific education in Breslau, when he worked under Purkinje, were rich in work and in success in various fields. The great value that Purkinje himself placed on collaboration with his pupil Valentin can be seen in a letter written in 1841 to Professor Wagner in Göttingen as reported by Heidenhain in *Allgemeine Deutsche Biographie* **26**: 721. Purkinje wrote there of the past years of productive study and research, saying: "It happened that I was able to make many fortunate discoveries, especially when I was associated with such remarkable talent as that of Valentin."

In 1835 Valentin's *Handbook on Comparative Embryology* (43), which he dedicated to his "Highly esteemed teachers, protectors and friends, C. G. Nees von Esenbeck and J. E. Purkinje," was published. His close relationship with his teachers is shown by the wording of the dedication in which he expresses his "esteem, thankfulness and love." This handbook of 658 pages was a landmark in the development of embryology. Valentin had already published a chapter, "Entwicklungsgeschichte" (Embryology), in the Encyclopaedic Dictionary of Medical Science in Berlin in 1834. In the introduction to his book Valentin now mentioned that from the beginning of his medical and physiological studies in 1829, he always had a special devotion for the field of embryology. It was this preference that led him in 1832, as mentioned previously, to choose as the topic of his doctoral thesis a study on the embryological development of the muscle system (40). Apparently this was the first time that the microscopic structure of muscles of insects was studied. This subject, subsequently investigated time and again, has up to the present remained of the highest interest for anatomists and physiologists alike.

In his handbook Valentin stressed the great value of *comparative* embryology, and also its importance for the study of the *development* of the different *tissues* from the point of view of comparative embryology, and not merely the development of a single organ, as had been done up to that time. Thus he created the field of *histiogeny*. His work in the embryological field was soon known far beyond the borders of Germany. In 1835 there appeared in the *Edinburgh Medical and Sur-*

[14] The wording in the introduction of the first publication on the ciliary movement leaves no doubt as to which of the two authors was the discoverer and which verified the correctness of the discovery.

[15] 1834: 160.

gical Journal (No. 127) an abridged translation of Valentin's embryological studies by Martin Barry, President of the Royal Medical Society of Edinburgh, under the title, "History of the Development of the Human Ovum with a Comparative View of the Development of the Ova of Mammalia and Birds."

Alexander von Humboldt, the outstanding scientist at this time, was most enthusiastic about Valentin's work. In Valentin's effects (B.B.B.) there is a letter from Humboldt dated January 30, 1835, containing flattering remarks about this book "which accompanies me for the past three weeks on all my travels." Unlike Robert Remak, Valentin was fortunate enough to be acclaimed from the very start of his research as an outstanding scholar and authority by the most prominent scientists in Germany and abroad as well. This fact, as Johannes Müller mentioned in an extensive letter to Valentin, may, indeed, have spoiled him somewhat and made him oversensitive to any kind of criticism.

Characteristic of the honest, though stubborn, personality of Valentin are his remarks in the introduction to his handbook on comparative embryology concerning his repeated quotations from the classical studies by von Baer. Valentin wrote that he preferred to do this, even though he himself had ample experience of his own in the matter, because he considered it fair always to give credit to the man who had first recognized a particular fact in natural science. He would not like to claim as his own discoveries that might turn out to be merely confirmation of the work of earlier scientists or minor additions to them. This attitude of justness and honesty toward other research workers, unfortunately not very common in our day, was emphasized time and again by Valentin and became a pronounced feature of his personality.

THE GRAND PRIX DES SCIENCES PHYSIQUES

Valentin's special interest in embryology and the universality of his knowledge in the most varied biological fields at the age of twenty-three enabled him to enter a contest sponsored by the Institut de France in 1833. The exact title of the contest, as given in the *Comptes rendus de l'Académie des Sciences*,[16] was: "Examiner si le mode de développement des tissues organiques, chez les animaux, peut être comparé à la manière dont se développent les tissues de végétaux." This was a problem of the highest interest before Schwann and Remak worked out the fundamentals of our modern cellular theory. There is no question that Valentin with his prize paper on this problem became the most outstanding forerunner of Schwann.

In 1835 Valentin submitted his manuscript of eleven hundred pages and forty-two tables drawn by him in quarto, under the title: "Histiogenia Comparata." In accordance with the rules of the contest it was filed

[16] 1: 5, 9, 1835.

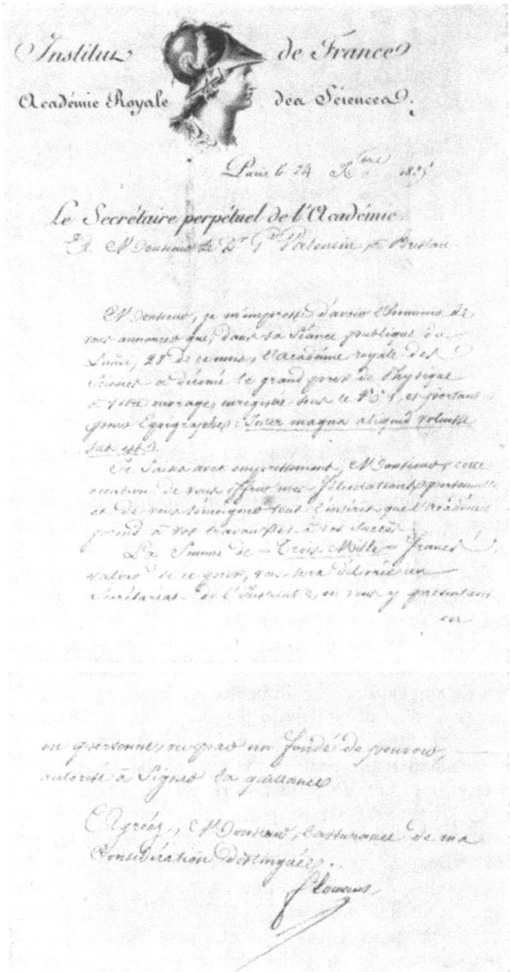
Institut de France
Académie Royale des Sciences

Le Secrétaire perpétuel de l'Académie

Inter magna aliquid voluisse sat est.

Flourens

FIG. 7. Letter of Professor Flourens in Paris informing Valentin of his having been awarded the Grand Prix of the French Royal Academy in the amount of 3000 francs. Courtesy of B.B.B.

anonymously under the motto, "Inter magna aliquid voluisse sat est" (in great endeavors it is enough to have tried to contribute a share). The judges of the contest were Mirbel, Magendie, Blainville, A. Brongniart, and Serres (65). Valentin received a prize of three thousand francs awarded for the best work on this topic, the Grand Prix des Sciences Physiques, which enabled him to travel through Europe, increasing his knowledge of foreign countries and scientific laboratories and his personal contacts with outstanding scientists. A substantial part of this paper was published in his *Comparative Embryology*, as mentioned in the Jewish

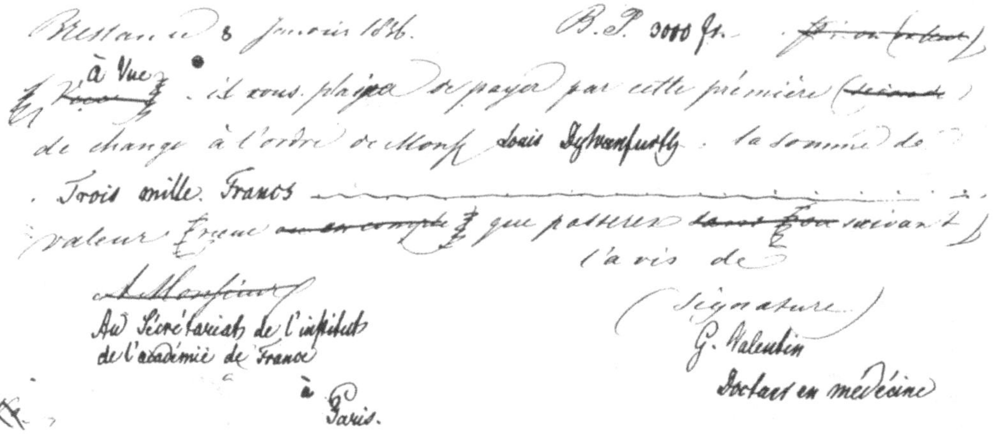
Breslau le 8 janvier 1836. B.P. 3000 fr.
à Vue il vous plaira de payer par cette première
de change à l'ordre de Monsr Louis [illegible] la somme de
Trois mille Francs
valeur reçue que passerez suivant
l'avis de
A Monsieur
Au Sécrétariat de l'institut
de l'académie de France
à Paris.
(Signature)
G. Valentin
Docteur en médecine

FIG. 8. Valentin's draught of the receipt of the amount of 3000 francs. Courtesy of B.B.B.

journal *Sulamith*.[17] The year of publication is there wrongly given, and the date of the award of the prize as December 2, 1835.

The Académie announced its decision at its meeting on December 21, 1835, somewhat incorrectly stating that the award was given to "M. Valentin, professeur à Breslau." At the following meeting of the academy, a detailed report was presented on the decision. The judges emphasized the difficulty of covering such an enormous field of biology in the short time of fifteen or sixteen months. They observed that none of the competitors had really reached the goal of the contest completely, but that Valentin's work was regarded as the best. They gave as the reason for their decision the enormous work done, and the "profonde intelligence des choses, de consciencieuses récherches, de savantes descriptions, d'excellentes figures," concluding with the remark that this work would be as valuable to the progress of science as it was "glorieux pour l'auteur" (65).

At the same meeting the topic of the next contest of the academy was announced, the closing date for the submission of papers being April 1, 1837, and the award of a gold medal of the value of 3,000 francs ("Le prix consistera en une medaille d'or de la valeur de 3000 fr."). There is no doubt, however, that Valentin received a sum of 3,000 francs, because a copy of his receipt is preserved in the archives of Bern (B.B.B.).

Alexander von Humboldt expressed his recognition of Valentin's stupendous work in flattering language (15). It was the famous Dutrochet who unofficially informed the twenty-five-year-old author of his success in the contest. He received official notification from Flourens (21).

Next to Purkinje and Nees von Esenbeck, both of whom were his teachers, Valentin counted among his protectors Alexander von Humboldt, the helpful friend and counselor of every promising talent in the field of science. To young Valentin also Humboldt extended his help and cooperation in a touching way. The draft of a letter of March 28, 1836, directed to Flourens in Paris is preserved (B.B.B.). It was written by Valentin and corrected with additional explanations in von Humboldt's handwriting. To von Humboldt Valentin and Purkinje gratefully dedicated their joint paper on the ciliary movement. Purkinje wished to dedicate it to the Prussian Minister of Education, von Altenstein, but Valentin insisted that this publication, which contained one of the most important discoveries of his lifetime, should not be inscribed to von Altenstein alone but jointly with von Humboldt (21).

The award of the Grand Prix was for Valentin not only a great moral success; it also helped in solving many personal problems. Valentin's financial situation was not at all good, especially in the years after his father's death, when he and his mother were forced slowly to consume the small estate left by his father (B.B.B.), on which the expense of his education was a heavy burden. A well-to-do sister of Valentin's father, Mrs. Sarah Samosch, and her husband were helpful and treated Valentin as their own child (32). Indeed, a few years later, in 1841, Valentin, by that time a famous professor, married their daughter, his cousin Henrietta Samosch. But all financial worries were over for the next few years when Valentin was awarded the prize of 3,000 francs, and before long his financial difficulties vanished forever with his appointment as professor.

The first pleasure the laureate of the Paris Academy, who had never before seen the world, gave himself was a trip to Berlin and its medical centers early in 1836.

THE REPERTORIUM

It was in 1836, when his work was still unrecognized by the German Government, that Valentin carried on his fruitful research steadfastly and devotedly. Shortly

[17] 8 (1): 167, 1836.

after he received the award of the Paris Academy, the *Transactions* of this institution reports the receipt of his above-mentioned *Manuel de l'histoire du developpement de l'homme.* He then announced that he would soon send two more papers, one on the ciliary movement, and the one on the nerve-endings in organs (68). In 1836 Valentin also published in Hecker's *Annals* an interesting study in the field of clinical medicine, viz., on the sensations experienced after amputation of an extremity, and in the same year he launched his *Repertorium* (46), a most extraordinary quarterly. It casts light not only on the universality of Valentin's knowledge and experience, but also on his responsible, honest, and scientifically stubborn character and his incredible diligence and assiduity.

At the time when Valentin began publishing his *Repertorium,* his reputation was distinguished enough for him to dare to undertake such a venture, probably unique in the field of medical literature, for this quarterly journal was written exclusively by Valentin. It was a one-man enterprise in which Valentin summarized all the published literature in the vast field of biology. These summaries resembled and soon were unquestionable competition for those published annually by Johannes Müller and his collaborators in his *Archiv.* But Valentin's reports were more extensive and, as Müller's annual reports, contained additional, sometimes unnecessarily strong, criticism. His judgment of other scholars' publications was occasionally very sharp and made him many enemies. Even Johannes Müller, the adored master of physiology and anatomy, complained about this kind of criticism (see p. 173). However, the striking feature of the *Repertorium* was that the original papers in it also were written exclusively by Valentin. The title of this journal was *Repertorium für Anatomie und Physiologie*; the subtitle explained that it contained a critical report on the work of other scientists and the results of his own research, all written by Valentin himself (46).

Valentin characterized his new journal in a letter to von Humboldt of August 4, 1836 (B.B.B.), when, shortly before his departure for Bern, he announced that the first (double) issue of his *Repertorium* would appear in a few weeks. He wrote:

> Besides a critical presentation of the most prominent contributions of our time in anatomical and physiological science [the journal] will also contain original contributions all exclusively by myself. It is not intended to be a common journal, but a continuous outlet for my own research. (B.B.B.)

Many of these original articles of Valentin were valuable contributions to physiology. The first volume, published in Berlin in 1836, featured Valentin's discovery of the presence of ciliary epithelium in the central parts of the nervous system in man as well as in vertebrates, as established at the same time by Purkinje, but this discovery is true in man probably only for the newborn (Kölliker, Dittrich, Gerlach). Valentin thought to be able to prove its existence there in man, mammals, birds, fish, and amphibians. In the third volume (p. 281), he published a method that, for the first time, permitted an approximate measuring of the blood volume. The ratio of blood volume to body-weight was found in dogs to be, 1:4.5, in sheep 1:5. In his journal also appeared Valentin's studies on pathological concretions and wound healing, and his observations on decapitated criminals. Up to 1843 eight volumes of the journal were issued. Beginning with the second volume, publication took place in Switzerland.

Only one similar enterprise appeared and that much later, when Gustav Retzius published at his own expense the periodical *Biologische Mitteilungen,* a splendid folio publication devoted exclusively to his own research, of which the first volume came out in 1890 and the nineteenth and last as a Gustav Retzius Memorial volume in 1921.

In the review section of Valentin's *Repertorium* each separate paper published concerning biological problems was carefully listed, reviewed, and criticized. When he was doubtful or not clear about a method or result, he would try to repeat the investigation and give the results of his own experiments in addition. This holds true not only for the field of his main studies, physiology and anatomy, but for plant physiology, as well as for pathology. In the preface to Volume 1, he lays down the basis and the final aim of this endeavor, making the very sound statement: "If our entire medical science wishes to have a reliable basis, it is necessary that this basis should be the most excellent knowledge of the physiological conditions of the body in health and in sickness."

He emphasized that he regarded it as his main task in life to contribute as much as possible to this endeavor, and that he had founded his journal in order to have at his disposal an outlet for his continuous studies in this field. With this declaration and announcement, and with his physiological research in clinical problems, Valentin became one of the outstanding leaders in the development of modern medicine, he and his ideas standing on a par with his friend, J. Henle, and the latter's ideas as expressed in Henle and Pfeufer's *Zeitschrift für rationelle Medizin,* and with the other protagonists of modern scientific medicine.

It was more than twenty-five years later that Valentin expressed clearly these ideas which had aided him through his entire scientific life in the preface and the introduction to his book, *Versuch einer Physiologischen Pathologie der Nerven.*[18] Here, and in the succeeding three volumes on physiological pathology, he emphasizes his further conviction that science and medicine should be approached with the mentality of a physicist or a mathematician, and quoted the Pythagorean saying:

[18] Leipzig-Heidelberg, C. F. Winter, 1864.

Ὁ Θεὸς ἀριθμητίζει.[19] This attitude was not generally accepted at that time and had earned for him in 1848 the nickname of a "yatro-mathematician," bestowed by Emil DuBois-Reymond. This scientific approach to medicine rules his *Repertorium* from the first to the eighth (and last) volume. Today medicine is accustomed to regarding exact physics and mathematics as indispensable tools of its research. And it owes this development to the early hard work of "yatro-mathematicians" like G. Valentin, A. Fick, K. v. Vierodt, and others. This great contribution should never be forgotten.

We know that in the early nineteenth century an endeavor was made by various pioneers in the field of physiology and medical science to establish certain new journals, mainly for the purpose of publishing their own and their pupils' work. Some of these journals soon disappeared, while others attained a remarkable age. Valentin's *Repertorium* was not only unique in its type, but to a certain degree it was also successful, as proved by its continuation through eight volumes. Its first part contained the literature, as a bibliography, then, in systematic order, a review and a criticism of the various new papers; the third part presented new experiments and investigations by the editor himself. The subdivision of the entire field was excellent and quite up to date and demonstrates that Valentin, in organizing the vast biological material, became the forerunner of all the following "review" journals and "Centralblatt" Archives.

In Volume 1, Valentin subdivided the material as follows: general physiology, plant physiology, human anatomy, comparative anatomy, embryology, and experimental physiology.

In Volume 2 the subdivisions were: normal anatomy, pathological anatomy, normal embryology, pathological embryology, normal zoochemistry, pathological zoochemistry, normal physiology, and pathological physiology.

In the second volume the reviewing of plant anatomy and plant physiology was omitted. Valentin intended to make a separate comprehensive review of this field, which was to be published in the Swiss *Bibliothèque Universelle de Genève.* But on the request of his friends, he again included this branch of biology in his *Repertorium,* beginning with Volume 3. More and more the reviews filled the pages until the seventh and last volume contained no original contributions, except those that were interwoven with the reviews.

We do not know why the *Repertorium* finally ceased to appear. Of course it did not bring its publisher the financial success hoped for. Probably, however, Valentin was not able to continue with such a time-consuming enterprise, in addition to all his research work and writing, especially his textbooks on physiology, which needed all his time and energy. It seems that Valentin could not go along with the modern way of review journals, already initiated at that time by Johannes Müller's *Archiv,* by Cannstadt's *Jahresberichte der gesammten Medizin,* and others, whereby different authors were put in charge of reviewing certain parts of the enormous field. This was done in the above mentioned *Archiv*; but apparently Valentin did not approve of thus dividing the field of his interest among different reviewers.

Much information about Valentin's work and personality is found in these volumes of the *Repertorium.* How deeply, for instance, the young romantic Valentin was influenced in the early years of his research by Goethe and his *Farbenlehre* is apparent from the first volume of the journal. Here, in the title of the chapter in which he reviews fibrillatory movement in vertebrates, newly discovered by him and Purkinje, he calls it "Morphologisches Urphaenomen." This, of course, is a typical expression and approach to science taken from Goethe's vocabulary and mentality.

Valentin's reviewing activities did not stop with the discontinuation of the *Repertorium.* In any case he had to follow up the latest publications on physiology because he had to keep his textbook on physiology abreast of developments in science and medicine. How conscientious he was in this respect is apparent from the reproduction of two pages (see fig. 9) from his personal copy of his book on the physical investigation of tissues. The pages of the personal copies of his books were printed with especially wide margins, and these margins, as can be seen, are covered with his own alterations of the text and with notes on the most recent literature.

When he stopped publishing the *Repertorium,* he accepted Cannstatt's invitation to take over the task of reporting on the physiological literature for his annual reports on the progress of medicine in all countries, known under the name *Canstatt's Jahresberichte.* From 1844 to 1865 he did this very conscientiously, and because he did not spare criticism, he again made many enemies. One of his targets, A. W. Volkmann, Professor at the University of Halle, published in 1847 a small booklet under the title *Excursions in the Field of Exact Physiology,* bearing the subtitle, *A Polemic against Herrn Professor G. Valentin.* In this booklet Volkmann attempts to show in the rudest manner that Valentin does not understand anything, either in the field of physics or mathematics. As absurd as such generalized statements may be, the author, in explaining why he takes the pains to publish the booklet, nevertheless makes an interesting remark (p. 4). Valentin's criticism has to be answered, according to Volkmann,

> Because the medical world knows that the professor of physiology at Bern is a champion of exact physiology in Germany. Herr Valentin has made physical experiments in all branches of physiological knowledge and has tried

[19] It has not been possible to find up to now the exact source of this quotation.

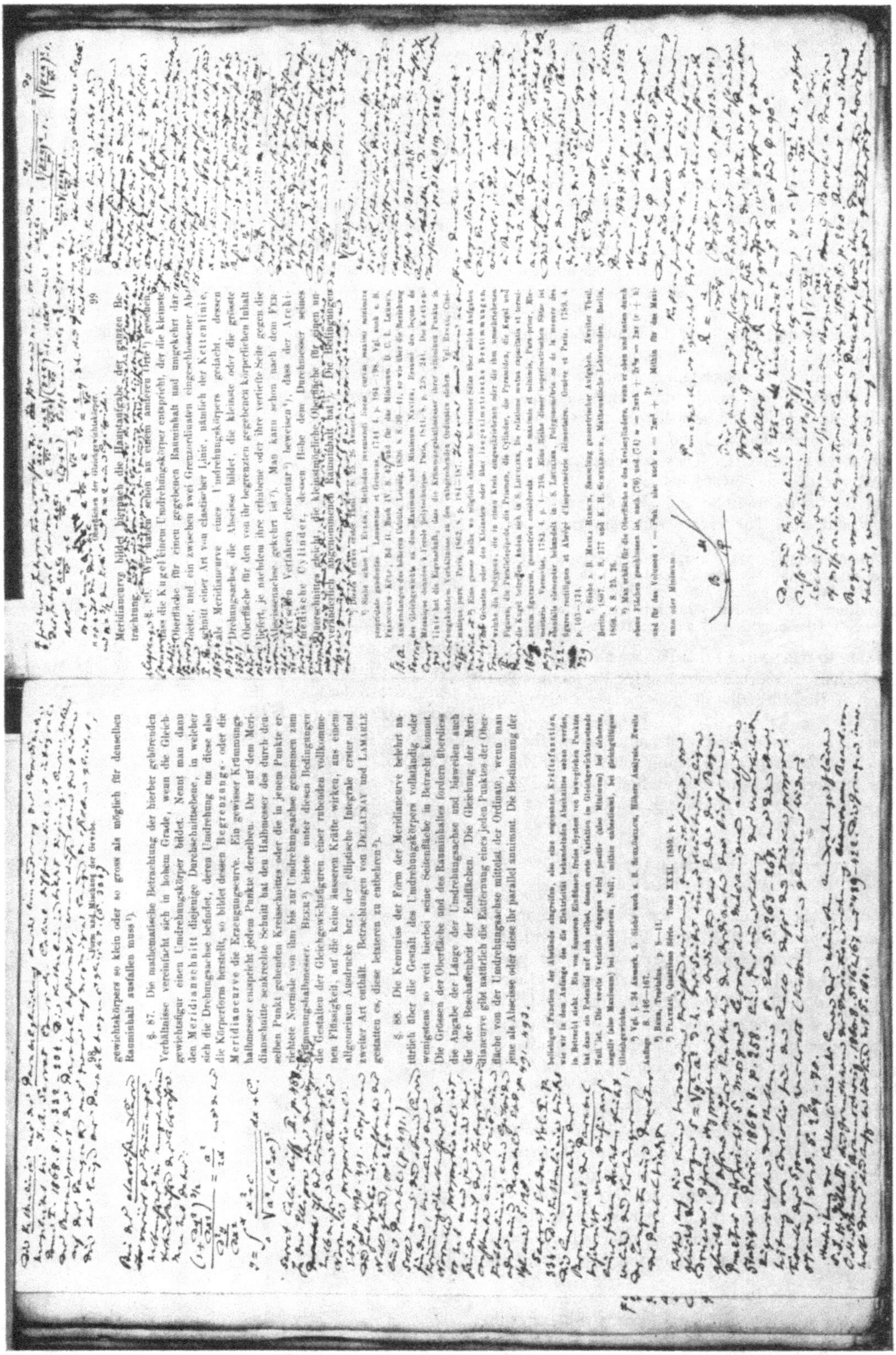

FIG. 9. Two pages from Valentin's textbook on the physical investigation of tissues, covered with his own annotations. From the author's collection.

everywhere to reduce the functions of life to figures and he has given us a textbook on physiology as richly furnished with formulae as a theory in astronomy.

Volkmann, who had a previous controversy with Valentin in the field of neurology, writes his booklet in a way that shows at a glance his personal animosity. In spite of this fact, however, it may be frankly admitted that Volkmann may have been right in objecting to certain of Valentin's statements.

In the manuscript biographical sketch which is extant in Bern in the handwriting of Valentin's son (B.B.B.) there is for the year 1848 a short remark on Volkmann's personality. I did not check on the reliability of the statements. They may be biased by the sentiment of the son toward his father. At least they present the family tradition and Valentin's feelings toward Volkmann. The entry reads (in translation):

> Volkmann from Dorpat,[20] dismissed demagogue and anti-Semite, was angry that the Physiology [Valentin's textbook] was twice published between 1845 and 1849. The Compendium (der Grundriss) ran into five editions in spite of Vieweg's [the publisher's] avarice and difficulties.

According to this source (B.B.B.) the stingy publisher, Vieweg, charged Valentin an extra fee for proofreading because of the allegedly illegible handwriting of the author.

There is no question that Volkmann was not the only one to fight back against Valentin's criticism. Nevertheless, between 1844 and 1865 we find Valentin eagerly busy reviewing the new physiological literature for *Canstatt's Berichte.*

FURTHER RELATIONS WITH THE PARIS ACADEMY

Meantime, in the name of the Paris Academy its secretary approached the busy Valentin[21] with the request that certain changes be made in his prize-winning paper and that it be adequately edited to make it possible to publish this 1,100-page manuscript. It was suggested that he omit parts that may have already been published and that he may reduce the number of figures and that he cite authors not only by name, but with the title of the quoted work and the pages. As a matter of fact, part of this manuscript had been published in the first volume of Valentin's *Repertorium.*

Valentin agreed to these changes, and Flourens, at that time "Sécretaire perpetuel," was directed to send the manuscript back to Valentin for this purpose, with instructions that a new revised manuscript be drafted and that the original manuscript be returned unchanged so that it might be preserved in the Archives of the Academy.

[20] Volkmann as well as Bidder was formerly professor at the University of Dorpat.

[21] *Compt. Rendu* 3: 435, 1836, and letter to Humboldt (B.B.B.).

At the meeting of April 16, 1838, Flourens was able to present Valentin's revised manuscript before the Academy for publication in the *Recueil des savants étrangers.* De Mirbel, one of the judges for 1835, received the manuscript for final judgment.

Later we find Valentin receiving honorable mention place, *aequo loco* with his teacher, Purkinje. At the meeting of February 4, 1839, he was nominated to fill a vacancy among the corresponding members in the section of Anatomy and Zoology, together with other world renowned scholars like Oken of Zürich, Carus of Dresden, Johannes Müller of Berlin, Owen of London, v. Baer of Königsberg, Rathke of Königsberg, and Delle Chiaje of Naples. Two ballots were necessary to reach an absolute majority for one of the candidates. The final vote was Owen of London, 24; Johannes Müller of Berlin, 17; and Oken of Zürich, 6. Owen was elected.

Valentin's name was proposed a second time when the section of Zoology and Comparative Anatomy had to elect a successor to the late Provençal. He was nominated July 30, 1845 together with Johannes Müller, Carus, v. Baer, Rathke, Purkinje, Delle Chiaje, Nordmann, Eschricht, and Newport, being named in fourth place, *aequo loco* with his teacher Purkinje. At the meeting of August 4, 1845 of the forty-two votes, forty-one were in favor of Johannes Müller and one in favor of Carus.

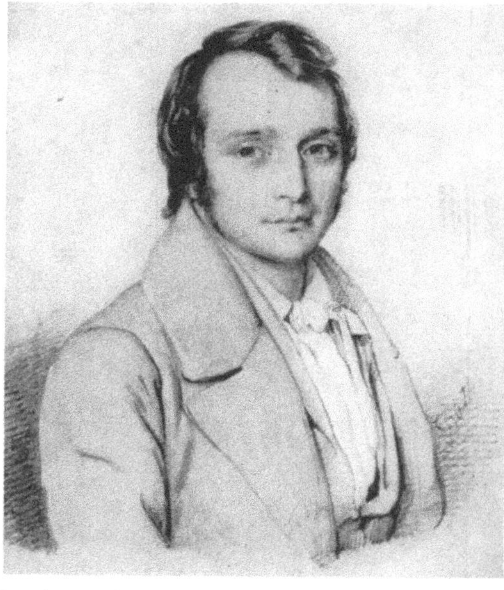

FIG. 10. Drawing of Valentin about 1840 made by Friedrich Dietler, a Swiss painter from Solothurn (1804–1874). Possession of Valentin's grandson, Dr. Hector Maillart. Courtesy of B.B.B.

PROFESSOR IN BERN

It was in 1835 when, finally, the day dreamed of by every young research worker came for Valentin. A university offered him a chair on its medical faculty with a generous salary of 1,500 thaler a year (B.B.B.), which meant independence, freedom from material worries and an opportunity to teach and to study to his heart's content. The University of Dorpat, re-established in 1801, invited him to join its medical faculty as a professor. Only one condition was imposed: he had to be baptized. Valentin rejected this offer (15, 21). The offer of a professorship could not persuade him to follow his master Purkinje's advice to the Jews, that they assimilate themselves to the point where recognition would be impossible. His father was already dead at this time, but his education and background had endowed him with a strong character and he refused to succumb to the great temptation of this offer or to a similar one that came from the University of Königsberg in Prussia at the same time. A short time later, in 1836, he was called as professor of physiology and zootomy to the young University of Bern in Switzerland. After his previous experiences, he first notified the University that he was a Jew (21 and B.B.B.) Only when Professor Rau's reply came stating that the head of the Bern Government, Schultheiss Neuhaus, did not see how Valentin's religion could interfere with his teaching, did he gladly accept the call, and he remained faithful to this small University in spite of the fact that later Brussels, Tübingen, Lüttich, and other universities repeatedly tried to win him for their medical faculties.

The University of Bern can, for all time, be proud of this unique, democratic decision, free of bias and prejudice. On the other hand, Valentin never did, as has been usual in Europe to the present, try to enhance his position in Bern by refusing calls to other universities. To him remaining in Bern was an expression of his attachment to the only place he liked warmly and thankfully all his life. Proof of this unselfish attitude is a letter from the Government of the Republic of Bern written on October 9, 1843 (B.B.B.), thanking Valentin for not accepting a call to the University of Tübingen in Germany, and also a previous call to the University of Brussels (Belgium), of which he himself did not even notify the Department of Education in Bern. When, in 1838, he refused a very distinguished and advantageous offer from the University of Utrecht in Holland, the grateful medical students of Bern serenaded him with a torchlight procession (71).

Before he decided, in 1836, to accept the professorship in Bern, Valentin asked the Prussian Minister, Altenstein, whether he could get even an assistant professorship (*Extraordinariat*) in Breslau, where he could remain with his teacher, Purkinje, or in Berlin,

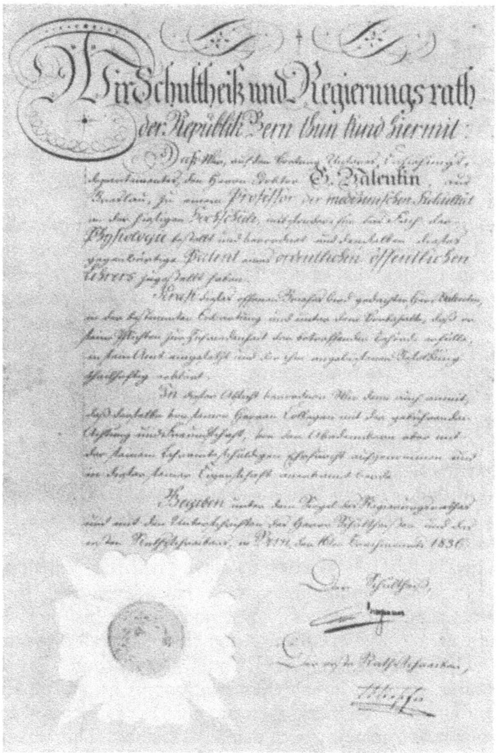
Wir Schultheiß und Regierungsrath der Republik Bern thun kund hiermit:

FIG. 11. Document appointing Valentin as full professor in the medical faculty "especially for the topic of physiology." This kind of wording indicates clearly that Valentin was obliged to teach not only physiology. See text p. 162. Courtesy of B.B.B.

where Johannes Müller was an attractive star on the faculty. This request was refused.

Shortly before this event and after he had received the Grand Prix, in March, 1836, Valentin went to Berlin and delivered a lecture there with demonstrations of his most recent discoveries. This lecture was given in the presence of a selected audience of outstanding physicians of Berlin on March 16, in the house of the above mentioned surgeon and professor, Dieffenbach (67: 237). He was hailed by teachers and students in Berlin (see p. 162). The minister of education, Altenstein, received him in a friendly way (32), but had no appointment for one who was not baptized. Johannes Müller told him very kindly that in the event of his baptism, he would immediately receive a professorship in Germany (see p. 163).

Rejected in Prussia as he knew he would be from his visit in Berlin (32), and refused a lesser university appointment, as a Jew, Valentin went to Switzerland to succeed Mohl, who until 1835 was professor of botany and physiology in Bern, and then left the university to follow a call to his home university, Tübingen (12).

The story of Valentin's call to Bern is worth reporting in some detail, not only because it was the first time that a non-baptized Jew was offered a chair on a German-speaking faculty, but because of the fact that some people later on tried to blame Valentin for having unjustly entered the field of anatomy in Bern whereas he was supposed to have been a physiologist. Fortunately, the correspondence concerning Valentin's call to the Bern faculty is extant (B.B.B.). Already in his first letter, that of April 25, 1836, Rau, professor of ophthalmology and pediatrics at Bern, asked Valentin whether he would be inclined "to accept a professorship in physiology and if possible at the same time in zootomy." Zootomy means literally dissection of animals; this would indicate that as early as Rau's first letter, Valentin was already asked to teach, not only physiology, but, if it would be possible for him, comparative anatomy also.

On that occasion Rau also stated that the University had two hundred students, fifty of them students of medicine.

In his first reply letter to Rau, (B.B.B.) Valentin, happy as he undoubtedly must have been over this great academic success, first mentioned his Jewish faith as a possible difficulty and then suggested as his weekly schedule for the winter term three hours lectures and one hour demonstrations in general anatomy and for the summer term four hours lectures in comparative anatomy with demonstrations. This leaves no doubt that from the very beginning and before his acceptance of the call to Bern, Valentin made it clear, at Rau's request, who spoke in the name of the faculty, that he would take over the duties of a physiologist as well as that of a teacher of general and comparative anatomy. That may also be the reason why his diploma of appointment mentions that he is appointed "especially for physiology"—peculiar wording that makes sense only in connection with the mutual agreement that he teach anatomy, too.

On May 5, Rau (B.B.B.) answered that Valentin's "religion will be no obstacle in the mind of any enlightened personality," and that this was also the attitude of the President of the Educational Department of the Government, but since some members of the faculty could be of a different opinion, he suggested that Valentin be anyway baptized before coming to Bern. This, of course, Valentin refused; nevertheless his appointment was unanimously recommended by the medical faculty to the Government on June 11, 1836, which appointed Valentin at its meeting on June 16, 1836.

Rau's letter of July, 1836 and his benevolent and well meant advice showed a complete lack of understanding of the importance of the religious question for the young professor, and caused the latter much uneasiness. To it Valentin wrote a very interesting reply concerning his moving to Bern and his acceptance of the call to this university (B.B.B.), the draft of which is preserved in Valentin's handwriting. It reads in translation:

My most esteemed friend and colleague, I leave up to you the decision concerning my apartment. I will bring with me bedding but not the furniture. I repeat only my wish to live with you in the same house, or in your neighborhood because you are the only one whom I know in Bern. It would be very desirable for me to have a separate working-room and bedroom. In any case I intend to hire a male servant.

Concerning my religious affiliations, I really don't know what to make of your latest letter. On the one hand, you say my religion could be offensive only to a few narrow-minded people; on the other hand, I should consider whether I would not rather be baptized before my arrival in Bern. May I take the liberty to explain why that cannot be done under any condition.

You know well that it is not bigotry which prevents me from being baptized but only the conviction that such a step, if connected with the attainment of any worldly goal, becomes despicable and discreditable. It means yielding to old prejudices, abandoning one's own people because one desires to join the group of better human beings. Especially we Jews are obliged to maintain our people's reputation, and I don't see any reason why I should bear this duty to a lesser degree than Meyer Beer, Halevy, Wilhelm Beer (the astronomer), Meyer (the jurist), Ruboni (the antiquary), Stilling (the physician), Levy, Weimars, Moser, Mendelssohn, and so many others. I have made great sacrifices for this idea, or better, for the consequence of this conviction. I report a few private experiences in my life to prove that, counting on your discretion as a friend when I mention events not proper to be made public. Of course, I mention without hesitation the names of the persons involved so that you may ask each of them whether there is the slightest difference between the facts and my report. Had I been inclined to receive baptism, I would have been professor in Dorpat a year ago with 1,500 rth. (3,600 Swiss francs) salary. Witness is Professor Erdmann in Berlin. If I had agreed to be baptized they would have offered me a professorship in Prussia on a silver platter (to use Prof. Johannes Müller's own words). A few weeks ago President Nees von Esenbeck was officially directed to tell me that I could have Rathkes' position in Königsberg with 1,200 rth (3,000 Swiss francs) salary. Here baptism is necessary for a teaching position at a university, because of a royal decree (*Kabinettorder*) which is definitely binding on the Ministry. Please ask those students from Switzerland now in Berlin about the kind of reception I received when I was there this March and you will find that my report is not exaggerated.

Again, two weeks ago the Curator of our University, Geheimer Oberregierungsrat Kleinke disclosed to me that the Prussian Ministry intends to offer to me everything that I have been offered abroad. I told him that I had given Bern my word and that I would keep it as an honest man. I don't like to be, so to speak, sold at auction, as is said to have occurred with the Danish and the Prussian Governments in the case of an esteemed theologian. I gave my word and I am decided to stand by it but only with the sure guarantee of my freedom of religion as I mentioned expressly in my letter to the Department of Education.

My dearest friend, you may ask each of our practicing physicians whether I am not making a great sacrifice economically by accepting the professorship in Bern and quitting my position as practicing physician in Breslau. I gladly do it to gain freedom of religion. Any violation of this principle and my quitting my new position in Bern would be inseparable. . . .

This letter, the original wording of which can be found on page 185, indicates how important the entire question of freedom of religion was for Valentin and his adamant and unselfish idealism. It also shows that he was busy and successful as a practitioner in Breslau, and we have proof of this fact also in his other correspondence, yet he was definitely not the over-busy, money-making type of practitioner (32).

Among the personalities he mentions as co-religionists refusing baptism, Meyerbeer and Halevy, the composers, are well known. The name, Meyerbeer, was originally written Meyer Beer. Otherwise, the spelling of the names mentioned by Valentin is not too exact. Wilhelm Beer, a brother of Meyerbeer, was a famous astronomer (1797–1850). His *Mappa Selenografica,* in particular, published in 1834–1836 together with Mädler was the first complete map of the moon, a standard work, which received an award from the Paris Academy. He was Prussian Geheimer Rath since 1837. A short biography of his was published in *Sulamith.*[22] The Meyer referred to unquestionably is the lawyer Marum (Max) Samuel von Mayer (1797–1862). Without being baptized he became, in 1829, lecturer and, in 1831, assistant professor (*extraordinarius*) at the University of Tübingen, and—but only after he received baptism in 1839—full professor at the same university. There is also a mistake in the spelling of the name, Ruboni. The scientist in question was Joseph Rubino (1797–1864). He was a legal historian who in 1832, without ever having taught at a university, received the title of professor and later lectured on ancient history and philology at the University of Marburg. After the death of his mother, he was baptized in 1842 and was nominated full professor in 1843. The anatomist and surgeon Benedikt Stilling (1810–1879) is famous for his investigations of the spinal cord, his pioneer work in abdominal surgery, and for performing, in 1837, the first extra-peritoneal ovariectomy. Because he remained faithful to his Jewish religion, he never achieved a position as an academic teacher. It is not clear which of the many famous men named Levy Valentin has here in mind. Perhaps the French mathematician and mineralogist, Armand Levy (1794–1841), at the University of Lüttich since 1828 and later professor of mineralogy at the Collège Royal de Charlemagne in Paris. The name, Weimars (or Levy Weimars), cannot be identified. Moser is probably Moses Moser (1796–1838), the friend of the poet Heine.

Later on neither Rau nor anyone else pressed the question of Valentin's baptism any more.

[22] 8: 363, 1838.

In September 1836 Valentin finally left Breslau by mailcoach for his wonderful new homeland. The Prussian police denied him (August 29, 1836) a passport for a projected trip to the various capitals of Germany and Switzerland but handed him, on August 30, a consent to his emigration (B.B.B. Mss.Hist.Helv. XXVIII/68). Such was his farewell from Germany. Valentin strongly resented this attitude of the Prussian Government. In a letter of August 9, 1836 he writes to Humboldt describing his departure from Germany: "To retain my citizenship was denied me by the Government in Breslau. I was advised to emigrate because, instead of being idle, I followed my unfortunate and inextinguishable inner vocation to do scientific research." Concluding his letter with the remark that he, like many others, knows well Humboldt's kind, understanding, and always helpful attitude, he says: "As long as my body does not break down and succumb, I will continue spiritual work. Perhaps this, my example, will one day have an effect, even when not an atom of me shall remain any longer" (B.B.B.).

It is understandable that after all these humilitating experiences, Valentin would want to make a dignified appearance for his new position in Bern. That is probably why he wrote Rau that he intended to hire a male servant. Also, before leaving Breslau, the twenty-six-year-old professor added some distinction by buying a seal ring for 3 thaler (account of his father's estate, B.B.B.).

His departure from his home town must have been celebrated by his friends and admirers in high spirits. As previously mentioned, his relations with old Purkinje, toward the end of his stay in Breslau, were less cordial than in previous years. However, some celebration took place before the young professor left Breslau, to participate in the meeting of the society of German physicians and scientists in Jena in September, 1836, where he demonstrated an apparatus for physiological optics,[23] before proceeding to Switzerland. A poem in Greek was printed (B.B.B.) in Breslau (Richter was the publisher) commemorating the occasion. It was written by one Adolph Levy, who a few years later, when he wrote a poem for Valentin's wedding, called himself a very close friend (Busenfreund). This poem, too, was printed.

The Jewish community of Breslau and the entire Jewry of Germany and Europe were proud of Valentin's success. When he was awarded the Grand Prix of the Paris Academy, he received a congratulatory scroll on January 8, 1836 of the Jewish community of Breslau (B.B.B.) and a diploma as honorary member of the historical Jewish Society for the Care of Sick People (Israelitische Krankenver-pflegsanstalt Chevra Kadischa), which had been in existence in Breslau since 1726. This certificate, also dated January 8, 1836, was the first honorary membership bestowed on Valen-

[23] *Repertorium* 1: 272, 1837.

tin, whose long scientific career was to be distinguished by many more such honors.

As mentioned before, Valentin was appointed on June 16, 1836 full professor (*professor ordinarius*) on the medical faculty of Bern University, with a yearly salary of 2,800 francs (12) and reimbursement for his moving and travelling expenses amounting to 400 francs (67: 544). After his refusal to accept a call to the medical faculty in Tübingen in 1843, his salary was increased to 3,000 francs (12).

The following year, 1837, Valentin was seriously considered for a chair on the medical faculty of Basel, but finally a Swiss competitor, Frederic Miescher, from Bern was appointed professor of physiology and pathology (5).

Valentin's domain as physiologist at Bern was, in the beginning, even less impressive than that of his former master, Purkinje, at Breslau. In the anatomy building there was one room for the physiologist, with a stove to dry his specimens, one large and one small table, a few chairs, a small desk, a locked cabinet, and a few shelves. He had a yearly budget of 100 francs for his laboratory (12). That was a modest beginning but he started out with enthusiasm and eagerness, and he brought with him an invaluable treasure in the form of a modern microscope made by Plössel in Vienna, at that time probably the only such instrument at Bern (64).

Shortly after he began his activities at Bern, in 1837, the young professor went to Paris to learn, by personal contact, about the leading new ideas of this world-famous school and to become acquainted there with people outstanding in the world of medicine and science, all of whom, when they met him, showed him kindness and respect, as the distinguished medical men in Berlin had done the year before. Among them were Magendie, Flourens, Blainville, and Arago, who became his new personal acquaintances (21). The draft of a letter to Magendie, dated November 15, 1837 (B.B.B.), still reflects Valentin's thankfulness for the "bien veillance que vous avez bien voulu m'accorder pendant mon séjour à Paris." Valentin's new friends in Paris tried to get him an appointment to the greater University of Lüttich (21, 12), but this University like Marburg (21), though very willing to acquire such a famous man, demanded that Valentin give up his Jewish faith in return for being admitted to their faculty, and this he refused decisively to do.

That Valentin's attachment to Judaism was really deep-rooted, we learn not only from his own letters, quoted above, but also from remarks in Ludwig Bamberger's autobiography (2: 210), recalling the time when the latter was a frequent guest in Valentin's house in Bern, as a German political refugee in 1849. Bamberger also tells there the story of how he introduced another political refugee to the Valentins, a physician named Loewe-Kalbe, the last president of the Frankfurt parliament (in Stuttgart). Valentin, mistaking Loewe-Calbe for a Jew, earnestly discussed Jewish problems with him all evening, and Loewe-Kalbe did not dare to dampen the enthusiasm of his kind host by revealing his true religion.

When Valentin took over the chair of physiology at Bern, he soon proved to be a most inspiring teacher. He taught in German as well as in French, mastering the latter language perfectly in spite of the fact that it was not his native tongue (15). In 1841 he also published a book on the anatomy of the echinodermata in French (1).

Valentin felt happy in his new activities as a professor, which had been denied to him in a biased Germany. Of course, his feelings were deeply hurt by his experiences in his native country, and that, too, may have influenced him later not to accept any call to a German university, such as he received repeatedly, for instance, from the University of Tübingen.

Among Valentin's letters to Andres Retzius, famous Swedish anatomist, there is one from 1837, about one year after he moved to Bern, from which we learn not only of his close attachment to Retzius, but also of his still lively resentment of German intolerance against a Jewish scientist and of his deeply-rooted feeling for the Jewish religion, also of his happiness over the working conditions in his very modest new realm in Bern.

This letter, as Valentin's personal report on his lot before 1837, is so revealing that it seems appropriate to reproduce it in its original form as well as in the following literal translation:

Esteemed Friend:

Since I was so fortunate to make your acquaintance at Purkinje's in Breslau, much has changed. Meanwhile she, good [Mrs.] Purkinje, my unforgettable friend, passed away, shortly after Purkinje's old mother had died. I myself am far away, separated from my old teacher; Providence designated me to the role of a "Refugié," not to a political one but a religious one. Refusing to handle my religion in a conscienceless way and to relinquish it for worldly goods, I had to part with my fatherland. Thank God! I found conditions here in Switzerland such that I can be satisfied with this change in every respect, and I may say I am better off than I would have expected and than I may deserve.

My sincerest thanks for your fine investigations about teeth! Permit me to send you enclosed my investigation of nerves. Its appearance already arouses some struggle, which may finally only help to foster the light of truth.

May I dare, perhaps, to ask you the favor to let me have for love or money, from time to time, the most outstanding papers on anatomy and physiology that appear in Sweden. I am almost entirely cut off from the Swedish literature.

Please write *soon, very soon*

to your

loving and admiring

Valentin.

Bern 1st of November 1837

The tone of this letter shows the close relationship between Valentin and Retzius, this closest friend of Johannes Müller, and the delight Valentin took in his

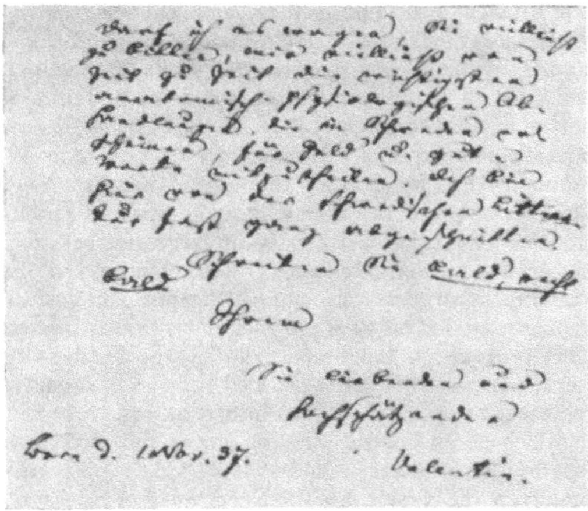

FIG. 12. Letter from Valentin to Professor Anders Retzius in Stockholm. Courtesy, The Royal Swedish Academy of Sciences in Stockholm.

small laboratory. He loved Bern and Switzerland, and time and again in his letters he invited Retzius to visit this wonderful country. Whoever has once visited the beautiful, romantic old town of Bern, situated in the most beautiful countryside, will understand very well Valentin's enthusiasm for his new home. He was delighted with his work and position in Bern, and the students as well as the Bern Government were greatly satisfied with their young and famous professor.

Valentin, with a natural gift for teaching, always felt happy when he was with his students. He was impressive as a teacher, loved by his pupils, and at the time, around 1840, he was unquestionably the outstanding personality on the faculty. A Berlin journal edited by Mundt under the title, *Der Freihafen,* in 1839 published a report signed "VR," concerning the young medical faculty in Bern and its various members. Valentin is described as the first personality among the professors. This report is literally quoted in the Berlin medical *Central Zeitung.*[24] The paragraph on Valentin reads as follows:

> Valentin, from Silesia, practiced previously in Breslau. It is an honor for the Government of Bern that it did not hesitate to appoint this efficient man, despite his profession of the Jewish religion, when he himself, before his appointment, asked them to consider this fact. He delivers his lectures in a quiet and contemplative way. His diction is flawless and easily understood. In company he is well-mannered and courteous, but he seldom associates with others. Valentin is small, with brown, curly hair. His forehead is high. His eyes are small and dark and down his cheeks he wears sideburns.

This description fits very well the drawing of young Valentin by F. Koska in Klein's almanac of 1845 and the drawing by Johann Friedrich Dietler from Solothurn (1804–1874), which we reproduce, and the lithograph which the firm Huber and Company published in Bern in 1845.[25] The entire report of the journal *Freihafen* conveys the favorable impression its writer received on attending Valentin's lectures and personally interviewing him. The author adds in the same article of 1839 that the anatomical theatre (lecture room) and "cabinet" (collections) were newly built and well-equipped under Theile and Valentin, and that there was even an assistant (*Gehülfe*) by the name of Schleu, with a talent and skill for modelling and castmaking, but that he did not have the necessary support. Besides the information on Valentin's personality, we learn from this article again that Valentin, from his early days at Bern, really was active in the anatomical department together with Theile, as well as doing his outstanding work in physiology.

In 1850 the governing body of Bern had to decide on Valentin's application for citizenship. The session turned into an occasion for the expression of warm appreciation for the contribution Valentin had made to the prestige of the Bern medical faculty. His naturalization as a Swiss citizen took place on May 1, 1850 at the Community Miécourt; the certificate is signed in the name of the President and *Grosser Rat* of the Canton of Bern (B.B.B. XXVIII/68).

According to Hirschfelder (21), Valentin was the first Jew to become a citizen of Switzerland (1850), just as he was the first unbaptized Jew to become full professor at a university using the German language.

Professor C. Vogt, who as a student shared, in close collaboration, Valentin's working place and problems in his first two years at Bern, gives the following description, as he remembered it sixty years later (64), of the place where Valentin was so content. This is what he has to say about the location of Valentin's first laboratory, and about its contents.

> Valentin found the collection of objects pertaining to comparative anatomy in a terribly neglected condition. They were kept, as badly as possible, together with the human anatomy and physiology, in an old powder magazine of the fortress. There were a few skeletons, and in addition, a series of miscarriages preserved in glasses whose alcohol content appeared very tasty to the drunken anatomy servant. From time to time, however, the alcohol had to be replaced, because this collection was of special attraction to the young couples who were to be married in the nearby church! There were, in particular, no preparations of soft tissues. Valentin instructed me in microscopical techniques and taught me how to prepare insects and other small animals under water. He also suggested that I should help him in the preparation of soft tissues for purposes of demonstrations in his lectures. . . .
>
> Theile, the professor of anatomy, approached his field mainly from the practical point of view of the physician

[24] *Central Zeitung* 1839: 856.

[25] Professor E. Hintzsche called my attention to an old Swiss book catalogue, which he found announcing the sale and year of publication but not the name of the artist of this lithograph, probably made from Dietler's drawing.

and surgeon. But Valentin asked continuously for new preparations for his lectures.

How much Valentin enjoyed the beauty of the Alps and the city is repeatedly expressed in his letters to Retzius. There he also took the opportunity to do scientific research on some matters that were new to him. His pioneer work in research on hibernation may have been inspired by the marmots, animals common in Switzerland. It resulted in not less then twenty-six publications by Valentin on this subject between 1856 and 1879.

Bern's coat of arms presents a bear, and live bears were always kept and are kept even now as heraldic animals of the town, in special bear pits for the amusement of the citizens. From this source Valentin probably got the material for a paper on the bear's spermatoza, published in 1837 in the *Proceedings of the Imperial Leopoldino-Carolina Academy.*[26] This paper is of great interest, showing how even an excellent microscopist like Valentin might become the victim of preoccupying ideas in science at a time preceding Schleiden and Schwann's cell theory. The old concept of the animalculists that the spermatozoön is, so to say, a little animal with animal organs was still so prevalent that Valentin describes, though hesitantly, the picture of what he observed on the bear's spermatozoa as follows:

> For the present the supposition may be expressed that the inner bubbles [he found in the head of the spermatozoa] may be explained as stomach bubbles, or as a liver-like organ, or, which seems most probable, as a microscopic presentation of a tortuous inner intestinal channel . . . the anterior dark circle would present the oral, and the posterior, the anal orifice.

Such an opinion was by no means unbelievable in 1837. Gerber, in his *General Anatomy* (p. 210), describes similar findings in the rabbit's spermatozoa, where he too thought he discovered the place of the sex organs. In 1841 J. Henle still reported these two observations seriously in his *General Anatomy* as contributions to our knowledge in biology. In spite of such grotesque misinterpretation of the microscopic facts, this paper of Valentin's made a new and valuable contribution in the introduction of the incineration technique into microscopic methods, a technique that to the present has played an important role in microscopy.

Valentin, of course, did not limit his activities, in the first year of his stay in Bern, to anatomical and microscopic investigations. Very soon the young professor of physiology also started experimental research in this field. He began with animal experiments to determine structure and function of the various nerves (cerebral n.n. and n. sympathicus) which, after a few years, resulted in his well-known book published in 1839 and in an Italian translation issued by G. J. Sacchero in Turin in 1843.

When Valentin took over his position in Bern, his first problem was to bring the anatomical collection up to the modern standard. He continued his microscopic studies, witness his paper on the bear's spematozoa, and tried to introduce interested students to this new field of medical research (64). He then started on new physiological experiments on dogs with a view to determining the function of the lingual nerves. Vogt (64) reports how this almost brought him into serious trouble. Valentin operated on a large butcher dog, but owing to the carelessness of the servant in the anatomy department, the animal escaped and with a gaping wound in his neck ran back to his former master. This provoked a tumultuous riot by the butchers of Bern, who were not easily placated. Swiss newspapers reported the incident. Valentin had to write a report, in which he blamed the careless porter and received a lengthy letter dated August 16, 1838, signed personally by the president of the Department of Education of Bern, C. Neuhaus, who urged Valentin "and the other teachers at the anatomical institution" to restrict for the future as much as possible all kinds of vivisections performed in the anatomical laboratory (B.B.B.).

From the beginning Valentin's teaching duties included anatomy, as mentioned above and established by Rau's and Valentin's letters. He later asserted (12) that from 1836 he was under contract as the director of anatomy, but apparently such a contract did not exist in writing. On the title pages of Volume 1, Nos. 3 and 4, Volume 2 and 3 of his *Repertorium,* he calls himself *only "o.ö Professor der Physiologie an der Universität zu Bern,"* and, beginning with Volume 4 (1839), only G. Valentin. However, from his appointment in 1836 until 1863, Valentin was the only full professor teaching anatomy at Bern. His *Traité de Névrologie,* translated into French by A. J. L. Jourdan in 1843, describes Valentin on the title page as *Professeur d'Anatomie et de Physiologie à l'Université de Berne* surely written with his consent, and the first printed biography of Valentin (32) calls him in 1845 *"Professor der Anatomie und Physiologie an der Universität Bern."* When, in 1845, the anatomist, Theile, left the Bern faculty, Valentin took over the directorship of anatomy officially. He discharged this duty successfully until 1862, when the faculty, against Valentin's wishes, decided to create a chair in anatomy independent of that in physiology.

THE CONTROVERSY VALENTIN *vs.* REMAK

Unfortunately, as mentioned before, Valentin did not realize the relationship of the constituents of the nervous system to each other, and when Robert Remak (1836–1838) made the fundamental discovery that the nerve fibers stem from the ganglionic cells, Valentin did not abandon his own misconception that both these parts of the nervous system are only in local contact and not really connected. In Valentin's opinion only a "juxtaposition" existed between ganglionic cells and nerve fibers, never and nowhere a real connection or fusion

[26] **19**: 239, 1837.

of these two parts of the nervous system. He still emphasized his point of view very strongly in 1838 and later, after Remak's fundamental discovery (69) had already been extensively published and recognized.

The entire controversy between Valentin and Remak, and Valentin *versus* Bidder and Volkmann concerning the histology of the nervous system, sheds a very strong light on Valentin's character, its strong points and shortcomings. The struggle really started in 1838 in Volume 3 of Valentin's *Repertorium.* It is clear from his remarks there that he, at that time already the twenty-eight-year-old famous professor, the recipient of the Grand Prix of the Paris Academy, was irritated and indignant because of the sure and apodictic statements in Remak's doctoral thesis of 1838, which he strongly resented. According to Valentin's letter to Remak, which appears on page 169, there must have been an exchange of letters between the two scholars between 1836 and 1838. Unfortunately, these letters are not extant, but they must have been written in a somewhat sharp tone. Valentin seems to have offered Remak some help, which offer Remak regarded as insolence, to which he replied with strong personal attacks. This may have put the spark to the powder barrel. In his *Repertorium* [27] where he only enumerates the outstanding new literature, adding a short description and often somewhat schoolmasterish remark to the most outstanding papers of the year, Valentine supplemented the citation of Remak's thesis, "Observationes . . . ," with the following statement: "Numerous partly very beautiful, partly wrongly interpreted observations proffered with deplorable arrogance." This is strong language for a reviewing editor.

As a matter of fact, there is nothing arrogant in Remak's thesis. Johannes Müller, from whose laboratory it was published, would not have permitted an arrogant paper as a doctoral thesis, and he himself definitely resented Valentin's sharp, attacking reviews. Valentin was apparently hurt by the fact that a young student of twenty-one (in 1836), and again when he was twenty-three years of age, dared to utter as incontrovertible truth observations that had escaped the attention of Purkinje and Valentin, and had frankly refused to accept any help offered to him by Valentin (see p. 170).

One fact, of course, must be admitted, which makes Valentin's reaction understandable, though it does not justify it. In Remak's doctoral thesis he refers repeatedly to Valentin and his outstanding publication on the nervous system and emphasizes repeatedly that statements made there by Valentin are wrong or cannot be confirmed by him or that Valentin had overlooked important facts. All this Remak did in a very objective manner and tone, without any "subjectivities," as his teacher Müller used to call reproaches and personal attacks. Apparently, just as his teacher on his own account demonstrated it to Valentin, Remak, too, was of the opinion that objective scientific criticism cannot be regarded as an irritating personal offense. At least, with respect to his own personality Valentin was, in his acute sensitivity, of a different opinion, and this accounted for his acid criticism of Remak's fundamental work.

In many pages of Volume 3 of his *Repertorium* [28] Valentin fights stubbornly against Remak's great discoveries. Nowhere does he mention any new thorough reinvestigation of his own, but, blinded by his emotional attitude, he makes the bad mistake of condemning new discoveries from the point of view of old convictions. We do not believe our eyes when we read that Valentin disputes the existence of Remak's nerve fibers (the organic nerve fibers of the sympathetic nerves), for that contradicts the modern trend in medicine. Nothing was known at that time about the influence of nerves on the nutritional processes in the body; consequently, such nerves cannot be found. This is approximately Valentin's reasoning, and it remained on this level for many years. Johannes Müller, Purkinje, Rosenthal, and Hannover, all fine scholars, agreed more and more with Remak's statements; only Henle, who worked in Müller's laboratory at the same time as Remak, joined Valentin in his fight. This may have been the beginning of the close friendship between Valentin and Henle, Valentin later being instrumental in Henle's appointment to a chair at the University of Zürich. Still, in 1840, Valentin was fighting in the Remak controversy against his own teacher Purkinje, yet even so with all due respect toward his "forever thankfully revered father in science." [29] It is only in 1842,[30] when doubt as to Remak's discoveries was no longer possible, that Valentin, in two footnotes, admits the existence of Remak's unmedulated nerve fibers and the central band (axis-cylinder). However, he does not yet concede Remak's basic concept of the connection of nerve fiber and ganglionic cell. On the other hand, it speaks in favor of Valentin's character that when Remak complained in a letter (B.B.B.) about Valentin's attacks, stressing his own poor health and expressing a longing for peace and quiet studying, he answered in a very kind letter.

Remak was the victor in all the points of the discussion, and Valentin lost a great opportunity to be helpful in verifying publicly the great revolutionary discoveries of a young scholar. Later, in 1843, in his textbook on neurology, Valentin conceded the possibility that Remak was correct in his discoveries. However, in the fourth edition of his outline of physiology in 1855, he was still not convinced of the anatomical origin of nerve fibers in ganglionic cells (p. 367). Thus, this great personality is a deplorable example of all the

[27] 3: 14, 1838.

[28] 73 ff., 76 ff.

[29] *Repertorium* 5: 8.

[30] *Ibid.* 7: 113, 115.

dangers of personal prejudice when introduced into scientific research.

There is no question that Valentin was a stubborn character. It was not Valentin's way to accept easily other scientists' opinions or even their objective findings, if these were opposed to his own. Of course, we should not forget that in his attitude toward Remak's discoveries he was supported by some of the best of his confreres and contemporaries: in some points by his teacher Purkinje, by Reichert, Bidder, Volkmann, his friend Henle, and, for a certain time, even by Remak's own master, Johannes Müller. Things were not so obvious in the early days of medical microscopy as they are today in the era of embedding of histological objects, of microtomes, staining, and high power magnification.

We may feel strongly about Valentin's attitude towards Remak's discoveries from the scientific point of view and we may condemn the rude form of his criticism. However, we feel differently about Valentin's character on reading the following letters by Remak and Valentin, which may represent the culminating point of their dispute. Valentin's reply to Remak shows in more than one regard similarities to Müller's letter (see p. 187) of December 31, 1837 (see next chapter) to Valentin and may even have been influenced by Müller's human kindness in this letter. Underneath all Valentin's belligerence and his derogatory remarks appears a warm-hearted personality and a strong drive to discover the real truth. He is eager to be helpful, is astonished to find that he has hurt other people's feelings by his criticism, and is really sorry for it.

In all probability Valentin met young Remak, at that time a student of twenty-one years and not yet graduated, when he visited Johannes Müller in his laboratory in Berlin in March, 1836. He met there Schwann and Henle, and both appear later in Müller's letters to Valentin in his reports on their well-being and as sending Valentin their regards. It would have been strange if on such a visit he had not met Remak, too. We know that Purkinje met him on a similar occasion, but Remak is never mentioned in Müller's letters to Valentin.

Remak, the easily irritated member of this group, already deeply involved in neurological research which yielded results, contrary to Valentin's, may have met the laureate of the French academy, when the latter visited Müller's laboratory, with more reserve and even critical suspicion than the others did. Probably on this occasion occurred the incident mentioned in Valentin's letter—he offered Remak his help, probably in research problems, perhaps also in questions of his career, and Remak took this as an insult and arrogance on Valentin's part, so that when Remak's paper came out in 1836 and 1838 Valentin criticized it as he did in a sharp, sarcastic way. That, of course, infuriated Remak still more; then good friends called his attention also to previous publications of Valentin, inferring that they were meant as attacks against Remak, too. That was finally the reason for an exchange of letters between the two men, which at least on Remak's side, must have been written in a very belligerent mood, attacking Valentin's character. Of this entire correspondence only two letters, one by Remak and two similar drafts of Valentin's answer, are extant.

Remak's letter is an apology for having wrongly taken as a further offense a passage in Valentin's previous publications, which proved, indeed, to have been printed before the time of Remak's publication and could not have been meant as an attack against him. Remak's letter of excuse is concluded not in a peaceful spirit, but with a threat to renew the war at the first disparagement by Valentin. Valentin's answer is very friendly indeed; he tries to restore peace and even offers Remak help again, once hinting that he is willing to assist Remak in securing an appointment at a Swiss university, a magnanimous gesture considering Remak's previous letter. Recalling Müller's letter of New Year's Eve of 1837/38 one cannot help seeing in the tone and spirit of Valentin's letter to Remak of October 1838 a sincere attempt to make good for the wrong he had done before to Remak and Müller himself. Remak's letter mentioned here dated September 8, 1838, is a reply to the not traceable letter from Valentin of the seventh of July, apparently a letter in which Valentin denied having attacked Remak in a certain case.

Remak's letter reads in translation:

Sir:

To your letter of July 7 I answer that my previous statement should be corrected in so far as the paragraph I mentioned is to be found not in your *Repertorium*, but in your paper on the ends of the nerves. There it reads. . . .

Here follows a quotation (see the complete text of this letter, p. 186) and Remak's explanation for the delay in his reply. He concedes that he may have been mistaken in believing that this paragraph was intended to attack his work, as friends had told him. The last paragraph of this letter is of interest. It reads:

I surely hope that our correspondence concerning this matter will now be finished; otherwise, I shall be compelled to protect myself in an appropriate manner against new invectives. The present condition of my chest organs is such that in all probability I shall not be permitted to take part in any more scientific investigations in the future. I therefore would have more reason than anyone else to live in peace with all the world. Through no fault of mine I was not able to do so in this case. At least I can quiet my conscience knowing that I have irritated no one purposely by my publications.

R. Remak

Berlin, September 8, 1838.

This letter from one of the most promising collaborators of Johannes Müller impressed Valentin very much. Müller's letter of December 31, 1837, reproaching Valentin for his teasing and caustic criticism of the work of

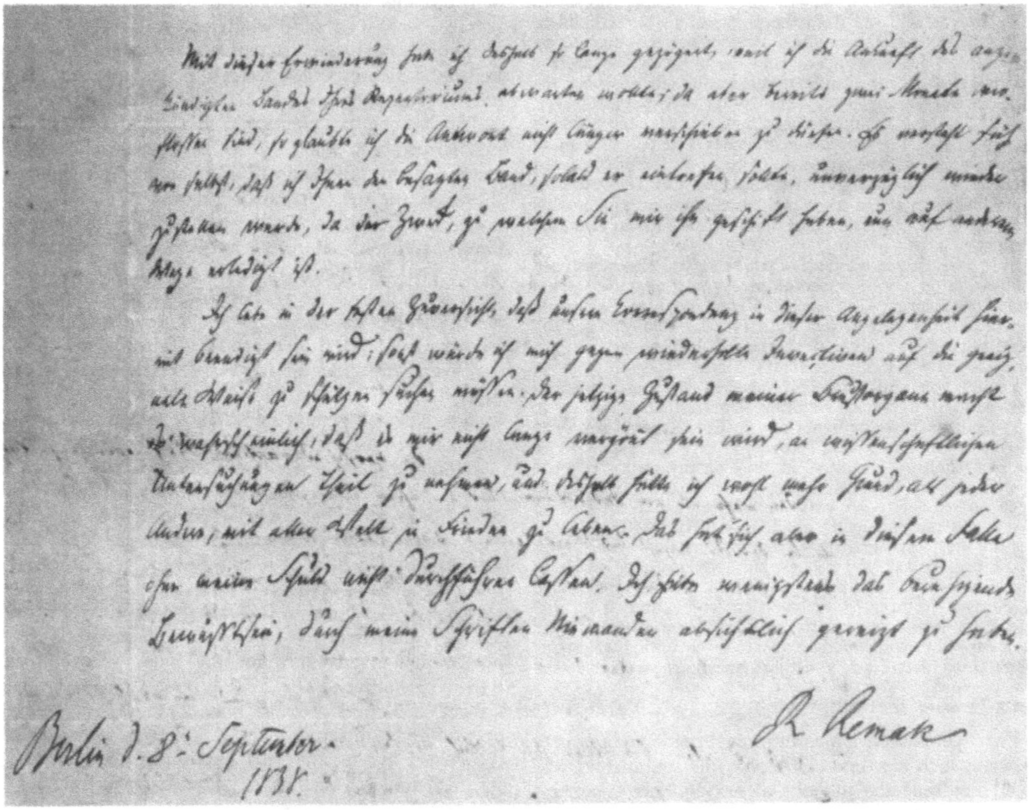

FIG. 13. Letter from Remak written to Valentin at the peak of their controversy. Courtesy of B.B.B.

others, was still well remembered and he was now really sorry to have hurt so deeply the feelings of a scientist who apparently was seriously ill. It was a time when tuberculosis still was the main killer of young people, and medicine was helpless against this enemy. Valentin's very kind answer must have been influenced by Müller's attitude towards him and the feeling that a scientist does not compromise his dignity by offering peace and a helpful hand to another scientist.

Two very similar, yet in significant details different, drafts of this letter are extant, both written on the same day, which shows how important this matter must have been for Valentin (see both on pp. 186–188). The following is a translation of one version, the final answer to a group of severely insulting letters from Remak:

Most esteemed Herr Doktor,

In your last letter you depict your disease of the chest in such dark colors that I am very sincerely sorry, in spite of what has gone before, which surely could only alienate me from you. I hope and wish that you regard your disease as more serious than it really is. In spite of your direct statement in your letters that you have no high opinion of my moral qualities and that you are convinced of my hatred toward you, I can definitely assure you that I feel the deepest sympathy with your bodily sufferings and that I am looking forward anxiously to receive better news concerning your health. Without going into details I can only tell you that I regard my feelings towards you as more sincere than those of the "denouncers" who call your attention to places in my publications, which, as you can see on the title page, were *printed* before your first paper came out in Müller's *Archiv.* I have long become accustomed to being misjudged by people and to be denounced is no longer new for me.

I myself formerly suffered most serious complaints of the chest. I therefore know very well the bad effect emotions have on such patients and feel it a duty to make peace with you. As sharp as was my thrust against you in the first issue of this year's *Repertorium*, it pained me to the heart when I received your latest letter. I am not reluctant to confess a mistake I have made, and I declare freely that I would have let the entire matter alone had I known anything about the condition of your health.

In a publication just off the press (*De functionibus sensoriis et motoriis N.N. cerebralium N. que Sympathici*), where I treat the same topic in the chapter, *De gangliorum fabrica*, as you will see, I first proffered my hand to make peace, because I now see clearly the relation between your organic fibers and the sheath of the ganglionic globules. Both, as you will see from the pictures, are entirely identical. In the N.N. mollibus presenting the connecting branches of the N. sympath. and the brain nerves are the continuations of the sheaths of the ganglionic globules, the main part of the material. The law is valid for all nerves, that an inverse relation exists between the processes of the sheaths of the ganglionic globules and the amount of cerebrospinal nerves present. You will learn from the publication that the N. sympathicus is a complete cerebrospinal nerve in so far as it can be checked experimentally. It is more than probable that also with regard to nutrition it belongs in this group.

Still during this winter I shall send you the mentioned publication as a gift presented in return for yours. Only please don't forget that packages from Bern to Berlin via bookdealers (a real detour, rather) take a long time, and from personal economic reasons no bookdealer is in a hurry to send out complimentary copies.

Should you still vaguely remember your previous letters, you will agree, on thinking it over, that according to the rules prescribed by honor and justice, I should not write to you at all any more. However, all that happened in the past shall be forgotten, at least on my part. When I offered you my services before, you regarded that as insolence and audacity. I may emphasize that even enemies who know me personally would not attribute these qualities to me. Trusting that you may change your opinion, I dare to ask you a question. Kronenberg, who was here for a few days this summer, told me that you intend to go as a lecturer to Wilna. To which branch do you intend to devote your activities? Do you speak French so fluently that you would be able to teach in this language? Don't think that I ask you these questions without a certain purpose.

Bern, October 27, 1838 G. VALENTIN

For a person like Valentin it must not have been easy to write such a letter. However, his sentimental soul could not bear the thought of having hurt a perhaps fatally ill younger colleague and he was disturbed by a guilty conscience. He apologizes and confesses a mistake. He pleads for forgiveness. He has meantime continued his studies and realizes that his judgment was hasty. In the other draft of his letter he even says: "I am very glad to be able to report that I now finally convinced myself of the correctness of your observation of your organic fibers." Of course, Valentin still regards Remak's fibers only as a continuation of the sheaths of ganglionic cells, but in his earlier review in the *Repertorium,* he had only sarcastic comments for Remak's "deplorably arrogant" assertion that these fibers existed beyond any doubt, and his resentment of Johannes Müller's criticisms was also connected with this statement, which he himself now had to revoke.

However, his letter to Remak is not a simple excuse and correction of a mistake made, but the expression of a real, warm, human sympathy, forgiving and asking for forgiveness; more than that, in spite of previous bad experiences, he offers Remak his help in securing a teaching position in Switzerland. Perhaps he was thinking of providing for him a call to Bern, as he did in 1855 for Moritz Schiff.

We do not know how Remak reacted to this offer of peace and friendship, and it took many more years before Valentin agreed that Remak was right in all his "deplorably arrogant" statements, but at no time after that did Valentin attack Remak in the rude manner of his first report on his work on the nervous system.

The Kronenberg mentioned in this letter was Heinrich Kronenberg who in 1836 had just graduated as a medical doctor in Berlin with an anatomico-physiological thesis on the nerve plexus. He was a pupil of Rudolphi and Johannes Müller, and his doctoral dissertation was part of a project for which he had won an award from the Berlin medical faculty. Born in 1813 in Warsaw and of the Jewish faith, he was unquestionably a friend of his compatriot and co-religionist, Remak. Perhaps his personal reports to Valentin also had a mollifying effect on the latter. Indeed, Remak's connections with and aspirations for Poland were soon to become of much greater importance than Kronenberger and Valentin had thought (see p. 239 ff.).

In our day it may not be understandable to a physician or even a layman that between scholars in the field of histology a conflict could be possible over the existence or non-existence of certain formations in the nervous system, which today are known to every student of medicine and are basic knowledge to be found in every textbook on histology. In the period between 1835 and 1840 microscopy was still in its infancy; the instruments, though advanced for the time, were still extremely primitive. The routine methods of today had not yet been developed, and even photography, invented only in 1839, did not yet exist. Only a few pioneers recognized at that time the importance of microscopy for medicine, and each of them had to learn for himself and by himself to see the details and to avoid the pitfalls of optical allusions, and to try to find a reasonable explanation for that which he was certain he saw.

RELATIONS WITH JOHANNES MÜLLER

Johannes Müller (1801–1858), since 1833 professor of anatomy, physiology, and pathology at the University of Berlin, was one of the leaders of European physiology and anatomy at the time of its modern development in the nineteenth century, ranking equally with Magendie in France and Bell in England. He was a painstakingly exact worker in every field of research, to which he brought a keen critical mind, a man who devoted his life and all his working power to his studies. His influence on the following generation in Germany was tremendous, his reputation in Germany and abroad was great, and his recognition in governmental circles in Prussia was as high as he deserved. His pupils, including Schwann, Henle, Remak, Helmholtz, Brücke, DuBois-Reymond, and Virchow, were among the creators of recent medicine as far as it developed in the second half of the last century.

There were, however, other great physiologists in Germany in the middle of the nineteenth century, contemporaries of Müller, and they too established important schools of research and teaching. There was, for instance, Purkinje in Breslau, Valentin's teacher, fourteen years older than Müller, who esteemed and revered him highly. In a letter to Valentin (see p. 172) in 1836 Müller characterizes him as follows: "Give my regards to Professor Purkinje, the excellent, highly esteemed man." There was also young Carl Ludwig, a rising star, teaching at the University of Marburg, fifteen years Müller's junior, the great methodical mind in the growing field of experimental medicine and especially of cardiology. Ludwig was the teacher of Bowditch, Kronecker, Luciani, Hammarsten, Pawlow, and many others. These contemporary leaders and their schools were, of course, in personal contact with each other, friendly, critical, and competitive. In his time at least from 1833, when he was called to Berlin, up to his death in 1858, Johannes Müller was respected and regarded as the outstanding representative of Germany's new, objective anatomy and physiology.

Valentin was as well known to Müller for his research and his teaching as Müller was to Valentin. Indeed, at this time every scientist felt a kind of personal attachment to every one of his confrères. The community of men of science was still a kind of family, and each member of it was sure to be a welcome guest wherever in the world he came to visit another member. Such was the relationship between Müller and Valentin up to 1836, when the latter began to publish his *Repertorium,* in which he had to report on Müller's as on every other scientist's work.

Müller's work, in spite of all its impressiveness and importance, was, of course, not flawless in its details and provoked criticism. One of Müller's pupils, Professor Th. L. W. Bischoff in Munich, in an eulogy he delivered shortly after Müller's death on November 27, 1858, before the Royal Bavarian Academy of Sciences expressed it in this way, characterizing Müller's new vistas in physiology: "The studying of Müller's *Arbeiten* does not lull you; it is not a comfortable armchair in which you may quietly relax; on the contrary, it troubles you, but it also makes you eager to contribute something to the solution of the problems in question. One not only admires his results, but besides that, one is encouraged to doubt them." This is exactly what Valentin did in his *Repertorium,* and he did it in a very outspoken way. His criticism may have been very justifiable, for instance when he rejected [31] Müller's classification of tumors into two groups—those that can and those that cannot be healed by surgery.

Valentin's criticism of Müller is time and again proffered in a somewhat rude manner. For instance, in commenting on Müller's classification of different kinds of lime, he simply says: [32] "The characterization of this classification is entirely false." Müller later called this kind of criticism "teasing" (Neckereien).

Probably these two great men met personally for the first time when Valentin, in March, 1836, was in Berlin and presented part of his research before a select audience at the home of the surgeon, Professor Dieffenbach. On that occasion, he, of course, visited Müller's institute and Müller personally demonstrated to him certain anatomical preparations.[33] There he met Müller's group of young scholars and pupils, among them Henle, Schwann, Remak, and there is no doubt that his personal contact with Müller was immediately a very friendly one. Müller, at that time dean of the medical faculty, in 1836 gave Valentin's reprints to the Prussian Minister of Education to influence him in favor of Valentin and his further career in Prussia. Valentin must have talked over his personal worries with Müller, too, as can be seen from Valentin's letter to Professor Rau in Bern (see p. 162). Müller apparently discussed the possibility of Valentin's becoming baptized, expressing the opinion that in this case a professorship would be offered him immediately "on a silver platter," but he probably understood Valentin's rejection of such a proposal, knowing very well this same attitude from his own collaborator, Remak. When in the same year, 1836, in June, Valentin was appointed professor at Bern, he announced it immediately in a letter to Müller, and the latter, in spite of his aversion to writing letters, answered at the end of August, excusing himself for the delay. This letter was written in a tone of friendship and tactful good advice to a younger colleague whose character Müller seemed to know very well. It reads in translation:

Most esteemed friend:

Late enough I answer your kind letter, being this year delayed with so many things. You know the reason [Müller was that year dean of the medical faculty] and will surely excuse me a little. Now the deanship will soon be finished and I feel relieved. I am sorry that you are going to leave us, but I have to congratulate you most heartily, because this is apparently the most favorable turn of events that could have happened.

You get the finest sphere of activity for which you are destined, and you will create a center of scientific life. Your relations with your colleagues will surely be most agreeable. This, of course, is necessary and indispensable, because for the stranger in Switzerland it is more difficult to create many-sided relations with the inhabitants. The neutrality he needs is, on the other hand, of advantage in a place where conditions are still new and many problems are approached from the point of view of factions. Kindly give my regards to Herr Professor Vogt with many thanks for sending me his reprints. Our Henle is now in Coblenz with his parents. His mother is suffering from an incurable disease; he will have to become accustomed to the idea that he will lose her. In his affairs nothing is as yet decided. We hope for a happy end soon, but at the moment no exceptions can be made. Many high-ranking personalities took an interest in the good outcome of his

[31] *Repertorium* 2: 117, 1837.
[32] *Ibid.* 2: 183, 1837.
[33] *Ibid.* 1: 189, 1836.

affairs, and it is not their fault if all is not yet decided favorably.

Please give my regards to Professor Purkinje, the excellent highly esteemed man.

The cordial regards of all of us accompany you on your travels.

Yours
D. Müller

Berlin, August 28, 1836

This letter indicates that Valentin must have made friendly contact in Berlin not only with Müller, but with his collaborators, too. The letter, written in a tone and spirit of friendship, also shows Müller's tact and fine psychological understanding of Valentin's personality in warning him to remain neutral in the rifts of the factions in small Switzerland to which he comes as a stranger, a foreigner. Müller also displays a good knowledge of conditions in Switzerland. The letter reveals the high opinion Müller has of Valentin whom he rightfully expects to create a new scientific center in Europe at Bern.

This mutual feeling and respect did not prevent Valentin from writing the above-mentioned sharp criticism of some of Müller's publications. At the same time, Müller in the annual review in his own *Archiv* criticized strongly some points of Valentin's work on the nervous system, which resulted in an acute crisis in the

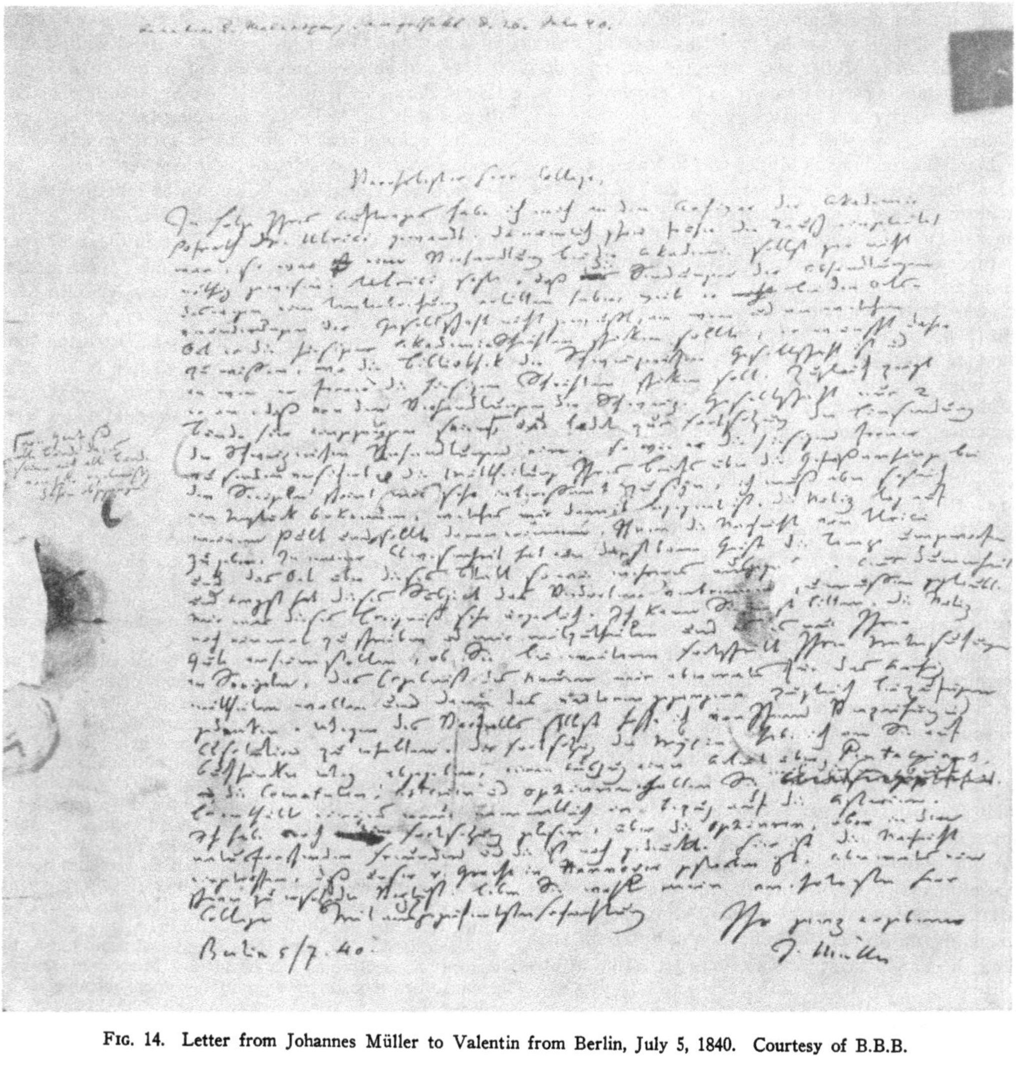

FIG. 14. Letter from Johannes Müller to Valentin from Berlin, July 5, 1840. Courtesy of B.B.B.

relations between the two men. Müller was as touchy and as easily hurt as Valentin was. His letter to Valentin shows that he has not forgotten any of the criticisms Valentin had ever made, but his temper was different. Then, too, he was nine years Valentin's senior and much wiser than the younger man, who used to lose his temper very quickly. This happened, for instance, when he read Müller's criticism of his work in neurology. He forgot that Müller was surely as well entitled to publish his judgment of other scholars' work as he, Valentin, was. He regarded such action by Müller as a personal insult, as evidence of a hostile attitude, and wrote Müller a letter of indignation accusing him of injustice and breaking their friendship. He also informed their mutual friend, Professor R. Wagner in Erlangen, about the letter and about his controversy with Müller. Unfortunately, no draft of Valentin's letter could be traced, but from Müller's reply to it (B.B.B.), its contents may well be imagined.

Müller's letter is dated December 31, 1837. It seems as though Müller would have liked to end the year by clearing up all misunderstandings. His letter is a classic document, indeed. It reveals as much of Müller's personality, his character and his attitude towards life, as it does of Valentin as Müller saw him. We learn from Müller's own words how much he disliked to write letters or to write anything at all which he did not regard as essential. We learn how he liked to be polite because politeness helps to make the life of a scientist easier. We see Müller's critical approach to man and problems, and the strict but at the same time thoughtful, understanding, and tactful way in which he paints before Valentin's eyes a picture of Valentin's own personality. This is a sharp but well-meant analysis of Valentin's faults. Only Müller's emphasis that he never expressed feelings of friendship for Valentin is contradicted by his own letter of August 28, 1836. But perhaps even this form and the content of the 1836 letter were chosen only to make life go smoothly for the Herr Geheimrat. At least for the future he avoided the word "friend" in every extant letter to Valentin, however warm the closing phrases of the following letters may have been.

After telling Valentin clearly his opinion of him and his own complaints ("because for that purpose a letter is better suited" than a publication), he closes the case in a really cordial way, stretching his hand out to make peace with the young adversary, and he does it in such a pleasant and charming way that Valentin (on January 9) immediately answered (draft of this answer could not be traced). This reply must have helped to restore the friendly relations between the two, because there are letters from Müller from the following years written in a very friendly spirit, and Valentin later published papers repeatedly in Müller's *Archiv* and on Müller's request, as before, in the encyclopedic dictionary of medical science, which was edited by Müller and other members of the Berlin medical faculty.

Müller's letter replying to Valentin's complaints and accusations reads in translation as follows:

Esteemed Herr Colleague:

Your letter was a surprise to me. Suddenly you are talking of discord, of attacks, of being persecuted by me, which I can't understand at all except that you try to justify by such accusations your usual teasing. Have you been spoiled by us to such an extent that you are no longer able to tolerate being contradicted? A right which you claim yourself against me year after year, ever since I have known you, whenever you find reason to do so and you are really entitled to do so. You did so in your first publications before I knew you personally and afterwards, and why not? I did not care about that when I had the pleasure to meet you here. I did not care about asking who you are and what kind of position you have. Even now that would be the last thing to ask; in fact I would not ask it. The comments on your neurological observations are now supposed to be attacks, whereas they are written in fullest appreciation of all that has been proved. I can vouch for every word. I checked them repeatedly, especially those concerning the description of the nervous system. I have to review it in the new edition of the physiology, where I shall record the facts and drop the polemics. Where you mentioned the present status of the physics of the nerves only indirectly I too answered in the annual report in the same way. On different questions which are my very close concern I had to defend myself and that is what you call attacks. That you informed Prof. Wagner about your letters is good; he may judge who is attacked there and should compare the teasing in your reports. I regard my remarks so little as attacks that if they had been written at the time of your visit in Berlin, I would have let you read them and would not have expected any disapproval on your side. First, you should become better acquainted with fault-finding and contradiction, and if you then for a period of time should experience this reproach and contradiction as we others have, you will lose this out-of-place touchiness. You see, most esteemed Herr Colleague, that I did nothing to produce a break in existing friendly collegial relations. I don't write letters. Yes, on this point I am always amiss and the fault is always mine. On this point, I need tolerance as I do of the many other acquaintances. I hate to write letters and I hate to write anything that just is not important.

You speak of the cooling of friendship. The kind of relationship that really existed between us did not change the slightest on my part. I did not take your interest in me, at the time you were here, for more than a colleague's friendly contact. Think of all that is needed to call a friendly and polite contact between colleagues friendship: years of acquaintence, years of youth, many mutual trials, compatibility of character and sentiment. Let it be what indeed it was from its start, a friendly and polite association between colleagues, and see whether it can still be that now. You came here as Purkinje's collaborator and as a scientist. In each of these capacities you, like every scientist without any exception, will find here the kindest reception, which is characteristic of our city and its scientists. Every natural scientist should expect it from professional colleagues and non-colleagues, and who would not enjoy it here? In this sense, I would have done for you everything one scholar can accept from another, without attaching any importance to it. For my part, no change took place in the pleasant collegial relationship that I started with you. In all this time I have taken no occasion to offend against it, except for my laziness in correspondence. On this point, as mentioned, I am always guilty even in the best relations.

Of course, you did not spare teasing and schoolmastering. My patience is great. I observe the forms as long as possible. They make scientific intercourse much easier. I find self-possession completely lacking in the arrogant and generalized remarks concerning the corps of scientists in your reports. To whom are these subjective remarks directed? To those whom you call your friends? They will advise you to apply them first to yourself and then see how much will still remain for us. If that is part of friendship, then the Lord save us from our friends, of our enemies we ourselves will dispose, but the friends—!

Now I have expressed to you sincerely and confidentially my "subjectivities," because such things are proper for letters. I wish to be and remain at peace with you and on good friendly collegial terms, and I will do my best with honest intention to reach that goal. You can be sure of that.

Your views concerning the vessels of the penis are a different thing. This kind of refutation can by no means be unpleasant to me. In science it has to exist, and everyone is entitled to it. After having read your article, I don't regard the art.helicinae endangered, but I accept with pleasure your friendly suggestion to reinvestigate this matter. I shall spend the next weeks on that. I thank you for sending your paper. Finally, after a long time, something from you. Every discovery must first pass through doubts before its recognition is sure, and in this way you serve the problem well. Your paper will be printed immediately. I received from Breslau a complete copy of your treatise on nerves. I thank you sincerely for it. The incomplete copy you were kind enough to send me before, I gave on your behalf to our Herr Minister when you still were in Breslau. It was not returned to me. I have sent you by the bookdealer a copy of my paper on the organic nerves of the penis. I don't have the paper on the *Wundernetze* any longer. Eschricht received many copies, and the few I kept were soon distributed here. My best wishes for the New Year, also for good light, it was so bad early this winter.

Yours faithfully,
Dr. Jo. Müller

Berlin, December 31, 1837

Valentin's answer to this gem of a letter from a great man with a kind heart could not be located. All the following correspondence between the two scholars, as far as it is extant, is written in the kindest manner and with a spirit of mutual respect and admiration. Müller, indeed, immediately published in his *Archiv* Valentin's polemic against his (Müller's) discovery of the so-called arteriae helicinae in the penis and added a very polite objective reply without any subjective disputations.

STRUGGLE WITH THE FACULTY

Feller (12), in his book on the history of Bern University, often expressed the opinion that the Bern faculty suffered considerable damage from Valentin's egotistic desire to keep both physiology and anatomy under his regime and thus to suppress younger collaborators. He is jubilant on reporting the separation of anatomy and physiology in 1863, considering it a case of poetic justice. This decision of the faculty, of course, was reached only a year after the death of Valentin's two best friends: Professor Vogt and Professor Rau. Both died in 1861. Valentin felt very strongly about this defeat in the year when he was Dean of the Faculty and his wife died. At first he made up his mind to resign his professorship, but was persuaded to remain as physiologist and Dean of the Faculty when Aeby was appointed Professor of Human and Comparative Anatomy in 1863.

Incidentally, in spite of the rapid development of physiology in the middle of the nineteenth century, it was not at all unusual at this time for the same professor to hold the chair of both physiology and anatomy, even in universities much larger and more renowned than Bern. The anatomist, Henle, was called to the medical faculty of Heidelberg, one of the outstanding medical schools of Germany, as Professor of Anatomy and Physiology and remained there in this capacity until 1852, when he went to Göttingen. The University of Tübingen twice offered Valentin the chair of both physiology and anatomy (21). Henle's successor in 1852, F. Arnold, also taught both anatomy and physiology at Heidelberg.

It is true that at Bern for a few years during pre-university times (from 1821) anatomy and physiology were taught by different teachers, physiology by Ith and anatomy by Albrecht Meckel, but this was a *faute de mieux* situation for there was no candidate at Bern who would have been able to teach both subjects adequately.[34] When Valentin was called to Bern, there was no full professor of anatomy, only the professor extraordinarius Theile, and from the beginning of the negotiations between Professor Rau and Valentin, Valentin had been asked and agreed to teach, not only physiology, but anatomy as well, and he suggested at the outset that he teach not less than four hours weekly of general and comparative anatomy (see p. 162).

The first university in Germany to create an independent professorship for physiology, separate from anatomy and zootomy, was apparently in Königsberg (1832: Burdach-von Baer). It was in 1858, when Carl Gegenbaur, at that time Professor Extraordinary of Zoology at Jena, was being considered a successor to the late Huschke both for anatomy and physiology. Gegenbaur, however, had neither experience nor interest in modern physiology and, therefore, could not take over any teaching in this field (14). The faculty, therefore, finally decided to appoint A. v. Bezold as physiologist and Gegenbaur as anatomist.

In Switzerland, in the nearby University of Basel, Wilhelm His was Professor of Anatomy and Physiology until 1872 (28). In that year he was called to succeed Ernst Heinrich Weber in the chair of anatomy at Leipzig. Weber himself resigned from teaching both anatomy and physiology only in 1866, in which year Carl Ludwig became physiologist of this famous uni-

[34] F. Haag, *Die hohen Schulen zu Bern*, Bern, 1903.

versity, while Weber remained as anatomist until 1872 (28). Berlin followed Königsberg's and Jena's example only after Johannes Müller's death (1858), when DuBois-Reymond was appointed physiologist and Reichert anatomist, and only in 1864 was physiology separated from anatomy at the famous University of Würzburg (27).

Not every university was fortunate enough to have a man for both anatomy and physiology as well-trained and as great a leader in both fields as Bern had in Valentin. He was not only a renowned physiologist, but his anatomical work, as published in his doctoral thesis (40), his book on comparative embryology (43), his book on the brain and the nervous system (50, 51), the book that won the Grand Prix of the Academy of Paris, and his various zoological studies, for instance, on the electric eel and echinodermata made him one of the outstanding anatomists of his time. He was the originator (1838) of the microtome with two knives [35] and, some years after he took over the directorship of the Anatomical Institute of Bern, he even published a valuable and interesting booklet on the technique of dissecting the viscera of a human body (58). His nomination for corresponding membership in the Academy of Paris in 1845, in the Section of Zoology and Comparative Anatomy, together with the most outstanding anatomists in Europe, proves how high his reputation as an anatomist was at that time.

Valentin's opposition to separating anatomy from physiology at Bern may have been rooted, first, in his clear insight into the fact that both these subjects are closely interwoven and should not be looked upon and taught as entirely different disciplines, a tendency that again assumed importance about one hundred years later, as evidenced by the way in which modern textbooks on anatomy and pathological anatomy are written nowadays. Valentin was himself fully convinced of his own ability to cover adequately both fields, anatomy and physiology, in teaching and in research, as indeed he did for twenty-seven years of his activities in Bern.

Besides this, however, there may have been other personal reasons for Valentin's attitude. All was not going so smoothly at Bern University at that time, as every unbiased reader will learn from Feller's own book (12). Working facilities were limited, and giving up anatomy meant for a research worker of Valentin's type and calibre, not simply a loss of prestige (as Feller would like to put it (12)), but what is more important, a loss of badly needed equipment and working facilities. Moreover, and despite the high esteem that Valentin had won in Bern, there is no question that reactionary tendencies in Switzerland at that time were very strong and were reflected in the life of the University. Bern University, like the Bern Government, had a definite unaristocratic and somewhat radical complexion when Valentin was called to the chair in 1836. That tendency was so articulate that the reactionary government of Germany was afraid to allow any of its students to come in contact with such a dangerously democratic place, full of subversive elements. On September 11, 1834, the German Bundestag decided, for the purpose of preventing psychological infections, that the various German governments should see to it that none of their subjects should dare to study at the new University of Bern (12).

In 1836 the same liberal and progressive spirit ruled Bern that offered a chair on the faculty in 1834 to a man like Wilhelm Vogt of Giessen (Carl Vogt's father), who did not feel safe in Germany because of his democratic sympathies, and who, on accepting the call to Bern, was not permitted by his government to remain a citizen of Hessen. Only by a coincidence did he escape being arrested in his homeland as a political suspect when he reached the border with his family while on his way to Bern (64).

The political trend changed however, in the middle of the century, especially in the canton of Bern, where a man like Jeremias Gotthelf (who died in 1854), a strong reactionary, was a widely read author with great influence over the people. He was strictly and militantly opposed to everything liberal, progressive, and non-Christian.[36]

The general attitude toward Jews and foreigners was, in the first half of the nineteenth century, still less enlightened in the other Cantons of Switzerland than in Bern. In 1843 Jews were not yet permitted to hold their religious services in the city of Geneva.[37] In 1845 the government of Graubünden proceeded to expel all the Jews living there; only one French subject was permitted to stay because the French government decided that, in the event of his expulsion, all citizens of Graubünden living in Paris would have to leave that city within two weeks time.[38]

This difficult political situation may also have been a factor in Valentin's hesitancy in voluntarily giving up important working facilities. It was surely not a pleasant prospect to put them in the hands of someone who might not be willing to cooperate with one not born in Switzerland and not of the Christian faith. Such situations were only too well-known to Valentin from the deplorable experiences of his teacher and friend Purkinje, who for many years suffered real martyrdom owing to the hostility of the Breslau anat-

[35] *Repertorium* 3: 30, 1837; 8: 55, 1843.

[36] See "Jeremias Gotthelf," written by Gottfried Keller, the Swiss poet (in *Nachgelassene Schriften*, 93 ff., Berlin, 1893). Jeremias Gotthelf was the pen name of a minister, Pfarrer Bitzius, in Lützelfluh in the Canton Bern. His son, Albert Bitzius, became head of the educational department in Bern in 1878.

A good picture of conditions and the attitude towards foreigners in Switzerland, especially in Bern, at that time is given by the German poet Gustav Freytag in his biography of Karl Mathy (Leipzig, 1872).

[37] *Sulamith* 8: 319, 1843.

[38] *Sulamith* 9: 65, 1845.

omist, Otto. Valentin's feeling that he had many enemies in the ranks of his colleagues at the University was definitely strengthened when, in 1842, the Senate chose the anatomist, Theile, and not Valentin as rector (the governing head) of the University, though Theile was not even a full professor, as Valentin was, but only professor extraordinary. As a matter of fact Valentin was never elected rector of the University. Valentin's qualities as teacher should also have been considered in the faculty's decision concerning anatomy, but they were not.

There was really no valid reason for limiting Valentin's activities on the faculty. Even in the matter of Feller's charge that Valentin mistreated his assistants, emphasizing especially the case of the physiologist, Moritz Schiff, who, on Valentin's suggestion, was called as assistant professor (extraordinarius) to Bern in 1856, we need only quote Schiff himself. After more than two years of working under the guidance of Valentin, who was thirteen years his senior, he wrote the following in the preface to his textbook on *Muscle and Nerve Physiology* (37): "Only a few chapters of this book were written while I was living in Bern, but these may be especially outstanding because I enjoyed the advice and the important help of my friend and colleague Valentin. To him goes the main credit for them." In a publication on a malformed frog, Schiff mentions in 1858 [89] how Valentin assisted him in his experimental observations and immediately volunteered to make an exact drawing of the preparation, which Schiff then published. Schiff was not the only one of Valentin's collaborators who felt this way about his former teacher.

E. Hintsche, as mentioned above, published extremely interesting letters from Valentin's former pupil, Alfonso Corti (18). Each one is written in a spirit of affection and admiration for his beloved teacher and friend. C. Vogt (64), who does not hesitate to condemn in the strongest fashion the behavior of Agassiz with whom he worked for five years, has not one word of complaint against Valentin, whose assistant he was for two years. But he does mention that Agassiz once visited Valentin in Bern and Valentin kindly called his attention to the abilities of Vogt, who in 1839 had just graduated with honors from Bern University. Finally, Agassiz appointed Vogt to the position he held for five years in Neuchatel.

In this author's collection is a most cordial letter written by Valentin on April 8, 1861, to the famous zoologist, Professor von Siebold, in Munich, highly recommending Duplehsis [?], his pupil and assistant in anatomy from the Canton Waadt. Duplehsis was especially interested in entomology and zoology and wanted to continue his studies under von Siebold. This letter shows deep sympathy of the great teacher toward an industrious pupil.

[89] *Ztschr. Wiss. Zool.* **9**: 454, 1858.

CONTINUED RESEARCH

Besides his teaching obligations, his efforts to build up a satisfactory physiological laboratory and a good anatomical collection, and his writing for his *Repertorium*, Valentin published several important books in the first years of his stay in Bern. In 1839 appeared his physiology of cerebral nerves and the sympathicus, written in Latin (47). In this book he gives not only a very careful report of all previous papers on this subject, but also his own observations on three hundred animal experiments which he performed. There he also tried to straighten out at least some of his differences with Remak. The book was soon translated into the Italian language by G. Sachero, Professor of Clinical Medicine at the University of Torino, Italy, and published as a volume of 264 pages in Torino in 1843 (36).

It is not intended to give here a report of all Valentin's findings. Among them the following may be mentioned here: the accelerator effect of the nervus sympathicus on the heart; the accleration of the heart after cutting the vagus nerve, a fact that had already been observed by Lower in the seventeenth century; the constrictor effect of nerve stimulation on arteries, veins, and lymphatic vessels and the intensification of the sensitivity of the heart muscle in cases of what is now called angina pectoris (36).

When Valentin published an extensive article on tissues in *R. Wagner's Textbook of Physiology* (**1**: 132), he even made certain claims with respect to having anticipated Schwann's cell theory. This, however, was not justified. Unquestionably, there are some pertinent observations reported by Valentin in his early publications. He even called attention to the similarities between animal microscopic globules and plant cells (45, 46). But he never comprehended, as Schwann did, the general idea of the cell theory and its fundamental importance for biology and medicine, until Schwann opened the eyes of every physiologist to the new concept. Consequently, Schwann is right in rejecting such a claim, and he does it in a most dignified and gentlemanlike way by reprinting verbatim, in an appendix to his book, the claims of Valentin (39).

Valentin was one of the main contributors to the first volume of Rudolf Wagner's *Handwörterbuch der Physiologie*. Completed in 1842, it contained several extensive articles by him on the following topics: secretion, electricity in animals, nutrition, fibrilatory movement, galvanism, tissues of the human and animal body. It may be remarked that Valentin here clearly differentiates between the reaction of living tissues to electricity and the electrical properties of living tissue. This distinction, highly important, received recognition from Du Bois-Reymond in 1848.

This kind of work, performed in Valentin's very conscientious and exact manner, must have been extremely time-consuming. It was not the case then as it is so often now, when, unfortunately, an eminent professor, to accomplish a similar purpose, has his assistants and secretaries collect and arrange the necessary material, to which he then contributes only slight finishing touches, his approval, and his name. Every single line of Valentin's articles for the handbook reveals his individual style, knowledge, experience, and personal opinion. He may have felt this kind of work, like the writing of the *Repertorium,* too great a tax on his time, for his name does not appear among the contributors to any of the subsequent volumes of Wagner's *Handwörterbuch.*

In 1840 Valentin at Johannes Müller's request published in the *Encyclopedic Dictionary of Medical Science*[40] an article on muscles and one on muscle movements. Here he tried to prove (against the opinion of Berzelius) that the red color of muscle fibers is due, not to their content of blood, but to a specific coloring matter contained in the muscle fibers. Today we know that he was right on this important point.

Finally, in 1841, a compendium of Valentin's encyclopedic knowledge and his many investigations and experiments in the field of neurology was published as the fourth volume of the new edition of Sömmering's work on anatomy. The editors of this classic treatise were Bischoff, Henle, Huschke, Theile, Valentin, Vogel, and Wagner. Valentin's neurological contribution (*Hirn- und Nervenlehre*) was a volume of 722 pages, and it is typical of this early period in medicine that it contains only one table of figures. A revised French translation of this volume by A. J. L. Jourdan was published in Paris in 1843.

Already in May 1840, Valentin had finished, for Louis Agassiz's *Monographs on Echinodermata,* a volume written in excellent French and printed in 1841 on the anatomy of this group of invertebrate animals. Here, in a book of 126 pages and 8 tables, Valentin again demonstrated the wide range of his knowledge in the field of comparative anatomy. As in the work that won him the Grand Prix of the French Academy in 1835, he again gave evidence of his outstanding talent in drawing. All the 188 figures in the book were drawn by Valentin himself from nature. To acquire the necessary experience for his study, Valentin, as mentioned above, had taken a trip at his own expense along the Mediterranean coast. In the same year he published a monograph on the electric eel (*Gymnotus electricus*).[41]

Of interest also are Valentin's experiments on the effect of cutting both nn. vagi in rabbits and cats, especially on rate and type of respirations. He published them in a book of 157 pages in 1857 (59).

[40] **24**: 175–203, 203–220.

[41] *Schw. Denkschr.* **6**, Neuchatel, 1841.

MARINE BIOLOGICAL INVESTIGATIONS

In the early nineteenth century such an expedition as Valentin undertook to study the echinodermata was by no means as easy and as comfortable as it would be today. When Valentin, in 1839, conducted his research by the Mediterranean Sea at Nizza, none of the wonderful marine laboratories existed like those at Naples, Woods Hole, Monaco, Trieste, Rovignio, and so on, which today, comfortable and well equipped, are at the disposal of every eager scholar in the world. Anton Dohrn, the German zoologist who established in Naples in 1870–1872 the most famous and exemplary of these marine research institutions, was not even born at that time.

More and more, however, it became clear to anatomists and physiologists that the rich living material inhabiting the sea should be used for research in comparative anatomy and physiology and not merely for food purposes. We find outstanding scholars at that time going out on marine research expeditions, even when they were not so fortunate as Andres Retzius from Stockholm to live near the seashore. Johannes Müller repeatedly made such research trips, as did R. Wagner, Rathke, Valentin, and others.

All the necessary instruments had to be brought from home to the headquarters, and the time allotted for such an expedition had to be spent fruitfully in order to compensate for the expense and effort. Consequently, some of the top men, on embarking on such an undertaking, took with them the best of their assistants. Such a trip involved not only weeks of hard, strenuous work and great expense, which sometimes had to be covered by the explorer personally, as in Valentin's case, but occasionally real personal danger too. We know that Johannes Müller, on such a research trip to Norway, narrowly escaped death in a shipwreck one night in September 1855 only by swimming. The ship on which he was travelling sank, and one of his most gifted students and companions, Wilhelm Schmidt, was actually drowned. Sometimes only an assistant or collaborator was sent out to collect and to send home rare material, which then was worked up by the chief and his staff at home and generously distributed to pupils for research purposes. We know from Müller's letters to A. Retzius that his assistant Peters was sent on such a collecting trip to far off parts of the world, and that Müller generously supplied his pupil Remak with rare material from the sea, such as sharks, from his own collection. Exchange of material was made or suggested between the scholars of various countries, like Retzius and Müller, Valentin and Retzius. Often scholars of different countries met at the same place for research, sharing their material and their experiences and enjoying the personal contact. Such a meeting of scientists at Nizza on the Mediterranean, which took place in the fall of 1839, is vividly described in the following letter from Valentin to A. Retzius, showing the delighted mutual interest of the scholars in each other's projects, withholding from each other neither the work intended nor that accomplished. Valentin writes (translated literally) to Retzius after his return to Bern from this trip:[42]

Esteemed Confrère:

I have to apologize for answering your dear latest letter so late and to thank you sincerely for your having kindly admitted me to your Societas medica. You would oblige me very much if you would kindly express my appreciation to your society for this undeserved courtesy.

I just returned from a little excursion to the Mediterranean Sea. In accordance with a previous agreement Prof. R. Wagner from Erlangen and some of his pupils, Dr. Erdl from Munich, and I met in Nizza. In spite of the fact that we were not favored by the season, we still obtained some new scientific results. Prof. Wagner was busy mainly with Medusae [jelly fish], especially investigating their cnidocils, which are probably exclusively or largely the cause of the nettling; furthermore he investigated the conditions of the muscle fibers, the circulation, and the digestive organs, the ciliary movement and so on in these peculiar creatures. Besides that, he was eager to continue his observations of spermatozoa and eggs and discovered some facts which turn out to be nice contributions to our present knowledge. Most interesting is the fact that the testicles of the rays don't have the peculiarities with respect to discharging the sperma which are now attributed to them. In fact, their spermatic vessels are built very much as they are in human testicles. Dr. Erdl mainly investigated the anatomy of polyp colonies and found among these animals two different kinds of polyp colonies: In one only male specimens are present, in the other only female. The latter type is found more often by far than the former. In the echinodermata, too, duality of the sexes could be found at least in part of the investigations. I got many male Holoturias with spermatozoa and also many females with eggs. I was less fortunate with echinus and asterias. Not in one single individual was I able to observe spermatozoa beyond a doubt. Dr. Will, in a series of investigations, measured the temperature of sea animals. The result was that the temperature of these animals corresponds approximately to the temperature of the sea water, but is found always to be just a little higher. Wagner investigated the chromatophors of Cephalopodes. Peters from Berlin, whom we met in Nizza, investigated their organ of hearing, and I myself the eyes of these animals. We hope to publish our findings in commemorative pamphlets of Nizza (*Erinnerungsblätter an Nizza*), and I shall surely not fail to send you at least the issue written by myself as a small token of my sincerest esteem and friendship.

Enclosed is Schuhmacher's small work. The doctoral thesis of C. Vogt on the nerves and the heart of reptiles probably reached you some weeks ago.

May I finally add, as a request to be granted as soon as possible, that you give me the pleasure of being able to welcome you in our mountains and of spending some days together with you.

In esteem and friendship
G. Valentin

Bern, October 1st 1839

Among the young scholars who met there in Nizza in 1839 for a happy and fruitful research trip, the oldest was the thirty-four-year-old Rudolf Wagner (1805–1864). He was at that time full Professor of Zoology at the University of Erlangen, Germany, but the following year he went, as successor to Professor Blumenbach, to Göttingen as Professor of Physiology, Anatomy and Zoology. He was outstanding in each of these fields, and especially well-known for his *Handbook of Physiology,* to the first volume of which (1842) Valentin contributed a great many articles.

The next one mentioned, Dr. Michael E. Erdl of Munich, was born in Munich in 1815; he was mainly interested in anatomy and comparative zoology. In 1844 he became professor in Munich, where he died in 1848.

Dr. Johann Georg Friedrich Will, born in 1815 in Baireuth, the same little German town from which Wagner came, accompanied Wagner on various research expeditions to Switzerland and also to Nizza. From 1848 on he was full professor at the University of Erlangen. He died in 1868.

Wilhelm Karl Harting Peters (1815–1883), successful African explorer, was, at the suggestion and the expense of his teacher, Johannes Müller, from July 1839 to the end of 1840 on the Mediterranean Coast to find the smooth shark described by Aristotle. In 1853 he became Professor of Medicine at Berlin and in 1858 Professor of Zoology at the same University.

Carl Vogt (1817–1895), mentioned in the above letter in connection with his doctoral thesis, was a pupil of Valentin and later famous as zoologist as well as for his activities as a radical, revolutionary politician.

THE TEXTBOOK OF PHYSIOLOGY

In the following years Valentin developed more and more the practice of summarizing his vast knowledge in monographs and textbooks, written partly for medical students and physicians and partly for the intelligent and interested layman. The rich experiences of the author himself were always the basis and backbone of such publications of his. This fact, together with his clear and excellent presentation of the material, created Valentin's reputation as the outstanding teacher of anatomy and physiology of his time. Already in his textbook of physiology and still more in his four volumes on physiological pathology (two of them devoted to neurology and two to circulation) Valentin emphasizes more and more the physical and especially the mathematical approach to biological and physiological problems. With this method of procedure he proved to be one of the leading pioneers in modern physiology.

In 1844 (54) Valentin's textbook on physiology, in two volumes, was published. In the year 1847 a second edition came out and in 1851 a volume of supplements appeared. Translations followed. This book and his outline (*Grundriss*) of physiology were an inspiration to his contemporaries. It was translated (1845) into Dutch by J. G. Rooseboom (54), and an English translation of the third German edition, by

[42] Letter preserved in the Library of the Royal Academy of Sciences in Stockholm.

William Briniton, was issued in London in 1853. It includes 684 pages and more than 500 illustrations on wood, copper, and stone.

Besides the textbook, Valentin published in 1841 a shorter outline of the human physiology entitled *For the First Study and for Self-Study* (52). When the fourth edition appeared in 1855, its contents amounted to 890 pages, 619 illustrations, and 7 tables. A Danish translation was put out in Copenhagen in 1857 by Valentin's friend, Adolph Hannover. This book emphasizes in the preface that it is meant not only for medical students, but also for the intelligent layman.

As in his textbook on embryology as well as all his other books, Valentin, in his textbook on physiology, brought out not only an eclectic compilation of other people's studies, but also his own investigations and his own as yet unpublished experiments. One of the most important among these was the announcement, in the first edition of his *Physiology* (1844), of the discovery of the diastatic properties of the pancreatic juice.

DISCOVERY OF THE PANCREAS DIASTASE

Already in Purkinje's laboratory in Breslau, Valentin became interested in problems of digestion. Purkinje was led by Beaumont's and Eberle's observations to these experiments, which he performed together with his pupil Pappenheim (70: 182). At the Jena meeting of the Convention of German Scientists and Physicians, Valentin reported on experiments on this topic (1836). He mentions especially the inhibition of the peptic protein-liquefaction by bile (66). In modern textbooks of enzymology Valentin's name will not be found, and, except for the scanty biographical notes on Valentin by Pagel and others (33), his role in the discovery of the diastase of the pancreas is entirely forgotten. After a detailed study of Valentin's original papers, this writer came to the following conclusions concerning the priority of the discovery of pancreatic diastase.

On pages 340 and 341 of the first edition of his textbook on physiology (54) Valentin reports (1844) on his own experiments on the influence of enteric juices and especially of pancreatic juice on starch. As the method used for his investigations he mentions the iodine test. He definitely and expressly states that bile does not have the same effect as pancreatic juice, and his conclusion (in a literal translation of page 341) is as follows: "As we see, these experiments [his own] do not yet permit any definite conclusions but are at most a clue that probably the pancreatic juice possesses the ability to make starch more soluble and sometimes starts its breakdown."

This statement contains two very important facts. First, Valentin thought of the possibility that the pancreas might enter into the digestion of starchy food, and he succeeded in performing the first rough experiments. In the fourth revised edition of Müller's *Handbook of Human Physiology* (1844), which was regarded as the storehouse of all the physiological knowledge of that time, we do not yet find any hint concerning the function of the pancreatic juice, and only in 1849 was Claude Bernard's pamphlet on the pancreatic juice published in Paris. Valentin wrote with all the caution that is characteristic of a serious research worker, saying that pancreatic juice probably is able to liquefy and to break up starch. It was a year after Valentin's publication (1845) that in Paris Bouchardat and Sandras (8) published different papers on the starch-digesting effect of diastase and of pancreatic juice.

To be fair to both sides, it can be said that Valentin's fame at that time was already international, and everyone interested in physiological problems must have been familiar with Valentin's textbook on physiology. Bouchardat was greatly interested in these questions, and it would be very strange if he did not know of Valentin's experiments. On the other hand, it must be admitted that the statements of the two French authors on the subject are much clearer and more definite and their experiments far more convincing. They tested the juice—collecting it from the main duct of the pancreas—mixed it with starch paste and found that its effect was to liquefy and to split starch. Literally, they say, "Il la liquefie et la transform en dextrine et en glucose." They found also that pure alcohol will precipitate a substance out of the pancreatic juice which has the same effect on starch as pancreatic juice itself. That is, in their opinion, the pancreas-diatase. "C'est la diastase."

These experiments were remarkable as a new trend of these French authors, especially if we consider that Bouchardat, only a short time before,[48] had published his own experiments in which the intestinal juice of a dog had practically no effect on starch even after a twenty-four hour incubation at 40°C.

Consequently, Valentin was to a certain extent justified when he mentioned on page 356 of the second edition of his physiology written, as the preface shows, in 1846 and published in 1847, that Bouchardat and Sandras had "continued on with his own experiments." He had apparently done the same, because his statement about the function of the pancreas (in the second edition, written with cognizance of the French papers) is also very clear and precise. On page 256, he says:

> The recent experiments made certain that this secretion (pancreatic juice) is, under favorable conditions, able to give a strong start to the self-disintegration of the loose carbohydrates. It liquefies starchy paste very easily and transforms it into dextrine, gum and glucose.

We must admit that none of these experiments—neither those of Valentin nor those of the French authors—would satisfy the demands of modern technique, especially with regard to the elimination of microorganisms. However, parallel experiments by Valen-

[48] *Compte Rendu* **20**: 107, 1845.

tin (1844) and the French scientists (1845) with other organs and gastric juice, which remained ineffective, gave the conclusions quoted above a certain validity. It can, therefore, be said that Valentin and the French authors should be regarded as the leading pioneers in the discovery of the diastatic properties of the pancreatic juice and its importance in the digestion of food. Valentin himself made no priority claims when, in 1846, he reprinted in Canstatt's annual reports (p. 173) the findings of the French authors. Summing up, Valentin is to be credited with the idea of the diastatic function of the pancreatic juice, the performance of the first experiments, and the correct conclusions, even if he was justifiably cautious in stating them. Bouchardat and Sandras must be credited with the first experiments showing strong evidence of the existence of the pancreas-diastase. Therefore, whenever the French scientists are cited as the discoverers of this important biochemical fact, Valentin's name, as a pioneer and forerunner, should not be omitted.

From the abundance of material accumulated in Valentin's textbook on physiology (53) as a result of his own observations, we should like to mention only the statements (page 409) concerning the valves of the heart and the nonschematic pictures he gives of the closed human mitral and tricuspid valve. They are proof of the clear observations he made in the field of human anatomy. In this book the first investigations were reported to measure the pressure of respiration. Here was stated for the first time that the center of respiration is stimulated to its automatic rhythm by insufficient supply with arterialized blood. Shortly before this textbook on physiology came out, Valentin rewrote his textbook on neurology, which was then published in a French translation by G. Jourdan (xxxii & 700 pages) in Paris in 1843 (53). In the following years of his activity, Valentin, even in his theoretical studies, never lost the clinical point of view. This can be seen in his book on the use of spectroscopy for physiological and medical purposes. The book appeared in 1863, the year of his defeat in his conflict with the faculty. It was again a pioneer work in clinical medicine as well as in research (62). Among other interesting facts, it contained Valentin's discovery of the presence of lithium in many parts of the human body. The close connection with clinical problems is also found in his two volumes on the physiological pathology of nerves (1864) and the two volumes on the physiological pathology of the heart and the blood vessels (1866 and 1867). It is noteworthy that his tendency strictly to apply physics and mathematics to physiological and clinical problems gave Valentin many practical suggestions. For instance, he strongly recommended taking the temperature rectally, because that would be the most exact method of measurement, a procedure not yet used at that time. Many of his early suggestions were later developed further and widely used. In his first volume (1866) on the physiological pathology of circulation he reports, for instance, his first attempts to record a pulse-tracing photographically, and gives the pictures of a sphygmograph making the tracings in a horizontal plane. This book, still very worth while reading, is one of the classic works on hemodynamics.

In 1861 Valentin suggested, in a book devoted to this subject, the most extensive use of polarized light for microscopic investigations of the tissues of plants and animals (61). This was a method applied for the first time for these purposes by Professor C. Boeck in Christiania in 1839.

SUMMARIZING PUBLICATIONS

In the decade between 1860 and 1870 Valentin wrote the voluminous books summarizing his life's work in various important fields. There he clearly differentiated (1869) between scientific and medical physiology. The main goal of these publications was to popularize and re-emphasize his leading ideas on how modern medicine should develop. He makes two main points in each of these books, points that Valentin emphasized from the start of his scientific career. First, he preached the importance of physics, and especially mathematics, for a real understanding of vital problems. He was thoughtful enough, even at that time in the late 60's, to write his books in such a way that the physician not interested in theory could easily omit the purely physical and mathematical part and still gain from reading the books. Those physicians, of course, who were interested and capable, like Valentin himself, of understanding a mathematical approach to problems, found profit and satisfaction and much information and inspiration in studying these books. For Valentin it was always a pleasure and a recreation to work on mathematical problems. His letters to his close friend, the mathematician Professor Moritz Stern in Göttingen, turn time and again to mathematical questions. So do letters of Vierordt to Valentin, and the latter accepts thankfully well-meant criticism of his own calculations. The intensity of this part of his work is well shown in two home-made notebooks of Valentin in the possession of this writer, page after page of them covered with mathematical calculations (see p. 181). DuBois Reymond, in spite of his rude criticism, calls Valentin in his textbook on electrophysiology (p. xxvi) the new yatro-mathematician of Bern.

It was Valentin's sincere conviction that if medicine was ever to become a real science, mathematics and exact physics were indispensable tools to foster and advance such a development. In this way Valentin became one of the early creators of what today is called biophysics.

This is the leading spirit of Valentin's book entitled *The Physical Investigation of Tissues* (*Die physikalische*

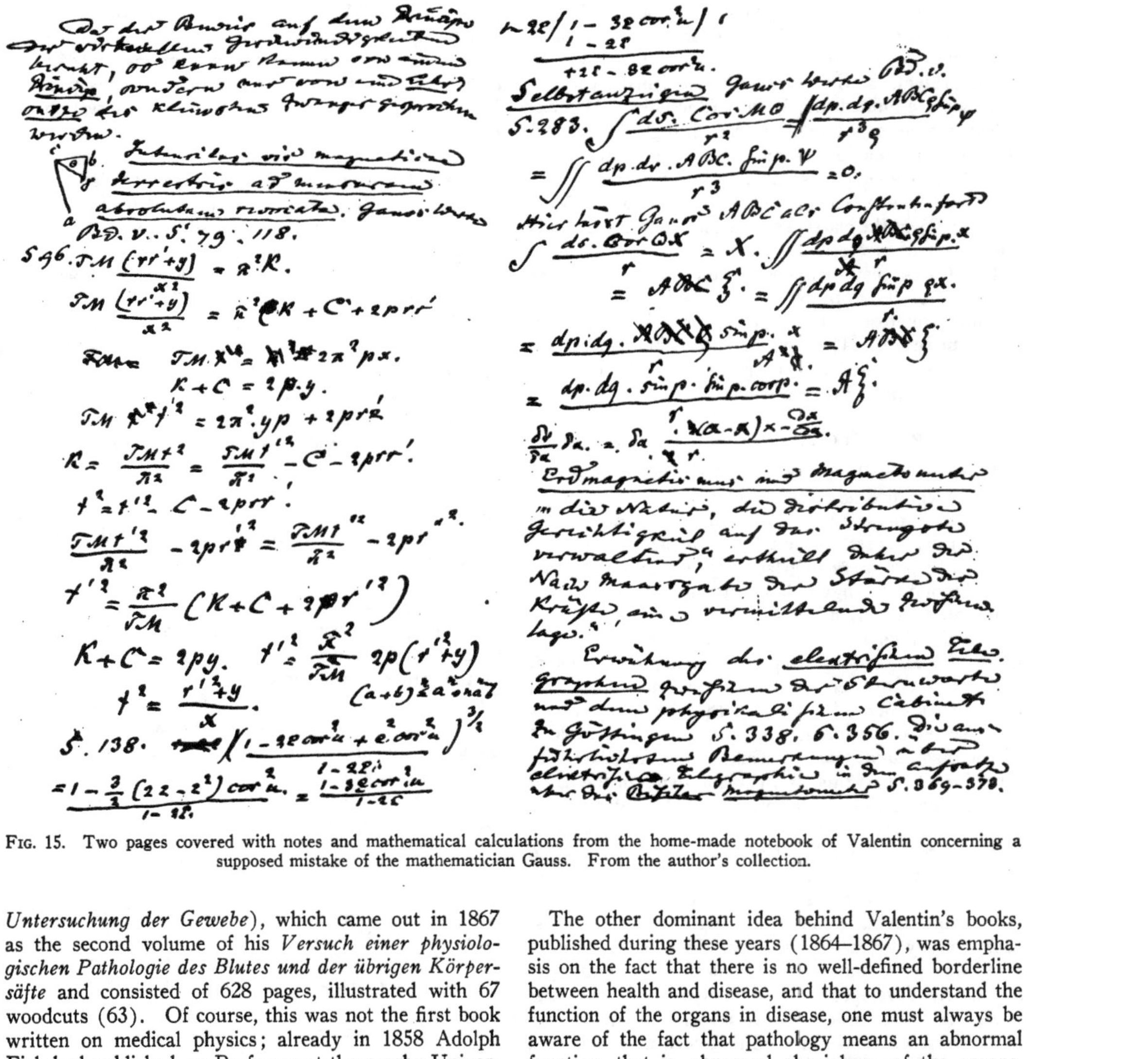

FIG. 15. Two pages covered with notes and mathematical calculations from the home-made notebook of Valentin concerning a supposed mistake of the mathematician Gauss. From the author's collection.

Untersuchung der Gewebe), which came out in 1867 as the second volume of his *Versuch einer physiologischen Pathologie des Blutes und der übrigen Körpersäfte* and consisted of 628 pages, illustrated with 67 woodcuts (63). Of course, this was not the first book written on medical physics; already in 1858 Adolph Fick had published, as Professor at the nearby University of Zürich, his classical textbook on "medical physics," as a supplement volume to Müller-Pouillet's textbook on physics. Fick's book was really the first in the field of what we would call today biophysics. However, in spite of its excellent content and in spite of the astonishing knowledge of physics and mathematics displayed by a medical man, Fick's book was apparently less suited to the practitioner and clinician than the research scientist. Valentin's book, on the other hand, was written page by page for the physician, to open his eyes to the new objective approach to biology as well as to clinical medicine.

The other dominant idea behind Valentin's books, published during these years (1864–1867), was emphasis on the fact that there is no well-defined borderline between health and disease, and that to understand the function of the organs in disease, one must always be aware of the fact that pathology means an abnormal function, that is, abnormal physiology, of the organs. Consequently, he used as a title for his books appearing at that time, *Physiological Pathology*. Virchow's similar expression, pathological physiology, has been used in Germany up to the present to designate the field of experimental medicine. In 1864 Valentin published the two volumes of his *Physiological Pathology of Nerves,* one of them containing 328 pages, and the other 400 pages (*Versuch einer physiologischen Pathologie der Nerven*). Two years later he published his book on the physiological pathology of the heart and the blood vessels. The first part (490 pages) is devoted largely to the physics of the circulation. Here in the introduction to the book he emphasizes on page 8, for all physiological processes and for the specific function of the various organs, the following rules: Whenever an organ presents a virtuosity of a particular type, its functions are limited mainly to that activity. This excellent concept of a limitation in each highly developed physiological function of an organ was, only a few years later, elaborated by Ewald Hering in his lecture on "Memory as a General Function of Organized Matter" (1870) in the classic remark that "one-sidedness is the mother of virtuosity."

The books just mentioned presented an excellent summary of those problems on which Valentin had expended interest and energy during a great part of his scientific life. They guided succeeding generations to new research and new progress, not only in physiology, but in medicine as a whole.

PARASITOLOGY AND TERATOLOGY

There are, finally, two more fields in which Valentin must be regarded as an outstanding pioneer, and these are modern parasitology and teratology. Already in 1839, in his studies on the function of nerves (47), he referred to the interesting fact (pp. 101 and 104) that he had found the Anguillula intestinalis parasite (a kind of nematode worm) in the vessels of the web membrane and in the fluid around the plexus chorioideus of the frog. A year later, he reported having seen eggs of Distoma, a trematode worm, in the cerebrospinal fluid of a sheep's embryo.[44] Then in 1841 he reported on a new species of protozoa, which he found in the blood of the fish *Salmo furio*. This was a flagellate, observed for the first time as a parasite living in the blood of a vertebrate (48). Valentin realized the importance of this discovery. Two years later a similar observation was reported by Dr. David Gruby in Paris, who then invented for this group of living beings the still generally accepted name of Trypanosoma (16).

It is interesting to note that even a great scientist cannot easily overcome the superstition of his time in cases where the knowledge of material facts is not yet adequately developed. In announcing this basic discovery of the presence of parasites in the liquor cerebrospinalis, Valentin observed that such parasites were found mainly in the region where the medula oblongata turns into the spinal cord and he added:[45] "Could it be that the proximity of the vascular plexus creates generally a disposition to produce such Helminths?" Johannes Müller accepted this manuscript for his *Archiv* without any objection to this notion of the spontaneous generation of parasites. His own mistake concerning parasitic snails inside sea animals and their alleged spontaneous generation is well known.

This survey of Valentin's research contributions should not be ended without mentioning certain papers, published in 1851 and 1853, on the embryology of fish and the gross malformations found. Valentin had already started the pertinent investigations in 1849, together with Corti, who was at that time his pupil at Bern (25). In this paper he described observations on twin malformations in fish of the type of Siamese twins, and he made the statement that in the cultures of fertilized fish eggs, which he investigated daily, there was a strikingly high number of such malformations. But he added: "It could be possible, therefore, that I have produced them unwittingly by pressing the fertilized eggs with the forceps." We remember that Valentin as a young doctor in 1833 had already published similar observations on chicken embryos at the meeting of German Natural Scientists and Physicians in Breslau. One of Valentin's manuscripts preserved in the Library of the Royal Academy of Sciences in Stockholm gives an exact description of an apparatus to hatch such eggs and is signed: "Valentin an Herrn Prof. Dr. Retzius d.24. September 1833." In the fertilized eggs of fish he found an object for his investigations that was much easier to handle. As we know now, he was entirely correct in his view on the artificial production of monsters. He proved in the paper mentioned above that this type of freak is not the result of growing together of two fertilized eggs, an opinion held then by scientists, but by the abnormal development of one single embryo. We may thus claim Valentin as the father of this branch of modern biology which Roux later called the mechanics of development. Quoting Valentin's own words, he pointed out that if his opinion were proved correct, "a physiological concept of teratology would thus be made possible." In this little paper he also discussed the idea that the embryologic development of certain organs is necessarily connected with the development of certain other organs. This was established experimentally in the twentieth century by Spemann. Valentin's short publication so impressed contemporary scientists that it was extensively reviewed (four pages) in 1852 in the *Proceedings of the Society of Biology* in Paris. Before this society Valentin read a paper on the same subject.[46]

CONCLUDING REMARKS

For more than forty-five years Valentin was a leading personality among the scholars and teachers at Bern University and among the physiologists of the world. In 1881 his activities in research and as a teacher came to a sudden end. He suffered a stroke, which paralyzed his left side completely. His speech, which was affected in the beginning, returned, but the paralysis remained, so that he had to retire from all his duties at the university. However, as Forster said in his eulogy, he did not stop working on scientific problems up to the very day of his death. He died on the twenty-fourth

[44] *Müller's Archiv* 1840: 317.
[45] *Ibid.*, 319.
[46] *Compte Rendu* 4: 99, 1853.

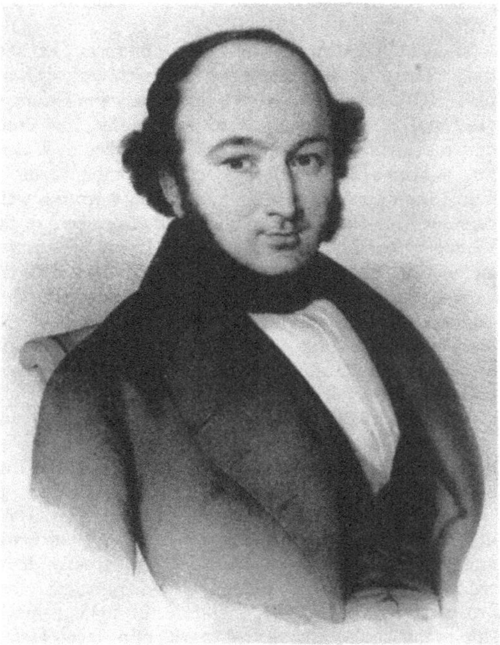

FIG. 16. G. Valentin. Lithograph by unknown artist. Published by Huber & Co. in Bern. Courtesy of Öffentliche Bibliothek der Universität Basel, Switzerland.

of May 1883 (75) in Bern and was buried there on the twenty-sixth of May.

Valentin was married on March 25, 1841 in Frankfurt am Main (B.B.B.); at that time his mother was no longer alive. She probably died early in 1839. A bill specifying the expenses of her burial is dated April 30, 1839. The bill for her tombstone is dated July 4, 1839, and the sale of her possessions is mentioned in the account book (B.B.B.) as having taken place on August 7, 1839. At that time, April 1839, Valentin was once more in his home town, Breslau. From the diary of Mrs. Henrietta Valentin we learn that of Valentin's three children, the eldest, Anna Caroline (named after Valentin's late mother), was born on August 18, 1843, the son, Adolf, was born on September 28, 1845, and the daughter, Ida, on February 2, 1849. This diary of Valentin's wife reveals the writer's high intelligence. She is very much concerned with the education and early bodily and mental development of the children. Professor Vogt (Carl Vogt's father) is mentioned as the Valentin family's physician.

Valentin's family life was apparently not a happy one. In later years, unfortunately, severe conflicts developed between the two fundamentally different personalities of Valentin and his wife, creating a difficult and tense atmosphere in Valentin's home. This may have been a factor why Valentin's son, Adolf, as a young student, was sent to Göttingen where he attended the higher schools up to his admission to the University (Hintzsche, 1953).

This son, Adolf Valentin, later became Professor of Otolaryngology at Bern. He was a pupil of Politzer in Vienna and died on May 17, 1911, in his sixty-sixth year. Anna Carolina, when she was fifteen years of age, was baptized on August 6, 1858, in Bern in the Church of the Holy Spirit. Witnesses were Professor Tonguiere of Bern and Mrs. Professor Studer-Hühnernadel, also of Bern. Later Anna married a man from Geneva by the name of Maillart. Their son, Dr. Hector Maillart of Geneva, was the owner of the portrait of Valentin reproduced on page 160. The other daughter, Ida, married a man by the name of Bodenheimer, who, in 1883, was editor-in-chief of the newspaper *Elsässer Journal* in Strassburg, where he is referred to as "ancient conseiller d'état." His eulogy on the death of his father-in-law, printed in the *Elsässer Journal* on May 26, 1883, is remarkable among all other eulogies for the personal knowledge of details it reveals. Bodenheimer acquaints us with the fact that Valentin was not a night-worker but rose every day, summer and winter, before four o'clock in the morning, undoubtedly a habit acquired during early youth. His favorite subjects were mathematics and history of fine arts. His vacations were spent on excursions into the Alps, and in later years on tours to Italy, Spain, and France (Paris) as well. Bodenheimer likewise mentions the fabulous retentive memory Valentin had.

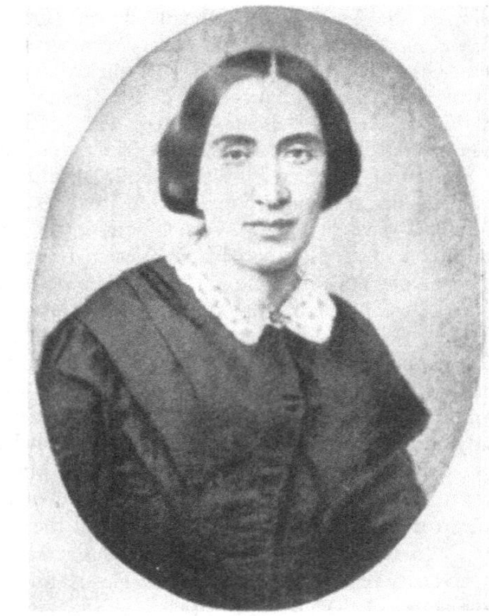

FIG. 17. Henrietta Valentin nee Samosch, Valentin's wife. Courtesy of Burger Bibliothek, Bern.

Many honors were bestowed upon Valentin from early youth, demonstrating his international reputation. Besides those already mentioned the following should be enumerated here:

In 1835 Valentin became a member and Secretary of the German Imperial Academy of Natural Scientists Carolino-Leopoldina; in the same year (October 15, 1835) membership in the Schlesische Gesellschaft für vaterländische Cultur in Breslau was conferred on him. On August 31, 1837, he was made a member of the Swiss Society of Natural Scientists (of which Agassiz was president), and in 1839 he was elected as a foreign member of the medical society in Stockholm, probably through the kind offices of Retzius. On January 2, 1841, Valentin became a corresponding member of the Medical Society at Hamburg; on May 12, 1841, of the Naturforschende Gesellschaft in Basel (Miescher, president); on October 14, 1842, of the Royal Medical Society of Buda-Pest (Hungary); on October 29, 1842, of the Royal Academy of Medicine in Belgium; on May 29, 1843, of the Royal Society of Sciences in Liège; on December 30, 1843, of the Società Medico-Chiurgica di Torino (Italy); and on February 17, 1844, he was elected to membership in the Society of Scientists and Physicians in Heidelberg (Germany). On October 3, 1844, he became a foreign member of the Royal Medical Society of Copenhagen (Denmark) (Eschricht was president). On October 2, 1845, Valentin was made an honorary member of the Russian Medical Society in St. Petersburg; on May 19, 1846, corresponding member of the Académie Royale de Médecine in Paris. He became an honorary member of the Naturhistorischer Verein für die Preussischen Rheinlande on June 26, 1847, and on August 13, 1847, honorary member of the Verein Grossherzoglich Badischer Medicinalbeamter. On November 18, 1848, La Société de Biologie in Paris voted him a Membre-Associé. Ruyer was president, Claude Bernard and Charles Robin vice presidents. The Society of German Physicians and Scientists in Paris made him an honorary member on July 23, 1849; the diploma was signed by Von Graefe. The same honor was conferred on him by the Verein Deutscher Ärtzte in New York on June 12, 1851. On December 15, 1861, Valentin became an Associé of the Académie Royale des Sciences, des Lettres et des Beaux-Arts de Belgique, and an honorary member of the Académie Royale de Médecine de Belgique on October 25, 1862. He was made a Commander of the Order of the Crown of Italy on November 6, 1882. The Philosophical Faculty of the University of Bern conferred upon him an honorary degree in the year 1876, on the occasion of the completion of forty years as a member of the University. In 1865, on the five hundredth anniversary of the University of Vienna, Valentin was elected an honorary member of the Viennese "Medicinisches Doctoren Collegium," together with his teacher, Purkinje, and E. von Baer, Helmholtz, von Liebig, Bunsen, Claude Bernard, and other celebrities of the scientific world (72).

This list of Valentin's honors is by no means exhaustive. There is a diploma in the archives of Bern (B.B.B.) from the Societas Physico Medica in Erlangen (Germany), on which the date was omitted, and other diplomas may have been lost. The number of Valentin's admirers was certainly great all over the world.

In 1845 Valentin and other outstanding scientists were suggested for election as corresponding members of the Viennese Gesellschaft der Aerzte.[46a] Every prospective member of this society had first to be submitted to the local government (The K. K. Niederoestereichisches Landesregierungspräsidium) which was supposed to discuss the case for political approval with the governmental Studienhofkommission and the Geheime Hof- und Staatskanzlei concerning the moral and political standing of the candidate. If such a candidate was living outside of Austria inquiries had to be made on these points through diplomatic channels. In the years before the 1848 revolution permission was given to elect a scientist a member of the Society of Physicians in Vienna only if all these inquiries proved his moral integrity and political reliability. Apparently these requirements could not be met by Valentin and other prospective members and, therefore, in 1845 membership in this society was denied to Valentin, Jacob Henle, David Gruby, and others. Valentin might have felt very comfortable on this occasion in the company of these other morally and politically suspicious characters.

On two solemn occasions a Festschrift was dedicated to Valentin by friends and colleagues, an honor which, from olden times has been regarded as one of the most outstanding academic awards for scientists. One was dedicated to him at the fortieth anniversary of his being elected professor in Bern in 1876; the other at the occasion of the fiftieth anniversary of his graduation as a doctor in 1882. At the latter occasion the University of Breslau renewed his doctoral diploma as is customary in German universities whenever a graduate reaches his fiftieth anniversary.

Like every outstanding man Valentin also had opponents in the scientific field. The controversy with Remak and Volkmann's polemic pamphlet have already been mentioned. In electrophysiology Du Bois-Reymond sharply criticized Valentin's publications. He did so in his standard work, where in the rudest way he also attacked the famous Italian pioneer in electrophysiology, Matteucci, as well as Valentin. P. Loewenberg wrote a polemic against certain parts of Valentin's studies on gas-metabolism in man.[47] All this is mentioned to show that Valentin's life, like that of every other pioneer, held, not only success and triumph, but also struggle and battle, and battle and polemics in the

[46a] *Geschichte der Gesellschaft der Aerzte in Wien 1837–1937*, Vienna, 1938.

[47] Traube's *Beiträge* 1: 201, 1846.

German literature of the nineteenth century were rough and brutal. But the magnitude of Valentin's contributions to modern medicine was not even touched by all the attacks on certain of his statements.

It should never be forgotten that the man who has the vision first to recognize the existence of a certain problem deserves no less and very often more credit than the one who finds final solution to the problem.

The affection felt toward this great teacher of generations of doctors was shown on the occasion of his golden jubilee as physician, October 10, 1882, when he himself was already a hopelessly ill man. His home University of Breslau sent him an honorary diploma and a printed testimonial; he received a printed congratulatory address from the Ordo Medicorum Universitatis Rostochiensis in Rostock (Germany). Other diplomas, addresses, and congratulatory cables came from universities in Germany (Bonn, Erlangen, Giessen, Heidelberg, Kiel, Königsberg, and Marburg) and Austria (Graz, Prague, Wien), from Pavia in Italy and Zürich in Switzerland, and elsewhere. His son had to thank them in the name of the paralyzed father.

When Valentin was buried, the Bundesrat of Switzerland and the Government of Bern were represented at the ceremony at the Bremgarten Cemetery and so were the citizens of Bern, as well as the teachers and students of the University. Professor Forster delivered a eulogy at Valentin's home and Valentin's successor as physiologist at Bern, Professor Grützner, spoke at the cemetery (73).

Just as in the Greek theatre, where tragedy was generally followed by satire, so here appeared as the last speaker at the open grave Valentin's old collaborator, friend, and colleague, Professor Maurizio Schiff, representing the neighboring University of Geneva. Schiff, at that time sixty years of age, after a dignified introduction, was soon carried away by his temper and scientific enthusiasm and, forgetting the place and the occasion and the solemn audience, started on a strong and lengthy criticism of certain of Valentin's publications which he deemed objectionable (74).

The really dignified finale to the life of this great man in medicine was presented by the students, who, at half past eight in the evening, started a last solemn torchlight parade through Bern to the last resting-place of their beloved teacher. There they piled all the torches together in a funeral pyre, burning as a last homage for Valentin.

Gabriel Gustav Valentin was one of the last of those rare personalities with an encyclopedic knowledge and the intuition and vision required for the application of new methods to old problems and for the perception of new, and as yet undiscovered, connections between facts. As a personality he earned not only the respect he deserved as a research worker, but, as Forster said of him, "In spite of his tendency to remain independent, he made, during his lifetime, innumerable friends and not a single

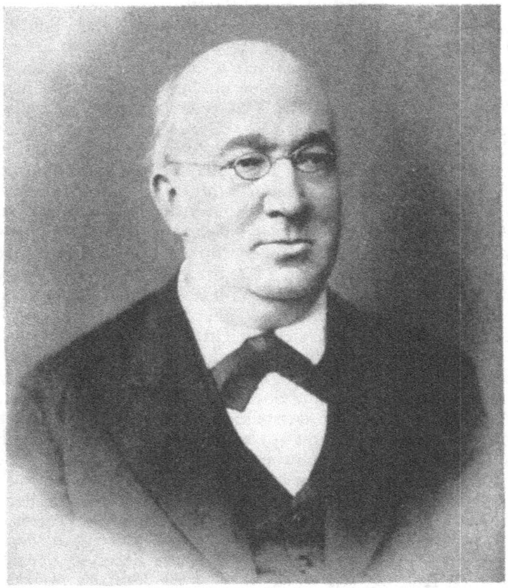

FIG. 18. G. G. Valentin about 1860. Original in the Stadtbibliothek in Bern. The same picture is hanging in the rooms of the Medical Faculty in Bern. Courtesy of Professor Dr. E. Hintzsche, Bern.

enemy." The famous historian of medicine, Pagel, said of him in the *Allgemeine Deutsche Biographie*: "Valentin was one of the most prominent physiologists of the nineteenth century." Such a statement means a great deal, considering the great historian who made it, and considering also the fact that the nineteenth century was the classical period of physiological research.

SELECTIONS FROM VALENTIN'S CORRESPONDENCE

DRAUGHT OF A LETTER FROM VALENTIN TO PROFESSOR RAU (BERN), OF JULY 1836

Verehrter Freund und College:

Die Bestimmung meiner Wohnungsverhaeltnisse ueberlasse ich Ihrem geneigten Gutachten. Betten werde ich mitbringen; Moebel aber nicht. Ich wiederhole nur meine Bitte, wenn moeglich mit Ihnen in einem Haus oder in Ihrer Nachbarschaft zu wohnen, da Sie der einzige sind, den ich in Bern kenne. Sehr lieb waere es mir, wenn ich Arbeitszimmer und Schlafcabinet geschieden haben koennte. Jedenfalls aber bin ich gesonnen, mir einen Bedienten zu halten.

Was nun aber meine religiösen Verhältnisse anbetrifft, so weiss ich nicht, was ich aus Ihrem letzten Brief in dieser Beziehung machen soll. Einerseits sagen Sie, dass mein Glaube nur bei wenigen Engherzigen Anstoss finden könnte; andererseits, dass es in Überlegung zu ziehen sey, ob ich mich nicht vor meiner Ankunft in Bern taufen lassen sollte. Ich erlaube mir auseinanderzusetzen, warum dies auf keinen Fall geschehen kann.

Sie wissen, dass mich nicht Bigotterie, sondern nur die Ueberlegung von der Taufe abhält, dass dieser Schritt, wenn er mit der Erreichung irgend eines irdischen Zweck [*sic*] verknüpft ist, verächtlich u. unwürdig erscheinet u. wird; dass es allen Vorurteilen huldigen heisst, wenn man deshalb, weil man sich der Klasse der besseren Menschen anschliesst, sein Volk verlässt. Gerade wir müssen seine Ehre aufrecht erhalten, und ich sehe keinen Grund, weshalb ich weniger diese Pflicht habe, als Meyer Beer, Halévy, Wilhelm Beer (der Astronom), Meyer (der Jurist), Ruboni (der Antiquar), Stilling (der Arzt), Levy Weimars, Moser J. Mendelssohn und so viele andere. Dieser Idee oder vielmehr der Konsequenz dieser Uberzeugung habe ich nicht wenig geopfert. Ich erzähle Ihnen, um dieses zu erhärten, einige Privatverhältnisse meines Lebens und rechne auf Ihre freundschaftliche Diskretion, wenn ich Dinge erwähne, welche sich zur Offentlichkeit nicht eignen. Ich nenne aber ungescheut die Namen der dabei agierenden Personen, damit es Ihnen freisteht, bei jeder von diesen nachzufragen, ob sich die Sachen um ein Haar breit anders verhalten als ich sie darstelle. Wollte ich mich taufen lassen, so war ich schon vor einem Jahre Prof. in Dorpat mit 1500 rth (3600 Schweizerfr.) Gehalt angestellt, wie Prof. Erdmann in Berlin bezeugen kann. Wollte ich mich taufen lassen, so würde mir (um mich Prof. Joh. Müller's eigener Worte zu bedienen) im Preussischen die Professur auf dem Präsentierteller geboten werden. Noch vor wenigen Wochen erhielt Präsident Nees von Esenbeck den officiellen Auftrag, mir zu sagen, dass ich Rathke's Stelle in Königsberg (mit 1200 rth = 3000 Schw.Fr.) Gehalt übernehme. Die Taufe ist bei uns zur Erreichung eines Lehramts bei der Universität deshalb unerlässlich, weil eine Kabinetsordre darüber vorhanden ist und diese auch das Ministerium absolut bindet. Erkundigen Sie sich bei denjenigen Schweizern, welche gegenwärtig in Berlin studieren, wie ich dort bei meiner letzten Anwesenheit daselbst im März dieses Jahres aufgenommen worden sey u. Sie werden meine Schilderung schon hiernach nicht utrirt finden.

Noch vor vierzehn Tagen erklärte mir der Curator unserer Universität, der Geheime Ober-Regierungsrath Kleinke, dass das preussische Ministerium Alles mir gern gewähren wolle, was mir von dem Ausland geboten werde. Ich erwiderte, dass ich nach Bern mein Wort gegeben u. als ehrlicher Mann es halten wolle. Ich habe keine Lust, mich, wie dieses ein geachteter Theologe zwischen der dänischen u. preussischen Regierung gethan haben soll, gleichsam versteigern zu lassen. Ich habe mein Wort gegeben u. will es sicher halten; doch nur unter völliger Garantie meiner Religionsfreiheit, wie ich auch in meinem Schreiben an das Erziehungsdepartement ausdrücklich erwähnt habe. Fragen Sie, verehrter Freund, jeden unserer praktischen Ärzte, ob ich nicht bei Annahme der Berner Professur in ökonomischer Beziehung durch die Aufgabe meiner Stellung als praktischer Arzt in Breslau sehr viel opfere. Ich tue dieses alles gern meiner geistigen Religionsfreiheit wegen. Verletzung dieser aber u. Kündigung miner neuen Stelle in Bern wären ganz identisch, da ich jeden Augenblick nach Preussen u. selbst nach mehrjähriger Abwesenheit leicht, leicht in meine alten Breslauer Verhaeltnisse zurückkehren kann.

Ich werde natuerlich kein Thor seyn, mich mit meinem Judenthum zu brüsten. Ich verlange nur, dass man es ignorieren, ebenso als es wenig interessieren würde, ob ich Katholik oder Protestant wäre. Ich verlange nur dieselbe Toleranz die unseren Collegen, Prof. Meyer in Tübingen, Prof. Ruboni in Marburg, Hauptmann Burg, Prof. an der Kriegsschule in Berlin, Prof. Aronssohn in Strassburg, Prof. Jacobsohn in Copenhagen—lauter israelitischen Universitätslehrern zu Theil wird.

Schreiben Sie mir, ich bitte Sie instaendigst, sogleich nach Empfang dieses Briefes, ob ich dies zu erwarten habe oder nicht. Schreiben Sie mir sogleich, damit ich sobald als moeglich in diesem wichtigen Punkt belehrt werde.

Interessant bleibt es, dass meine Vocation als Israelit mit mehreren Auszeichnungen zusammenfiel, welche anderen Israeliten gleichzeitig zu Theil geworden. Ich meine Halévy's Ernennung zum Mitgliede der Akademie der Künste in Paris, Levi Weimars Vocation nach St. Petersburg, Aronssohn's ehrenvolle Ernennung in Strassburg u. Riesser's Anstellung als öffentlicher Advokat. Alle diese haben ihres Glaubens halber nichts zu leiden.

ROBERT REMAK'S LETTER TO VALENTIN

Auf Euer Wohlgeboren Schreiben vom 7. Juli finde ich zu erwiedern, dass meine frühere Angabe insofern zu berichtigen ist, als die von mir angeregte Stelle sich nicht in Ihrem Repertorium, sondern in Ihrer Schrift über die Enden der Nerven befindet. Dort heisst es p. 51 (101.)

"Gäbe es einen leicht wahrnehmbaren materiellen Unterschied der sensiblen und motorischen Nervenfasern, den auch Ehrenberg J. Müller schon vergeblich gesucht haben, so müsste er auch an den verschiedenartigen varikösen Fäden des Gehirns und Rückenmarkes, als den unmittelbaren Fortsetzungen der Primitivfasern des Gehirns, existieren. Auch hier habe ich nichts der Art wahrnehmen können, da in dieser Rückicht selbst die verschiedenartigen Durchmesserverhältnisse den mehr als *ein* Individuum und *ein* Thier untersuchenden Forscher verlassen.

Um bei der Dunkelheit und Vieldeutigkeit dieser Stelle weiteren Erörterunge vorzubeugen, will ich zu Ihrem Vortheil annehmen, dass sie dabei nicht an meine Beobachtungen gedacht haben, und will in Bezug auf diesen Fall den Vorwurf des Mangels an Offenheit zurücknehmen. Der Angeber dieser Stellen, der darin eine unfehlbare Beziehung auf mich erblickte, glaubte lange, sie im Repertorium gesehen zu haben, und dies verhinderte mich, sie selbst zu sehen, bis jener sie endlich an dem citirten Orte auffand. Bei deren Anblick erinnerte ich mich wohl, vor 2 Jahren bei der Lesung der Schrift das Mystische dieser Stelle mit Befremden bemerkt zu haben; doch vergass ich damals bald daran, weil ich unbefangen genug war, keinen Groll bei Ihnen Vorauszusetzen. Mit dieser Erwiederung habe ich deshalb so lange gezögert, weizich die Ankunft des angekündigten Bandes Ihres Repertoriums abwarten wollte; da aber bereits zwei Monate verflossen sind, so glaubte ich die Antwort nicht länger verschieben zu dürfen. Es versteht sich von selbst, dass ich Ihnen besagten Band, sobald er eintreffen sollte, unverzüglich wieder zustellen werde, da der Zweck, zu welchem Sie mir ihn geschickt haben, nun auf anderem Wege erledigt ist.

Ich lebe in der festen Zuversicht, dass unsere Correspondenz in dieser Angelegenheit hiermit beendigt sein wird; sonst würde ich mich gegen wiederholte Invectiven auf die geeignete Weise zu schützen suchen müssen. Der jetzige Zustand meiner Brustorgane macht es wahrscheinlich, dass es mir nicht lange vergönnt sein wird, an wissenschaftlichen Untersuchungen Theil zu nehmen, und deshalb hätte ich wohl mehr Grund, als jeder Andere, mit aller Welt in Frieden zu leben. Das hat sich aber in diesem Falle ohne meine Schuld nicht durchführen lassen. Ich habe wenigstens das beruhigende Bewusstsein, durch meine Schriften Niemanden absichtlich gereizt zu haben.

R. Remak

Berlin d. 8 September. 1838

TWO DRAFTS OF A LETTER FROM VALENTIN TO REMAK

Verehrtester Herr Doctor,

In Ihrem letzten Schreiben, welches, da es erst nach

St. Gallen wanderte, mir vor 14 Tagen zukam, schildern Sie mir Ihr Brustleiden so bedeutend, dass es mich trotz der Antecedentia innigst betrübte. Ich will hoffen und wünschen, dass Sie es vielleicht selbst als bedeutender ansehen, wie es in der That ist. Und obgleich Sie von mir, wie Ihre Briefe aussagen, moralisch wenig halten und von meinem Grolle etc. fest überzeugt sind, so seyen Sie doch versichert, dass ich mich vielleicht mehr interessiere, ob es Ihnen wohlergehe oder nicht, als mancher, der Ihnen schöne Worte, aber nichts als dieses giebt. Lernen Sie Ihre "Angeber" dann kennen, wenn es sich darum handeln sollte, etwas für Sie zu opfern, und Sie werden überhaupt, bei mehr Welterfahung auch über Menschen besser urtheilen.

Doch abgesehen von allen diesen pensönlichen Umständen, freut es mich sehr Ihnen melden zu können, dass ich mich jetzt endlich von der Richtigkeit der Beobachtung Ihrer organischen Fasern überzeugt habe. Sie sind Fortsetzungen der Scheiden der Ganglienkugeln, finden sich in allen Ganglien des Körpers und vermischen sich mit den Cerebrospinalnerven, so dass nun dieser Punkt durch unseren gegenseitigen heftigen Widerspruch nun um einen Schritt weiter gekommen und Sie hatten in Betreff der Fasern eben so Recht, als ich in Betreff der auf den Fasern hier, wie überall aufliegenden Epithelialformationen. Inwiefern die Substanz der Scheiden der Ganglienkugeln und deren Fortsetzungen (Ihrer organischen Fasern) mit anderen Gewebtheilen der Nerven und der übrigen Systeme des Körpers werde ich bald ausführlicher zu entwickeln. So viel ist sicher, dass, sie, wie anatomisch, so auch chemisch, sowohl von den Ganglienkugeln, als den Primitivfasern der Nerven, sehr weit verschieden fand. Dass sie aber einen eigenthümlichen Bestandtheil enthalten, hoffe ich andeuten, wenn auch nicht beweisen zu können. Es ist ein Brief nicht geeignet, über die speciellen Verhältnisse der Scheiden und deren Fortsetzungen detailliert zu sprechen, da Abbildungen zu deren Erläuterungen unumgänglich nothwendig sind. Sie werden die ganze Sache ausfürlich in einer Schrift von mir: de functionibus sensoriis et motoriis nervorum cerebralium nervique sympathici die noch im Laufe dieses Winters in Ihren Händen seyn wird, finden. Der N. Sympathicus ist, wie dort experimentell gezeigt wird, ruecksichtlich seiner sensiblen und motorischen Kräfte ein reiner N. cerebro-Spinalis und zeigt dieselben Grundgesetze der Leitung, wie jeder andere Körpernerve, wie sich experimentell strictissime nachweisen lässt. Welches der specielle Nutzen der Ganglienkugeln, deren Scheiden u. deren Fortsetzungen sey, lässt sich experimentell nicht sicher bestimmen. Doch werde ich auch versuchen, ebenfalls, eine mit den neuesten anatomisch-physiologischen Details verbundene Theorie zu geben. In dieser Beziehung wird Sie das Capitel de fabrica et usu gangliorum rücksichtlich der Anatomica speciell interessieren.

So werden die Scheiden der Ganglienkugeln mit Ihren organischen Fasern ausgesöhnt, und ein wissenschaftlicher Streit hat, wie es überall ist, wo beide Partheien die Wahrheit, [suchen] um einen Schritt vorwärts gebracht. Ich werde als Gegengeschenk für Ihre Arbeit Ihnen meine Schrift über die Funktionen der Nerven zusenden. Allein vergessen Sie gefälligst nicht, dass die Verbindung zwischen der westlichen Schweiz und dem nördlichen Deutschland nicht die lebhafteste ist, und dass es daher etwas lange dauert ehe auf Buchhändlerwege (oder vielmehr Umwegen) eine Sendung nach Berlin gelangt.

Wenn Ihnen Ihre früheren Briefe nur irgendwie im Gedächtnisse sind, so werden Sie bei einiger ruhigen Überlegung bald einsehen, dass ich nach einfachen Gesetzen der Ehre und Billigkeit gar nicht mehr an Sie schreiben sollte. Allein von den Leuten verkannt zu werden, ist mir nichts Neues und überdies halte ich es bei der mich betrübenden Schilderung Ihres Brustleidend für meine Pflicht, Ihnen wenigstens meinerseits jede Ursache des Grolles zu nehmen. Als ich Ihnen früher meine Dienste anbot, fanden Sie darin statt guten Willens nur Hochmuth. Obgleich diese Deutung wenig einladend ist, so muss ich mir doch erlauben, Sie wegen Ihrer Stellung zu befragen. Kronenberg, der diesen Sommer mehrere Tage hier war, sagte mir, dass Sie nach Wilna als Privatdocent gehen wollten. Für welches Fach wollten Sie sich speciell ausbilden? Sprechen Sie so geläufig französisch, dass Sie auch in dieser Sprache Vorträge halten könnten. Glauben Sie nicht, dass ich Sie deshalb in die Luft hinein befrage.

Mögen Sie übrigens aus *meinem* Benehmen ersehen, dass ich persönliche Beleidigungen vor Ihrem wissenschaflichen Eifer vergesse. Seyen Sie aber auch versichert, dass ich grob zu seyn, nie, ungerecht oder verkennend zu seyn, stets scheue.

G. Valentin

Bern d. 27. Oct. 38

Verehrtester Herr Doctor,

In Ihrem letzten Schreiben schildern Sie mir Ihr Brustleiden mit so trüben Farben, dass es mich trotz der Antecedentia, welche sicher geeignet waren, mich Ihnen nur zu entfremden, innigst betrübte. Ich hoffe und wünsche, dass Sie selbst Ihre Krankheit für bedeutender ansehen, als sie in der That ist und obgleich Sie in Ihren Briefen geradezu sagen, dass Sie von mir moralisch wenig halten, dass Sie von meinem Hasse gegen Sie fest überzeugt sind, so kann ich doch Sie ruhig dessen versichern, dass ich gewiss den schmerzlichsten Antheil an Ihrem körperlichen Leiden nehme und besseren Nachrichten über Ihren Gesundheitszustand sehnlichst entgegensehe. Ohne in das Nähere einzugehen, muss ich Ihnen nur so viel sagen, dass meine Gesinnungen gegen Sie mir aufrichtiger scheinen, als die jener "Angeber," welche Ihnen Stellen meiner Schriften zeigen, die, wie Sie aus dem Titel sehen können, früher *gedruckt* waren, als Ihre erste Abhandlung in Müllers Archiv ausgegeben worden. Von den Leuten verkannt zu werden, bin ich längst gewohnt und "angegeben zu werden" ist mir auch nichts Neues mehr.

Da ich, der ich selbst früher an sehr ernstlichen Brustbeschwerden gelitten, nur zu sehr weiss, welchen üblen Einfluss Gemüthsaffecte auf Kranke der Art haben, so wird es mir zur Pflicht, mit Ihnen Frieden zu schliessen u. so scharf auch mein Auftreten gegen Sie in dem ersten Hefte des diesjärigen Repert. war, so that es mir herzlich weh, als ich Ihr letztes Schreiben erhielt. Da es mir nichts macht, einen begangenen Fehler zu bekennen so gestehe ich ganz frei, dass ich die ganze Sache auf sich beruhen haben lassen würde, wenn ich Ihren Gesundheitszustand gekannt hätte. In einer eben dem Drucke übergebenen Schrift, (de functionibus sensoriis et motoriis N.N. cerebralium N. que Sympathici) wo ich in dem Kapitel De gangliorum fabrica et usu auf denselben Gegenstand zurückkomme, habe ich auch, wie Sie sehen werden, zum Frieden die erste Hand wieder geboten, da mir jetzt das Verhältnis Ihrer organischen Fasern zu den Scheiden der Ganglienkugeln vollkommen klar ist und beide, wie Sie auch aus den Abbildungen sehen werden, durchaus identisch sind; während in den N.N. mollibus, welche Z.B. die Verbindungsäste des N. Sympath. aus den Hirnnerven darstellen, diese Fortsetzungen der Scheiden der Ganglienkugeln den relativ grössten Theil der Masse bilden, da in allen Nerven das Gesetz gilt, dass die Fortsetzungen der Ganglienkugelscheiden mit der Menge der enthaltenen Cerebro-spinalnerven in umgekehrtem Verhältniss stehen. Dass übrigen der N. Sympathicus ein completer Cerebrospinalnerve ist, so weit dieser Gegenstand experimentell verfolgt werden kann, werden Sie aus der Schrift ersehen; dass er sich rücksichtlich der Ernehrungsverhältnisse auch als solcher verhalte, wird mehr als wahrscheinlich.

Ich werde Ihnen noch im Laufe dieses Winters meine eben genannte Schrift als Gegengeschenk für die Ihrige zusenden. Nur muss ich Sie bitten, nicht zu vergessen, dass die Sendungen von Bern nach Berlin auf Buchhändlerwegen (oder vielmehr Umwegen) etwas lange dauern und dass jeder Verleger aus persönlichen öconomischen Rücksichten sich mit der Zusendung von Freiexemplaren nicht allzusehr beeilt.

Wenn Sie Ihre früheren Briefe nur irgendwie im Gedächtmisse haben, so werden Sie bei einiger ruhigen Überlegung bald einsehen, dass ich nach einfachen Gesetzen der Ehre und Billigkeit gar nicht mehr an Sie schreiben sollte. Allein alles frühere seÿ wenigstens meinerseits vergessen.

Als ich Ihnen früher meine Dienste anbot, fanden Sie nur Hochmuth und Vermessenheit darinzwei Eigenschaften, die, wie ich frei behaupten kann, mir selbst Feinde, die mich persönlich kennen, nicht zuschreiben. Im Vertrauen dass Sie vielleicht diese Ansicht änderen dürften, erlaube ich mir, an Sie eine Frage zu richten. Kronenberg, der diesen Sommer mehrere Tage hier war, sagte mir, dass Sie als Privatdozent, nach Wilna gehen wollten. Welches Fach wollen Sie speziell betreiben? Und sprechen Sie so geläufig französich, das Sie auch in dieser Sprache Unterricht erteilen könnten? Glauben Sie nicht, dass ich in die Luft hinein diese Fragen an Sie richte.

G. Valentin.

Bern d. 27. Oct. 38.

FIVE LETTERS FROM JOHANNES MÜLLER TO VALENTIN AND ONE FROM VALENTIN TO JOHANNES MÜLLER

Verehrtester Freund: [48]

Spät genug erwidere ich Ihren gütigen Brief, in diesem Jahr bin ich so manches schuldig geblieben. Sie kennen die Ursache und werden mich gewiss ein wenig entschuldigen. Nun das Dekanat zu Ende geht, atme ich wieder auf. Dass Sie uns verlassen, empfinde ich schmerzlich, und doch muss ich von Herzen Glueck wünschen, da diese Wendung offenbar die glücklichste ist, die eintreten konnte. Sie erhalten den schönsten Wirkungskreis, für welchen Sie bestimmt sind und werden einen Mittelpunkt des wissenschaftlichen Lebens bilden. Ihre Stellung zu den Collegen wird Ihnen gewiss die angenehmste werden. Dies ist allerdings notwendig, und unentbehrlich, da der Fremde in der Schweiz schwieriger sich vielseitige Beziehungen zu den Bewohnern schafft. Die Neutralität, auf welche er angewiesen ist, ist ihm aber auch wieder nützlich an einem Ort, wo die Zustände zum Teil noch neu sind und manches sich parteilich gegenueber steht. Empfehlen Sie mich gütigst Herrn Prof. Vogt,[49] dem ich für die Zusendung der Abhandlung verbindlichst danke. Unser Henle [50] ist dermalen in Coblenz bei seinen Eltern. Seine Mutter leidet an einem unheilbaren Übel; er wird auf ihren Verlust sich vorbereiten müssen. In seinen Verhältnissen ist noch nichts entschieden; es steht aber nahe bevor und es ist zu hoffen, wenn auch vor der Hand keine Ausnahme gemacht werden kann, dass es doch ein gutes Ende nimmt. Gar manche hochgestellte Personen haben sich für eine gute Wendung dieser seiner Angelegenheit interessiert und ihre Schuld ist es nicht, dass die Sache nicht jetzt schon im Guten für ihn entschieden ist. Grüssen Sie Pr. Purkinje, den trefflichen hochgeehrten, und nehmen Sie viel herzliche Grüsse von uns allen auf die Reise.

Ihr ergebener
D Müller

Berlin 28 8. 36.

Verehrtester Herr Collega,

Ihr Brief hat mich sehr befremdet. Sie sprechen plötzlich von Unfrieden, Angriffen, Anfeindungen gegen Sie durch mich, was mir völlig unverständlich ist, wenn Sie nicht durch diesen Vorwurf Ihre gewohnten Neckereien rechtfertigen wollen. Sind Sie so sehr von uns verwöhnt, dass Sie den Widerspruch nicht mehr ertragen können? dessen Gebrauch Sie seit Jahr und Tag und so lange ich Sie kenne, gegen mich, wie billig, in Anspruch nehmen, wo Sie dazu Ursache finden. Sie taten es ehe ich Sie kannte, in Ihren ersten Schriften und nachher und warum nicht? Ich fragte Sie nicht danach, als ich das Vergnügen hatte, Sie hier zu sehen. Ich fragte nicht danach, wer Sie sind, und welche Stellung Sie einnehmen. Diese Frage würde auch jetzt die letzte sein und nicht stattfinden können. Nun sollen gar die Bemerkungen im Jahresberichte über Ihre Nervenbeobachtungen Angriffe sein, während sie mit der vollsten Anerkennung dessen, was sich bewährt, geschrieben sind. Jedes Wort kann ich vertreten. Ich habe diese Sache wiederholt nachgesehen, besonders in Beziehung auf die Darstellung vom Nervensystem, die ich in der neuen Auflage der Physiologie zu geben habe, wo ich das factische anführe und die Streitfragen auf sich beruhen lasse. Wo Sie sich indirect über den gegenwärtigen Zustand der Nervenphysik ausgesprochen, hatte ich auch nur ganz indirect im Jahresbericht erwidert. In mehreren Punkten, die mich näher angehen, hatte ich gar mich meiner eigenen Haut zu wehren und das nennen Sie Angriffe. Dass Sie Prof. Wagner von Ihren Briefen Notiz geben, ist gut, der soll urteilen, ob hier einer angegriffen ist und soll die Neckereien Ihrer Berichte vergleichen. Ich halte jene Bemerkungen so wenig für einen Angriff, dass waeren sie zur Zeit Ihrer Anwesenheit in Berlin geschrieben gewesen, ich sie Ihnen zu lesen gegeben hätte, ohne dass ich irgend eine Missbilligung von Ihnen erwartet hätte. Werden Sie erst mit dem Tadel und Widerspruch vertrauter, und wenn Sie Tadel und Widerspruch erst länger, so wie wir andern erfahren haben, so werden Sie diese übel angebrachte Empfindlichkeit schon verlieren. Hieraus sehen Sie, verehrtester Herr Collega, dass meinerseits nichts schehen ist, einen Bruch bestehender freundlicher collegialischer Verbindung herbeizuführen. Dass ich nicht Briefe schreibe, ja in dem Punkte lasse ichs immer fehlen, und der Fehler ist immer auf meiner Seite. Hier bedarf ich Ihrer so wie mancher anderen Bekannten

[48] Attention is called not only to the tone of this letter, but also to its heading, for in the German language it means more than convential politeness to address someone as "my most esteemed friend." Valentin was therefore justified if he really thought that his relationship with Müller was that of a friend.

[49] The Vogt mentioned here, Professor of Medicine at Bern, came there from Giessen, Germany, became friend and family physician of Valentin. His son, Carl Vogt, later Professor of Zoology and well known through his radical political activities, was a pupil and assistant of Valentin.

[50] The Henle referred to was the famous anatomist, Jacob Henle, close friend and assistant of Müller. He was imprisoned for his political activities in the *Burschenschaft,* and his reinstatement as assistant and admission as lecturer was, for political reasons, difficult. Among those who were helpful in his final restoration, the principal figure was Alexander von Humboldt, who spared neither time nor trouble to help others. Henle was approximately of the same age as Valentin, and both later became close friends. Purkinje was Valentin's teacher and head of the Department of Physiology in Breslau at that time.

noetigen Entschuldigung. Ich schreibe sehr ungern Briefe und schreibe alles ungern was nicht gerade nöthig ist.

Sie sprechen von erkalteter Freundschaft. Diejenige Beziehung, die zwischen uns wirklich bestand, hat sich meinerseits auch nicht im mindesten verändert; und für mehr als collegialisch freundliche Berührung habe ich Ihr Interesse zu mir als Sie hier waren, auch nicht genommen. Bedenken Sie, wie viel dazu gehört, dass man eine freundliche und höfliche collegialische Verbindung Freundschaft nennen könne, jahrelange Bekanntschaft, Jahre der Jugend, vielfache gegenseitige Prüfung, Übereinstimmung des Charakters und der Gesinnung. Lassen Sie es also, was es auch in der Tat war, von Anfang an freundliche und höfliche collegialische Berührung gewesen sein und sehen, ob es das auch jetzt noch sein kann. Sie kamen hierher als Mitarbeiter Purkinje's und Naturforscher. In beider Eigenschaft finden Sie, wie jeder Gelehrter ohne Ausnahme hier die freundlichste Aufnahme, wie sie unserer Stadt und den hiesigen Gelehrten eigen ist. Jeder Naturforscher hat sie bei Fachgenossen und nicht—Fachgenossen zu erwarten, und welchem ist sie nicht hier zu Theil geworden? In diesem Sinne hätte ich Ihnen gern jeden Dienst geleistet, den ein Gelehrter von dem anderen empfangen kann, ohne dass ich darauf den mindesten Werth gelegt hätte. Von meiner Seite hat nun keine Veränderung der collegialisch gefälligen Berührung, in welche ich zu Ihnen trat, stattgefunden; auch hatte ich selbst in Jahr u. Tag keine Gelegenheit hiergegen zu verstossen, die faule Korrespondenz abgerechnet, in welcher ich wie gesagt, immer etwas verschulde bei dem besten Verhältnis.

Sie liessen es freilich nicht an Neckereien und Schulmeistereien fehlen. Meine Geduld ist gross. So lange es geht, halte ich an den Formen, weil sie fuer den wissenschaftlichen Verkehr so sehr erleichternd sind. Alle Sicherheit des Benehmens vermisse ich in den anmassenden allgemein gehaltenen Bemerkungen ueber das Corps der Naturforscher in Ihren Berichten. Wem sind diese subjectiven Bemerkungen zugedacht? Etwa denen, welche Sie Ihre Freunde nennen? Die werden Ihnen raten sie zuerst auf sich selbst anzuwenden und dann zu sehen, wieviel fuer uns andere noch übrig bleibt. Wenn das zur Freundschaft gehört so bewahre uns der liebe Gott vor den Freunden, mit unseren Feinden werden wir schon fertig, aber die Freunde.

Nun habe ich aufrichtig und vertraulich meine Subjectivitäten gegen Sie geäussert. Denn zu Briefen eignet sich dergleichen. Ich wünsche mit Ihnen in Frieden und in gutem freundlich collegialischem Vernehmen zu sein und zu bleiben und werde das Meinige in redlicher Absicht zur Erzielung desselben tun. Das können Sie versichert seyn.

Ihre Ansichten über die Gefässe des penis sind eine Sache für sich. Der Art Widerspruch kann mir in keiner Art unangenehm seyn. Er muss in der Wissenschaft seyn und Jeder nimmt ihn in Anspruch. Halte ich gleich die art. helicinae nach Lesung Ihres Aufsatzes nicht für gefährdet, so nehme ich doch Ihre Aufforderung, die Sache nochmals zu untersuchen, als freundschaftliche mit Vergnügen an, ich werde die nächsten Wochen dazu verwenden. Für die Mittheilung des Aufsatzes sage ich Ihnen meinen Dank. Doch einmal wieder etwas von Ihnen nach längerer Zeit. Jede Entdeckung muss erst durch den Zweifel durch, ehe ihre Anerkennung sicher ist, und so erzeigen Sie der Sache jedenfalls einen Dienst. Ihr Aufsatz soll unverzüglich gedruckt werden. Von Breslau aus erhielt ich ein vollständiges Exemplar Ihrer Abhandlung ueber die Nerven. Ich danke Ihnen dafür bestens; Das unvollständige Exemplar, welches Sie mir früher zu schicken die Güte hatten, hatte ich zu seiner Zeit in Ihrem Interesse an unseren Herrn Minister abgegeben, als Sie noch in Breslau waren. Ich hatte es von dort nicht zurueck erhalten. Ich habe hinwieder ein Exemplar meiner Abhandlung uber die organischen Nerven des penis an Sie durch Buchhandel abgegeben. Die Abhandlung über die Wundernetze habe ich leider nicht mehr. Eschricht hatte viele Exemplare erhalten, und die wenigen, welche ich behielt, waren hier bald verteilt gewesen. Meine besten Wünsche zum neuen Jahr, auch fur gutes Licht, das im Vorwinter so schlecht war.

Ihr ganz ergebenster
Dr Jo. Müller

Berlin. 31/12.37 [51]

Verehrter Herr Collega:

Empfangen Sie zuvörderst meinen wenn auch verspäteten, doch nicht nicht minder herzlichen Dank für die in Ihrem freundlichen Briefe enthaltenen Mittheilungen und den Beitrag zum Archiv, welcher gedruckt ist. Ich traf nach unserem Zusammentreffen an dem von Ihnen bezeichneten Tage die von Freiburg kommenden Naturforscher in Basel. Prinz Bonaparte reiste bald nach Neuchatel ab, wo dann später nochmals ein Zusammentreffen zwischen ihm, Agassiz und Henle stattfand und die Lieblingsangelegenheit der Fische besprochen wurde. Agassiz und Henle blieben zunächst noch in Basel, da gab es dann in ihrer und der Baseler Gesellschaft manche frohe und genussreiche Stunde, und ich hatte wieder Gelegenheit mich des liebenswürdigen Naturells der Süddeutschen zu freuen. Ich traf die Meinigen wohl am Rhein und eilte hierher. Der Wintercursus hat unterdes begonnen. Henle ist mit seinen Vorlesungen viel beschäftigt. Was uns an Zeit übrig bleibt, ist der Fortsetzung der Haifische bestimmt. Meine Geschäfte sind weniger zeitraubend als ich es für diese Zeit erwartete und ich habe Hoffnung, auch an der Fortsetzung des abgebrochenen zu arbeiten, wovon mir sehr die Myxinoiden am Herzen liegen. In der Angelegenheit der Wiederbesetzung der Bartelsschen Stelle ist immer noch nichts entschieden. Eine rechte Angelegenheit ist mir, Sie zu fernerem Anteil an dem encyclopaedischen Wörterbuch zu gewinnen. Ich wünschte sehr, dass Sie den Artikel *Muskel* (histolog.) und *Muskelbewegung* übernehmen möchten. Auch stelle ich die Artikel *Leben* mit *Lebenskraft* und *Menschenrassen* anheim. Haben Sie Lust einzugehen, so erlaube ich mir, Ihnen nächstens fernere Vorschläge zu machen. Der Buchstabe K ist bald abgesetzt. Bis der Artikel Leben zum Druck kommt, werden aber immer noch 2 Monate vergehen. Das Honorar ist nach dem neuen Satz 14 Thaler. Doch glaube ich dass sich die Verleger für Ihren Antheil zu grösserem Honorar, etwa 15 Thaler Gold verstehen würden, wenigstens haben sie sich einmal gegen mich geäussert für Mitarbeiter ersten Ranges grössere Zugeständnisse machen zu wollen. Es sollte mich herzlich freuen, wenn Sie Antheil nehmen. Ihren letzten Gruss durch Dr. [name illegible] habe ich erhalten. Ihre hiesigen Bekannten und meine Familie lassen freundlichst grüssen.

Ihr verehrungsvoll ergebener
Jo. Müller

Berlin d. 24. November 1838

Verehrtester Herr Collega:

Herzlichen Dank für Ihre Zusage des Antheils an dem encyclop. medicinischen Wörterbuch. Mit den von Ihnen übernommenen Artikeln hat es bis auf 4–5 Monate Zeit. Früher werden sie in keinem Falle nöthig. Ich danke auch bestens für den Aufsatz zum Archiv, gleich nach Empfang trug ich Sorge, dass er unverzüglich gedruckt

[51] In the upper left hand corner of the letter Valentin made the note, "response d. 9. Jan. 38."

und die Zusendungen gestochen werden. Ihre Haller betreffende Mittheilung interessierte mich lebhaft. In seinen persönlichen Beziehungen müsste man ihn sich als durchaus nobel (?) denken, er war ja auch in Hinsicht seines Characters ein Mann von grossartigstem Styl. Henle und Schwann lassen freundlichst grüssen. Letzterer wird wohl bald von hier abgehen. Er steht mit Löwen in Unterhandlung. Empfehlen Sie mich Herrn Prof. Theile, gelegentlich bitte ich ihm zu sagen dass alles besorgt sei. Beiträge zur Anatomie des Bären hat er versprochen. Erinnern Sie ihn daran. Neulich untersuchte ich die Lymphherzen beim Crocodil frisch am eben verstorbenen Thiere. Die Muskelfasern waren auch mit Querstreifen. Diese Organe sind sehr gross und liegen an der Stelle wo ich sie bei lebenden Eidechsen sah. Sie stehen mit den Beckennerven in Verbindung. Glück und Segen im neuen Jahre!

Mit hochachtungsvoller Ergebenheit

Berlin 19. Januar 1839 [52]

Ihr

Jo. Müller

LETTER FROM VALENTIN ADDRESSED TO JOHANNES MÜLLER

Verehrtester Herr Professor!

Unsere Allgemeine Naturforschende Gesellschaft hat mich beauftragt, bei der Berliner Akademie die Anfrage zu stellen, ob dieselbe geneigt wäre, mit unserer Societät in Tauschverkehr ihrer Drucksachen zu treten. Wir besitzen schon in unserer Bibliothek einzelne frühere Bände der Berliner Denkschriften, welche wir der gütigen Zusendung der Akademie verdanken.

Von unserer Gesellschaft wird jährlich ein Oktavband Bericht u. ein Quartband Denkschriften ausgegeben. Von den letzteren befindet sich der 4. Band eben unter der Presse. Da ich nicht weiss, an wen ich mich zur Erledigung dieser Sache speciell zu wenden habe, so erlaube ich mir, Sie ergebenst zu bitten, diese Anfrage selbst gütigst besorgen oder mir gefl. denjenigen Akademiker anzeigen zu wollen, an welchen ich zu schreiben hätte.

Die von Rathke im letzten Hefte des Archiv mitgeteilten Bemerkungen über Syngnathus aequoreus veranlassen mich, auf die Discussion über die Brutverhältnisse dieser Fische wieder zurückzukommen. Schon unmittelbar nachdem Rathke in seinen Reisebemerkungen den ersten Zweifel gegen den Ausspruch, dass die Männchen die Bruttasche tragen, rege gemacht, bemerkte ich, dass ich bei einem mit einer Bruttasche versehenen Tiere Eier mit Dotter darneben gefunden habe (repert. III. 193). Seit jener Zeit hate ich durch Agahsiz mehrere Bruttaschen und Embryonen führende Exemplare von S. Aphidion, Rondoleti u. pelagicus erhalten und in einem grossen Teil derselben das Vorkommen von Eiern in den keimbereitenden Genitalien bestättigt. Umso mehr verwirrte mich eine Erfahrung, welche ich vorigen Herbst in Nizza machte. Ich erhielt einen s. pelagicus oder wenigstens eine dieser species sehr nahe Form, in deren Bruttasche sich eine gallertige aus unregelmässigen Brocken bestehende Masse befand. Wider Erwarten zeigte sich bei dem Öffnen waare Genitalien, welche ganz das Aussehen von Hoden dem freien Auge darboten, nach der mikroskopischen Untersuchung aber Resultate lieferten, welche mich bis auf den heutigen Tag in Unwissenheit lassen, ob ich ein männliches oder ein weibliches Individuum untersucht habe. Statt Eier oder statt Samentierchen fanden sich sehr zierliche Körper, meist von spindelförmiger, oft auch von mehr oder minder kugeliger u. einseitig geschwänzter Gestalt, welche innerhalb einer durchsichtigen, gesonderten, feinen Wandung eine Menge runder Körnchen enthielten. Nach Ruptur der Wandung traten die runden hellen scharf begrenzten Körperchen frei heraus, zeigten jedoch weder die charakteristischen Spermatozoen Bewegungen noch Schwänze u. dgl. Ebenso wenig liess sich aber in dem ganzen Organ auch die geringste Spur eines Eies u. eines Keimbläschens auffinden.

Sie werden sich erinnern, dass Krohn im vorigen Jahre in Frorip's Notizen sehr schöne Erfahrungen über die Venenanhänge, die in ihnen, vorkommenden Entozoen u. die an ihnen sich vorfindenden Crystalldrusen aus den Dintenfischen mitgeteilt hat. Nach meinen Erfahrungen glaube ich annehmen zu können, dass auch die Seeigel solche eigentümliche Venenanhänge besitzen. Es sind diese bei E. Lividus u. E. Eskulentus in der Unterfläche der Laterne befindliche Organe, welche ich noch nirgends beschrieben sehe. Geht man nämlich von demjenigen Teile, welchen Tiedemann als Herz u. Della Chiaje als Polische Blase bezeichnet, aus, so verläuft längs der Speiseröhre ein arterieller Stamm, welcher an der Unterfläche der Laterne (das Tier in der seiner Stellung im Leben entgegengesetzten Position, mit dem Munde nach oben, dem After nach unten gedacht) einen arteriellen Kreis bildet. Nach aussen von diesem befindet sich dann ein sehr dünnhäutiger Kreis, welcher auf den ersten Blick aus der sich hier hinüberschlagenden dünnen Laternenhaut anzugehören scheint. Allein bei genauerer Prüfung sieht man, dass in diesem Kreis ein dünnwandiger Kanal, wahrscheinlich eine Kreisvene verläuft. Mit diesem Gebilde hängen dann die fünf (?) Organe, welche ich als Venenanhänge deuten zu müssen glaube, zusammen. Jedes von ihnen liegt in einem Zwischenraume der Unterfläche der Laterne und zwar in demjenigen, der seitlich von beiden Balken und den beiden y-förmigen Stücken begrenzt wird, haftet an seinem unteren Ende an dem genannten Kreisgefässe, während sein äusseres Ende frei ist, zeigt schon dem unbewaffneten Auge regulär verteilte Punkte oder rötliche bis rötlich braune Pigmentflecke u. besteht aus einem mit dem Kreisgefässe zusammenhängenden Hauptgange, der sich in wenige Nebengänge sondert. An dieser hängen dann Träubchen von Blindsäckchen, an welchen vorzugsweise jene Pigmentkugeln sich finden. Diese letzteren bestehen aus runden rötlichen Flecken. Crystalldrusen oder Crystalle konnte ich nicht finden. Allein leider habe ich diese Beobachtungen nur mit wenigen Exemplaren vornehmen können, da ich auf die hier erwähnten Organe erst, nachdem ich die Meeresküste verlassen, aufmerksam wurde. Jedoch andererseits kann ich anfüren, dass ich an den ebenso drüsigt gebaueten Venenanhängen von Sepia officenalis ganz die gleichen roten kugelförmigen Gebilde bei Weingeistexemplaren vorfand.

Die eben beschriebenen Organe sind nicht mit denen von Monro schon abgebildeten ovalen Säckchen, in welchen die Enden der weicheren Teile der Zähne stecken, zu verwechseln. Man sieht sie vielmehr erst, dann aber auf der Stelle, wenn man die ovalen Säckchen zurückbiegt. Ob diejenigen Gebilde, welche Della Chiaje unter dem Namen der Grappoli Vessicolosi anführt auch hierher gehoeren oder nicht, vermag ich nicht zu bestimmen. Es dürfte wohl auch wahrscheinlich sein, dass sie als Venenanhänge funktionieren.

Es wäre mir lieb, wenn Sie diesen Bemerkungen einen Platz im Archiv gönnen würden,[53] damit Forscher, welche

[52] A note on this letter, made by Valentin, says that it was answered the twenty-seventh of January, 1839.

[53] Valentin's letter to the editor, could not be printed immediately because, unfortunately, it was lost through the fault of Müller's servant (*dienstbarer Geist*) and in the following letter he confesses to Valentin this little tragedy.

das Glück haben, an den südlichen Küsten Europas zu wohnen, vielleicht Krohn selbst, angeregt würden, nach Beobachtung frischer Exemplare zu bestimmen, ob ich irre, wenn ich jene Organe für Venenanhänge zu erklären geneigt bin.

Genehmigen Sie die Versicherung meiner hochachtungsvollsten Ergebenheit.

G. Valentin

Bern 2. 6. 40.

Verehrtester Herr Collega:[54]

In Folge Ihres Auftrages habe ich mich an den Archivar der Academie, Hofrat Dr. Ulrici gewandt. Da nämlich schon früher der Tausch eingeleitet war, so war eine Verhandlung bei der Academie selbst garnicht nötig gewesen. Ulrici sagte, dass die Sendungen der Abhandlungen deswegen eine Unterbrechung erlitten haben, weil er bei den Ortsveränderungen der Gesellschaft nicht gewusst, an wen und an welchen Ort er die hiesigen Academieschriften schicken sollte; er wünscht daher zu wissen, wo die Bibliothek der Schweizerischen Gesellschaft ist, und an wen er ferner die hiesigen Schriften schicken soll. Zugleich zeigt er an, dass von den Verhandlungen der Schweiz. Gesellschaft nur 2 Bände hier eingegangen seien. Von Genf sind alle Bände da. Es seien auch alle Bände von hier regelmässig dahin abgegangen, und ladet zur Fortsetzung der Einsendung der Schweizerischen Verhandlungen ein, sowie er die hiesigen ferner zu senden versichert. Die Mitteilung Ihres Briefes über die Gefässanhänge bei den Seeigeln scheinen mir sehr interessant zu sein, ich muss aber sogleich ein Unglück bekennen, das mir damit begegnet ist. Die Notiz lag auf meinem Pult und sollte daran erinnern, Ihnen die Nachricht von Ulrici zu geben. In meiner Abwesenheit hat der dienstbare Geist die Lampe umgeworfen und das Öe über dieses Blatt sowie Mehreres ausgegossen. Aus Dummheit und Angst hat dieses Subject das Verdorbene verbrennen zu müssen geglaubt. Mir war dieses Ereignis sehr ärgerlich. Ich kann Sie nicht bitten, die Notiz noch einmal zu schreiben oder mir mitzuteilen und es es [*sic*] nur Ihrer Güte anheimstellen, ob Sie bei weiterem Fortschritt Ihrer Untersuchungen mit Seeigeln, das Ergebnis des Neuen mir abermals für das Archiv mitteilen wollten und dann das verloren Gegangene zugleich beizufügen gedenken. Wegen des Vorfalls selbst hoffe ich, von Ihnen Verzeihung und Absolution zu erhalten. Die Fortsetzung der Myxin. habe ich an Sie auf Buchhändler Weg abgegeben, einen Auszug einer Arbeit über Pentacrinus und die Asterien und Ofiuren erhalten Sie mit diesem Brief. Er enthält einiges Neue, namentlich in Bezug auf die Asterien. Ich habe noch eine Forsetzung gelesen über die Ofiuren, aber in den naturforschenden Freunden, und die ist noch [nicht] gedruckt. Hier ist die Nachricht eingetroffen, dass unser F. v. Graefe in Hannover gestorben ist. Abermals ein schwer zu ersetzender Verlust.

Leben Sie wohl, mein verehrtester Herr College. Mit ausgezeichnetster Hochachtung

Ihr ganz ergebener
J. Müller[55]

Berlin 5.7.40

[54] At the top of this letter Valentin wrote: "Beantw. u. Mitteilungen eingeschickt d.26.Juli 40."

[55] This means that Valentin, who had the above draft of his letter to Müller in his file, had to send a new manuscript for publication and reply to Müller on July 26, 1840. The loss of the first manuscript was due to the fact—as Müller describes so dramatically—that his servant threw over the lamp, spilling its oil on the manuscript. Afraid of being scolded, he simply burned the manuscript. It was not published in the volume referred to in the letter nor in the following volume of Müller's *Archiv.*

This is the last of the extant letters from Müller to Valentin (B.B.B.). It is written, as can be seen from the concluding remarks, with the sincerest and most respectful sentiments, and no sign of the old resentment can be detected in his previous letters.

Von Graefe, whose death is mentioned, is the famous Professor of Surgery in Berlin, Karl Ferdinand von Graefe (1787–1840). He was the father of Albrecht von Graefe (1828–1870), the outstanding ophthalmologist and ophthalmic surgeon.

REFERENCES

1. Agassiz, Louis. 1838. Monographies d'échinodermes vivaux et fossiles. Neuchâtel.
2. Bamberger, L. 1899. Erinnerungen. Berlin, G. Reimer.
3. Bastholm, E. 1952. Zwei Briefe von Ad. Hannover an Gabriel Gustav Valentin. *Acta Med. Scand.* **266**: 29–37.
4. Brann, M. 1913. Die schlesische Judenheit vor unf nach dem Edict vom 2. März 1812. *Jahresber. d. jüdisch-theologischen Seminars.* Breslau, Th. Schatzky.
5. Burckhardt, A. 1917. Geschichte der Medizinischen Fakultät zu Basel 1460–1900. Basel, F. Reinhardt.
6. Burdach, Karl Friedrich. 1848. Rückblick auf mein Leben. Leipzig, L. Voss.
7. ——. 1848. Die Physiologie als Erfahrungswissenschaft. 2nd Ed. 1. Band mit Beiträgen von Ernst Meyer, Heinrich Rathke, and G. Valentin. Leipzig, L. Voss.
8. Bouchardat and Sandras. 1845. Des fonctions du pancréas et de son influence dans la digestion des féculents. *C. R. Acad. Sci. Paris.* **20**: 1085–1091.
9. Callisen, A. C. P. 1830–1845. Medicinisches Schriftstellerlexikon der jetzt lebenden Aerzte, Wundaerzte, Geburtshelfer, Apotheker und Naturforscher aller gebildeten Völker. 33. v. Copenhagen u. Altona.
10. Dieffenbach an Stromeyer. Briefe aus den Jahren 1836–1846. 1934. Leipzig, J. A. Barth.
11. Du Bois Reymond, Emil. 1848–1884. Untersuchungen über tierische Electricität. Berlin, Reimers.
12. Feller, R. 1935. Die Universität Bern 1834–1934. Bern und Leipzig, Paul Haupt.
13. Fontana, F. 1787. Abhandlungen über das Viperngift, die amerikanischen Gifte, das Kirschlorbeergift und einige andere Pflanzengifte, nebst einigen Beobachtungen über den ursprünglichen Bau des thierischen Körpers, über die Wiedererzeugung der Nerven und der Beschreibung eines neuen Augenkanals. Berlin, C. F. Himburg.
14. Gegenbaur, Carl. 1901. Erlebtes und Erstrebtes. Leipzig, W. Engelmann.
15. Graetzer, J. 1889. Lebensbilder hervorragender Schlesischer Aerzte aus den letzten vier Jahrhunderten. Breslau, Schottländer.
16. Gruby, David. 1843. Recherches et observations sur une nouvelle espèce d'hématozoaire, Trypansoma Sanguinis. *C. R. Acad. Sci. Paris.* **17**: 1134–1136.
17. Heppner, A. 1931. Jüdische Persönlichkeiten in und aus Breslau. Breslau.
18. Hintzsche, E. 1944. Alfonso Corti. (1822-1876.) Bern, P. Haupt.
19. ——. 1944. Ein neuer Brief von Alfonso Corti (1822–1876). *Gesnerus.* **1**: 137–146.
20. ——. 1952. Aus Briefen skandinavischer Naturforscher an G. G. Valentin. *Acta Med. Scand.* **266**: 93–99.
21. Hirschfeld, J. 1876–1877. Gallerie berühmter Kliniker und hervorragender Aerzte unserer Zeit. Wien, M. Perles.

22. His, Wilhelm. 1903. Lebenserinnerungen, Leipzig. Als Manuskript gedruckt. [No publisher.]
23. Kahn, R. H. 1932. Aus Goethe's Purkinje-Zeit. *Lotos.* **80**: 1–27.
24. Kalisch, M. 1860. Die Judenfrage. Leipzig, Veith & Co.
25. Kisch, Bruno. 1950. Ein Beitrag zur Kenntnis von Corti's Tätigkeit in Bern. *Gesnerus.* **7**: 74–76.
26. Kisch, Guido. 1949. In search of freedom. London, E. Goldstone & Son.
27. Koelliker, A. 1899. Erinnerungen aus meinem Leben. Leipzig, W. Engelmann.
28. Kollmann, J. 1904. Wilhelm His. Worte der Erinnerung. *Verh. Naturforsch. Ges. Basel.* **15**: 434–464.
29. Mayer, Robert. 1893. Kleinere Schriften und Briefe. Stuttgart.
30. Moleschott, J. 1894. Für meine Freunde. Lebenserinnerungen. Giessen E. Roth.
31. Müller, Johannes. 1844. Handbuch der Physiologie des Menschen. 4th ed. Coblenz. J. Hölscher.
32. Neumann, M. 1845. *K. Klein's Jahrbuch des Nützlichen und Unterhaltenden für Israeliten.* **4**: 87–95.
33. Pagel, J. Valentin, G. G. 1895. *Allg. Deutsche Biographie.* **39**: 463–464.
34. Purkinje, J. E., and G. Valentin. 1834. Entdeckung continuirlicher durch Wimperhaare erzeugter Flimmerbewegungen, als eines allgemeinen Phänomens in den Klassen der Amphibien, Vögel und Säugetiere. *Müller's Archiv.* **1834**: 391–400.
35. Purkinje, Johann Evangelista, and Gustav Valentin. 1835. De Phenomeno Generali et Fundamentali Motus Vibratorii Continui. Wratislaviae, Sumptibus Aug. Schulz et Socii.
36. Sachero, G. J. 1843. Delle Funzioni dei Nervi spinali e cerebrali e del nervo sympathico. Libri quattro del Professore G. Valentin da Berna. Torino.
37. Schiff, J. M. 1858–1859. Lehrbuch der Muskel und Nervenphysiologie. Lahr, M. Schauenburg & Co. (see p. XI).
38. ——. 1859. Untersuchungen über die Zuckerbildung in der Leber und den Einfluss des Nervensystems auf die Erzeugung des Diabetes. Würzburg, Stahel.
39. Schwann, Theodor. 1839. Mikroskopische Untersuchungen über die Uebereinstimmung in der Struktur und dem Wachstum der Tiere und Pflanzen. Berlin, Sander.
40. Valentin, Gustav. 1832. Historiae evolutionis systematis muscularis prolusio. Doctoral Thesis. Wratislaviae Typis Fritschianis.
41. ——. 1833. Zur Anatomie des Foetusauges der Säugetiere. *Ammons Zsch. f. Ophthalmologie.* **3**: 302.
42. ——. 1834. Ueber die Dicke der varikösen Fäden in dem Gehirne und Rückenmark des Menschen. *Müller's Archiv.* **1834**: 401–409.
43. ——. 1835. Handbuch der Entwicklungsgeschichte des Menschen mit vergleichender Rücksicht der Entwicklung der Säugetiere und Vögel. Berlin, A. Rücker.
44. ——. 1836. History of the development of the human ovum with a comparative view of the development of the ova of mammalia and birds. Translated and abridged from the German by Martin Barry. Edinburgh, J. Starck.
45. ——. 1836. Ueber den Verlauf und die letzten Enden der Nerven. Breslau, Grass, Barth & Co. Repr. from *Nova Acta Acad. Leop. Carol.* **18**; part (1): 51. See also *Repertorium* **1**: 264.
46. ——. 1836–1845. *Repertorium* für Anatomie und Physiologie. **1–8**. Berlin 1836, Bern & St. Gallen 1837–1843.
47. ——. 1839. De Functionibus Nervorum Cerebralium et Nervi Sympathici. Bernae et Sangalli Helvetiorum, Huber et Soc.
48. ——. 1841. Ueber ein Entozoon im Blute von Salmo Fario. *Müller's Archiv.* **1841**: 435–436.
49. ——. 1841. Beiträge zur Anatomie des Zitteraales Gymnotus electricus. Neuchâtel.
50. ——. 1841. Hirn- und Nervenlehre. v. 4 of Th. von Sömmering's Vom Baue des Menschlichen Körpers. Leipzig, L. Voss.
51. ——. 1844. Trattato di nevrologia. Italian translation by M. G. Levi. Venezia, G. Antonelli.
52. ——. 1841. Grundriss der Physiologie des Menschen. Braunschweig, F. Vieweg u. Sohn.
53. ——. 1843. Traité de nevrologie. Traduit par J. L. Jourdan in *Encyclopedie Anatomique* v. 4. Paris.
54. ——. 1844. Lehrbuch der Physiologie des Menschen. 2 v. Braunschweig, F. Vieweg u. Sohn.
55. ——. 1845. Naturkunde van den Mensch. Transl. by T. G. Roosebloom Gouda.
56. ——. 1850. Zur Entwicklungsgeschichte der Fische. *Zsch. wissenschaftl. Zool.* **2**: 267–270.
57. ——. 1851. Ein Beitrag zur Entwicklungsgeschichte der Doppelmisgeburten. *Arch. f. Physiol. Heilkde.* **10**: 1–39. See also 1837 *Repertorium* **2**: 161.
58. ——. 1857. Die Kunstgerechte Entfernung der Eingeweide des Menschlichen Körpers (Exenteratio viscerum). Ein Leitfaden für wissenschaftliche Leichenöffnung. Frankfurt, a.M., Meidinger Sohn & Co.
59. ——. 1857. Die Einflüsse der Vaguslähmung auf die Lungen-und Hautausdünstung. Frankfurt, a.M., Meidinger & Sohn.
60. ——. 1866. Hydraulische Hilfslehre. Blut im Allgemeinen und Kreislauf desselben. Leipzig und Heidelberg, C. F. Winter.
61. ——. 1861. Die Untersuchung der Pflanzen-und Tiergewebe in polarisiertem Licht. Leipzig, W. Engelmann.
62. ——. 1863. Der Gebrauch des Spectroscopes zu physiologischen und ärztlichen Zwecken. Leipzig und Heidelberg, C. F. Winter.
63. ——. 1867. Die physikalische Untersuchung der Gewebe. Leipzig und Heidelberg, C. F. Winter.
64. Vogt, Carl. 1896. Aus meinem Leben. Stuttgart, E. Nägele.
65. 1835. Prix décernés. *C. R. Acad. Sci. Paris* **1**: 519–520.
66. 1836. *Froriep's Notizen* **50**: 209.
67. 1836. *Berliner Med. Central Ztg.* **20**: 237 and 544.
68. 1836. Correspondance. *C. R. Acad. Sci. Paris.* **2**: 83.
69. 1838. *Froriep's Notizen.* **110**: 341.
70. 1838. *Ber. über d. Vers. Deutscher Naturforscher und Aerzte in Prag.* 1837. Prag.
71. 1838. Note. *Berliner med. Zentralztg.* **17**: 147.
72. 1865. *Oesterr. Zsch. für prakt. Heilkunde.* **11**: 748.
73. 1883. *Berner Stadtblatt.* May 28.
74. 1883. *Intelligenzblatt für die Stadt Bern.* May 28.
75. 1883. *Breslauer Aerztliche Zeitschr.* p. 118.

II. DAVID GRUBY

1810–1898

INTRODUCTION

In the same year in which the physiologist Valentin was born in the city of Breslau, in German Silesia, a child was born in southern Hungary to a poor Jewish farmer by the name of Gruby. He was called David and was destined to have a very extraordinary life. Highly gifted intellectually, emotionally very sensitive, with a tender and kind hearted sympathy for all his suffering fellowmen, for suffering mankind at large, and for suffering animals too, he showed himself to have all the prerequisites for an outstanding physician and contributed much of importance to the development of modern medicine.

His early adolescence was marked by a hard struggle against innumerable obstacles, including physical starvation and the difficulties existing at that time in the way of a poor Jewish boy who wished to gain access to sources of knowledge. In later years, a successful though never adequately recognized scientist, Gruby finally was materially successful too, as a practicing physician. This fact gave him the opportunity to arrange his life independently of other people's benevolence or approval, according to his own intentions and inclinations. From its very beginning to the day of his death, Gruby's life was extremely interesting, extraordinary, and also somewhat extravagant and bohemian. As an anonymous eulogist put it in the *British Medical Journal* (page 1705, 1898): "Gruby was one of the most eccentric as well as one of the most successful physicians in Paris."

This may be the reason that many writers during Gruby's lifetime and later too, were attracted to the task of writing biographical sketches and even voluminous biographies about him. There is probably no other person in the medical world who has had so many biographers and yet is so utterly forgotten and unknown to the layman as well as to most members of the medical profession as is Gruby.

For a short biography, such as is intended here, there were various sources available from which the facts of Gruby's life were assembled. The first of his biographies, written when he was still a rather young man, was a short sketch that appeared in 1850 in the *Wiener Blaetter* (79).[1] This was a Jewish weekly, published in Vienna in 1850 and 1851, edited by Dr. M. Letteris. Another such biographical sketch appeared in Hungarian in *Orvosi Hetilap* in 1859 (80). These two were followed by a biography in *Beth El,* a periodical edited and written by Ignaz Reich, a Hebrew teacher in Pest (64). The first edition of this now rare book in three volumes was published in 1859. This author of Gruby's life story refers to the two previous biographical sketches and some personal information received from a student, who visited his famous compatriot in the year of revolution 1848 in Paris and made some notes in his diary about his personal impressions. Apparently these early sources and the very early German publications of Gruby were not known to his two outstanding biographers, namely, Blanchard and Le Leu. It is due to the physician Blanchard's brief but excellent biographies (5, 6) that, shortly after Gruby's death, his scientific achievements were for the first time thoroughly studied and justly evaluated.

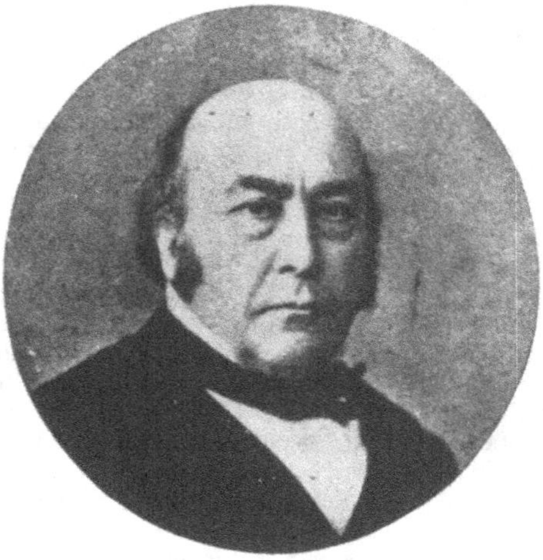

FIG. 19. Picture of Gruby from Le Leu's Book.

Gruby's other principal biographer was his secretary, Mr. L. Le Leu (57), who held this position from 1885 until the death of Gruby in 1898. While we owe to Blanchard important information on some documents from the archives of Vienna and Paris pertaining to the early days of Gruby's career, to Le Leu we are mainly indebted for the picture of the last years of a person very intimately known to him. He even published a short autobiographical report which Gruby dictated to his secretary.

Both these biographies were published after Gruby's death, but other minor publications concerning him appeared during his lifetime. Some newspaper articles were already mentioned in a letter written by Gruby's father to his son in 1841, reporting on the scientific achievements and excellent reputation of the latter (57).

[1] Numbers in parentheses indicate references at end of chapter, p. 224.

While Gruby was still alive, a twelve-page pamphlet written by Count Montemerli (61), was published in Paris in 1875 entitled, *Biographie du Docteur Gruby.* Another source of information on Gruby's personality is an article by Count Witzthum entitled "Le Sphinx," published in 1888 in *Les Lettres et les Arts,* also published in quarto as a de luxe edition and reprinted in Le Leu's book. Count Witzthum, an Austrian court counsellor who lived in Paris for a long time, conveys a very vivid picture of his friend Gruby, whom he introduces by the name of Prospero, (the powerful sorcerer, persecuted in his homeland, in Shakespeare's Tempest). Immediately after Gruby's death there appeared many obituaries in medical and other journals and, later, many authors were tempted to outline Gruby's biography, for example, Rille (66), Ebstein (13), and in recent times, Beson (3), Rosenthal (67), Zakon and Benedek (77), and A. P. M. Salaün who, in 1935 in Bordeaux, wrote a doctoral thesis on the life and achievements of David Gruby (68). A bibliography of most of Gruby's medical publications was collected by Blanchard (6), by Le Leu (57), and recently by Salaün (68). Last but not least this writer was fortunate enough to receive from the achives of the Vienna University Library photostats of very valuable documents concerning Gruby. These documents are as follows: (1) Päge 1119 of "Reversalien Protocoll der an der hiesigen Universität graduierten Doctoren" containing the names of the candidates for graduation as medical doctors, dates of their graduation and their own signatures (see fig. 23). (2) One page of the year 1836 of the "Matrikel," the list of all students of Vienna University. (3) One page of the list of all students of Professor Joseph Bernt, of the year 1836 containing detailed data about the students in their fifth academic year. (4) One page with the list of graduated "Doctores Medicinae" with detailed report on their examination, disputation, and graduation. The help of Direktionssecretär Dr. Hugo Alker in providing this material is highly appreciated.

Further information may be found in contemporary publications by people who met Gruby in Paris and were impressed by his personality. We find remarks about him in Alexander Dumas' *Notes et Souvenirs;* he is mentioned in Ludwig Bamberger's *Autobiography* as the physician of the poet Moritz Hartmann (1), and in various letters and publications of friends and contemporaries of the poet Heinrich Heine, whose physician Gruby was in Paris until the day of Heine's death. Many stories on the relationship of Heine and Gruby were carefully collected by Houben (50). All these sources and, above all, Gruby's original publications have been used for the present biography.

The early years of Gruby's life were effectively devoted to study and research in anatomy, histology, physiology, comparative zoology, parasitology, and experimental pathology. Toward the middle of his life he apparently did not cease these studies, but refrained from publishing in the proceedings of the scientific academies of Paris, where formerly he had reported most of his outstanding discoveries.

About forty years of Gruby's life were devoted to an extensive and highly lucrative practice which left him apparently not the time, needed for intense continuation of scientific research, that in the nineteenth century developed more and more to a full time occupation, absorbing all energy of those who became the leaders of modern theoretical medicine.

Gruby's vivid interest in the suffering patient, his excellent psychological approach, and therapeutic originality was thankfully enjoyed by many patients, and regarded by others and by many physicians as pure charlatanism. Gruby was not much impressed by the scorn and grudge of some of his colleagues. Their derogatory remarks as well as the enthusiasm of successfully treated patients contributed equally to make him soon one of the most famous physicians in Paris. At the same time he studied new fields of practical medicine, astronomy, and military medicine. Here Gruby proved to be a successful pioneer in a still much neglected field.

The end of his life was the tragedy of an isolated and invalid bachelor.

EDUCATION IN THE HUNGARIAN STEPPE

Gruby repeatedly mentioned to his secretary Le Leu that he was born August 20, 1810 in Kis-Kér in the comitate of Bascka in South Hungary. We have no reason to doubt this statement (57) in spite of the fact that various sources offer conflicting information on the year and place of his birth. For instance, Ignaz Reich in his biography mentions the year of Gruby's birth as 1809 (64). An examination entry of his graduation as doctor medicinae in the archives of the medical faculty of Vienna gives it as 1813, but one in the list of Vienna's medical students of 1836 mentions Gruby in this year as being twenty-five years of age. Von Wurzbach, in his *Biographical Lexicon,* reports 1814 as the birthdate and Grosswardein as his birthplace, and so do Hirsch and Pagel in their biographical dictionaries. Gruby's biography in the *Jewish Encyclopedia* mentions him as having been born on October 10, 1810 in Neusatz (Ujvidek). In all the documents concerning Gruby in the Archives of Vienna University his birthplace is mentioned as Kis-Kér.

David's father, Menachem Mendel Gruby, was a Hungarian Jewish farmer who owned a small farm and a large family of seven or eight children. That he must have been an intelligent man and a sincere, religious Jew can be gathered from one of his letters, dated 1841, published by Le Leu (57). The very fact that it was sealed with a neat personal seal bearing a Hebrew inscription speaks for a certain level of culture. Gruby's mother died at an early age and his father remarried. In the list of matriculated students of 1836 in the archives of the University of Vienna the profession of Gruby's father is given as merchant. That does not contradict his having been a small farmer too.

The first education the child received, except for that which he was given at home, was in a cheder, the Jewish school traditional to large and small Jewish communities in olden times. We do not know anything about special conditions in Kis-Kér, but as a rule the teaching of Jewish youth in little places, like that in Hungary in the early nineteenth century, was restricted mainly to Hebrew and religious subjects. From the point of view of modern pedagogics they were not very good, but the children did learn to write and to read Hebrew and to a great extent also to understand the Hebrew of the Bible and of the prayer book. When a child reached his thirteenth year, he was free to continue his studies, but in most cases at this age he had to begin to work for a living and very often also to help support his family. The possibilities for finding work were plentiful for a healthy boy in the home of a farmer. However, to the dissatisfaction of his father and stepmother, young David showed no inclination for the life and work of a farmer. He preferred to spend all his time in reading and studying. Nor did he wish to confine his reading to Hebrew books in the cheder.

It is difficult to understand how it happened that early in the nineteenth century in this remote little place in Hungary a Jewish child became eager to gain secular knowledge. Kis-Kér's non-Jewish population, as we know, did not have a very high intellectual standard and offered no intellectual inspiration to its young people. Gruby himself in later years shuddered to remember how in his youth, for example, it was still customary in Kis-Kér to punish minor offenses by breaking the teeth of the delinquent. This sentence was carried out by the farrier with the same instrument he used for his horses.

The later biographies of Gruby give no hint of how and who awoke in the child an interest in modern science, but we find a few pertinent remarks in J. Reich's biography, written in 1859 (64). Reich's report differs from the more or less romantic pictures given by later biographers. However, by giving the names of the personalities involved, who probably were still alive in 1859, it has a high degree of credibility, even though some of the dates, like the date of Gruby's birth or the date of his arrival in Paris, given as 1836, are wrong.

According to Reich, it was a student by the name of Jaegerndorf who furnished young Gruby with his first instruction in secular knowledge. Jaegerndorf himself was a young Jew studying at the University of Pest in Hungary. He needed to earn money for his graduation fees and therefore accepted a position as a substitute teacher in Kis-Kér and found hospitality in the home of the elder Gruby. As compensation for his board and lodging he supervised the Talmudic studies of little David, of whom he was very fond and to whom he liked to teach in the evening subjects that were extra-curricular in a Talmudic school in Hungary. This instruction lasted for two terms, by which time Jaegerndorf had accumulated enough money to pay for his examination and graduation fees and so returned to Pest. However, he remained in contact with the elder and younger Gruby. It was he, according to Reich, who tried to persuade Gruby's father to send his son to Pest, in order to start the young man on a career more suited to his talents than that of a small Hungarian farmer. Salaün asserts that Gruby was first sent as an apprentice to a watchmaker and optician in his hometown and that his interest in lenses and microscopical work may have originated there (68).

We do not know exactly when father Gruby finally agreed to part with his son who insisted on following Dr. Jaegerndorf's advice, but it was unquestionably not before David's thirteenth year. According to Reich, the young man remained until 1828 in Pest, where he was studying. He may have left his home in Kis-Kér in 1824 or 1825. Salaün (68) says that he left for Pest at the age of fifteen. A friend of the elder Gruby, Elchanan Schindler, a merchant in Pest, promised father Gruby to take care of his son (64), and so, finally, one morning David Gruby started out for a life in the world of science.

Whether all the stories in later biographies about the hardships the boy had to endure during his travels on foot from Kis-Kér to Pest are literally true cannot be ascertained. Even Le Leu, who may have heard this from Gruby himself, mentions that young Gruby received from his father only a 50-Kreutzer bill (approximately 25 cents) and a loaf of bread when he left for Pest. These two treasures were not great resources for a hungry boy to start a career with. The touching story of his trip was written in Hungarian about 1858 by Auguste de Gerando, nee Comtesse of Teleky, and published as an inspiration for Hungarian youth. Mrs. Gerando, a close friend of Gruby, had her information from Gruby immediately. She was a political refugee from Hungary, enjoying the help and encouragement of Gruby during her early stay in Paris (57). Whatever may have been the case—whether he, as most biographers including Mrs. de Gerando agree, travelled the long distance on foot, earning his money by working or, as Reich states, Mr. Schindler took him to Pest in his carriage, he finally arrived there, and started on his own.

HIGHER STUDIES IN PEST AND VIENNA

Pest (Pesth), the capital of Hungary, was not yet at that time combined with the nearby town of Ofen (Buda) into what is now known as Budapest. Here the young boy looked for a livelihood and found it, probably with Mr. Schindler's aid, as bookkeeper in a small kosher Jewish eating place on Waitzener Street (6). Reich (64) mentions that Mr. Schindler was the owner. Gruby worked there evenings, sometimes as a bookkeeper, sometimes as a waiter, while he devoted the hours of the day to his studies at school or sitting in a corner of the noisy, busy place concentrating on his books. In Pest the outstanding school for education in the humanities at that time was the Piarist Gymnasium (Piaristenschule), a Catholic institution, which had no room for a poor Jewish student. Since 1784 Pest had also been the seat of a university, but Gruby was not yet able to meet the requirements of such a school. We know that Gruby's compatriot, Ludwig Mandl, born in 1812, later professor at the University of Paris as a child of wealthy Jews from Pest attended this Piarist Gymnasium, but Gruby's biographers emphasize unanimously that he was not admitted to classes because he was a Jew (6). By a decree of Emperor Joseph II, Jews were entitled to attend the Latin Schools of Higher Learning (Gymnasiums). However, tuition had to be paid, and apparently little David could not afford such expense. He therefore tried to obtain at least some of the knowledge available to other pupils there and denied him as a poor Jew by standing at the door of the classroom listening attentively to what was taught inside.

There is no question that the child listening there at the door was reminded of the story of the famous legendary Rabbi Hillel, who became one of the most outstanding Talmudic authorities and whose life story was well known to every Jewish child. As a young man this rabbi was so poor that at one time he was not able to pay even the small nominal fee required to enter the house of Jewish learning. However, he was not willing to give up his studies even for one day, and so he tried to acquire his knowledge in a similar way to that which Gruby now used.

Little Gruby was finally discovered learning by eavesdropping by one of the professors, whose interest was aroused by such unusual perseverance and eagerness to learn. He approached the young Jewish boy, learned his personal and financial situation, his plans and his decision to obtain by any means the basic knowledge needed to enter a university. The teacher, who had never before met such a stubborn and determined will to learn, was deeply impressed and, though it was against the rules, admitted Gruby on his own responsibility to his classes.

It is not clear whether Gruby was rejected by the Piarist school for financial reasons alone or whether religious reasons, too, played a role. As mentioned, Mandl, two years younger, was admitted there and already in 1820 so was another Jewish boy, Josef Hauser from Altofen (Ofen-Buda, near Pesth), who later became a physician (64: **2**: 33 and 296).

Doctor Jaegerndorf, who was instrumental in Gruby's leaving Kis-Kér for Pest, helped at the beginning by giving young David private lessons and instruction to enable him to pass the first examinations (64) in school. That was the start of Gruby's regular studies. Soon he was making such good progress that he was recommended to supervise the studies of less gifted children of well-to-do parents and thus he was able to earn the money necessary for his room and board and all the other needs of a modest young student.

According to Reich, Gruby left Pest in 1828 for Vienna with the intention of studying medicine there. The list of matriculated students of Vienna University mentions Gruby in 1836 to be in the fifth year of his studies, and so does a catalog of students in 1836. Of course, the University of Pest also had a medical faculty, but its standard was so low that even ten years later Gruby's famous compatriot, Ignaz Philipp Semmelweis, could not endure its atmosphere as a student for more than one year, returning then to Vienna. Gruby's family did not live in Pest, as Semmelweis's did, so there was nothing to bind him to this city, where he acquired his first secular education in such a difficult and humiliating way. Having the prerequisite for entering a university, he hurried to the splendor of Vienna's school and life. Since Emperor Joseph II's famous Tolerance Act (1782), many prejudices and much bias had been abolished in Austria, and in Vienna Jewish students were admitted to the University.

Medical students in Vienna, at the time of Gruby's arrival in the Austrian capital, were obliged to attend classes and clinics for a period of five years. The professors had to examine their pupils every week, and, in order to go on to the next class, the student had to pass final examinations at the end of each term. At the end of the fifth year two case reports of patients treated by the candidate had to be submitted. Two examinations followed. A doctor thesis had to be presented and defended in public. These were the requirements for a medical doctor's degree (62). The degrees conferred by the University of Vienna were those of Doctor of Medicine and Doctor of Surgery but lesser degrees, such as Master of Surgery and even Patron of Surgery, were also awarded. Each physician and surgeon was eligible for the degree of Obstetrician, but only a graduate medical Doctor or Master of Surgery was permitted to work for the degree of Master of Ophthalmology.

In 1828 when Gruby came to Vienna, the height of the renowned first Viennese Medical School with which such teachers were connected as Van Swieten, Boer, de Haën, von Stoerck, and Johann P. Frank, had passed, but Vienna's clinics were still very famous and attracted students and physicians from all over Europe. However, in 1828 none of the great masters of medicine and founders of the second Viennese School were teaching yet. It was not until 1831 that the first of them, Joseph Berres, came from Lemberg to Vienna as Pro-

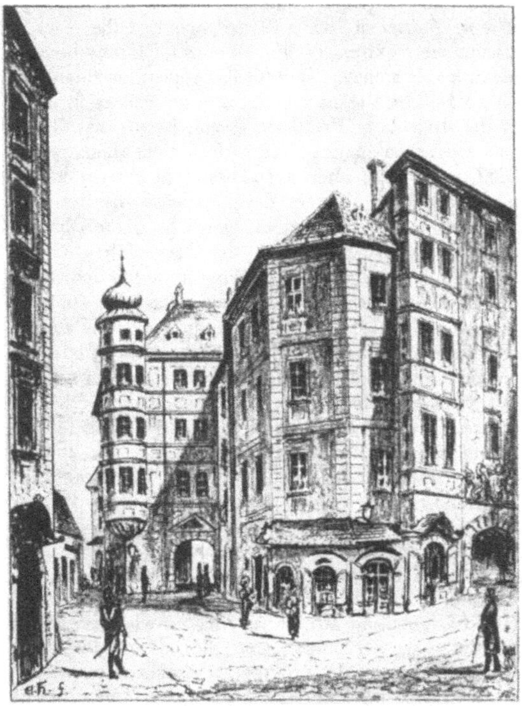

FIG. 20. Küssdenpfennig in Adlergasse in Vienna, the house with the little turret, of alleged Paracelsus fame. Gruby lived here as a student. From W. Kisch, *Die alten Strassen und Plätze Wiens,* Wien, M. Gottlieb, 1883.

fessor of Anatomy. He was a pupil of the anatomist Prochaska and became Professor of Anatomy at Lemberg at the age of twenty. He had already published an important textbook on anatomy in 1821–1827, the German edition of which appeared in Vienna in 1834. The first portion, of his textbook on the microscopical parts of the body, *Anatomie der mikroskopischen Gebilde des menschlichen Körpers,* was issued in 1837 (52). Rokitansky, the leader of the second Viennese school, who just graduated from Vienna in 1828, became assistant to Johannes Wagner, the pathological anatomist, in the year 1831. In 1833 he succeeded his teacher Wagner as Prosector (chief pathologist) at the General Hospital. He became Professor Extraordinarius in 1834, but full Professor only in 1844. This "Linnaeus of pathological anatomy" as he was called by Virchow, initiated the new era of pathological anatomy and microscopy. It was mainly Rokitansky, Berres, and the clinician Skoda who justified Wunderlich in writing in a book on medical Vienna (76) in 1841: "Today Vienna is the city in Germany most frequently visited by foreign physicians."

The savings which the eighteen-year-old Gruby had been able to accumulate in Pest were not large, and in Vienna he had to look around again for opportunities to earn a living by tutoring young students. That may have been one reason why he did not join Vienna's medical faculty until 1831. He lived in a sort of Latin Quarter in Vienna, on Eagle Street (*Adlergasse*) in the house "Zum Kuessdenpfennig," where many poor students of the University stayed. This house was the place where Paracelsus once was supposed to have lived when in Vienna. It is reported that Paracelsus, when urged by his landlord to pay his rent, gave the man a penny. When the landlord indignantly refused to accept this trifle, Paracelsus, the alchemist, transformed the penny into gold, and the delighted landlord kissed the miraculously transformed money. This story gave the house its name. There is, however, no historic proof that Paracelsus had anything to do with this

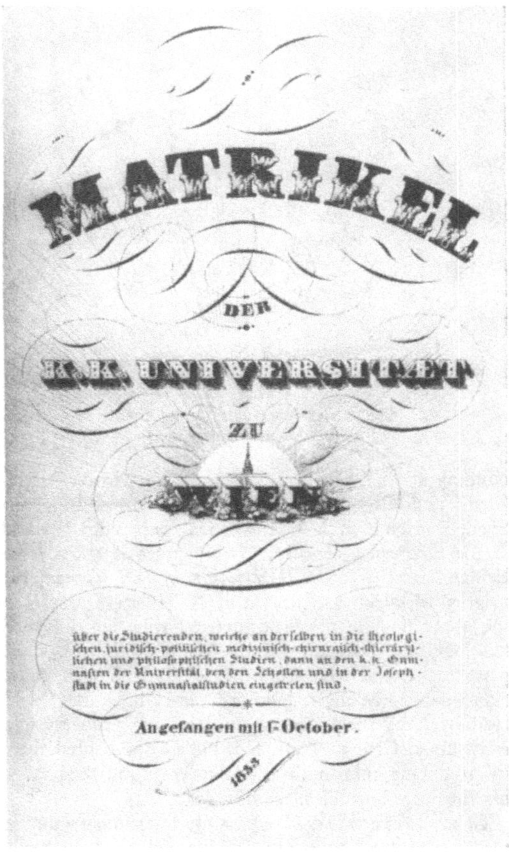

FIG. 21. Title page of the Matrikel of the University of Vienna with the detailed information about the students. Gruby is registered here in 1836 as being in his fifth year of academic studies.

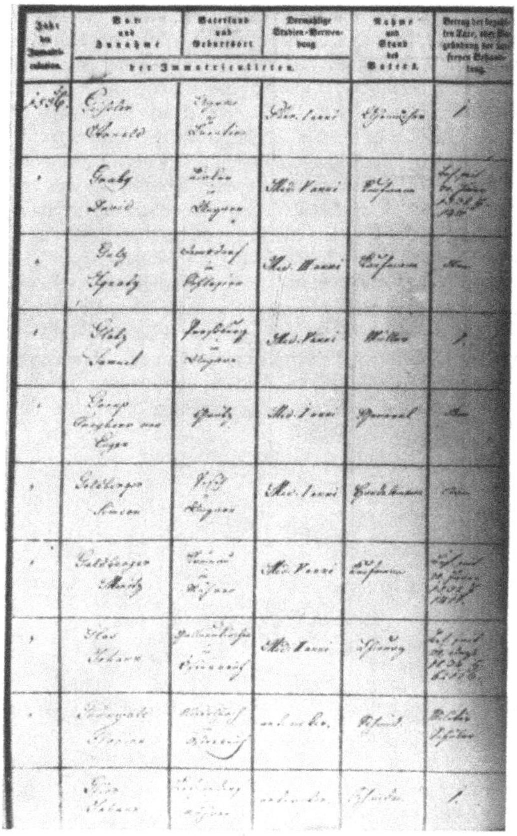

FIG. 22. The entries concerning Gruby in the Matrikel of the Vienna University.

building at all. The house with the little tower, where Gruby and allegedly also the famous chemist Berzelius lived, was built in 1741 and stood there until the end of the nineteenth century. Our picture is taken from William Kisch's (54) *Description of Old Vienna,* the original of which was drawn by A. Huetter. Here on the upper floor of the little turret, Gruby not only had his lodgings, but had turned the place into a small private chemical laboratory (79). It is reported that once, when Gruby's landlord had difficulties with creditors, the sheriffs came to seize the property and went up to Gruby's floor, too, but Gruby routed them by producing chlorine in his laboratory and thus saved his furniture and his place of work.

Gruby's time was devoted mainly to chemistry and to medical studies, especially in the fields of anatomy, microscopy, and as pupil of Rokintansy to pathological research. At least in the last years of his studies, he worked under the guidance of the anatomist, Berres, and under Rokitansky.

His first biographer, the anonymous writer in the *Wiener Blätter* of 1850 (79), reports that the years in Vienna were extremely difficult ones for Gruby because of lack of money. Indeed it is mentioned in the "Matrikel" of Vienna's University as well as in a list of the students of Professor Joseph Bernt, that Gruby was exempt of paying tuition fees since January 30, 1832, apparently after a successful first term in the medical faculty. To cut down expenses he lived for weeks at a time on potatoes, which he himself had to cook. This writer also tells the story of how Gruby saved himself the trouble of looking for a new apartment by the above mentioned chlorine trick. By applying himself assiduously to his studies he soon was able to teach chemistry and anatomy to the less gifted ones among his colleagues, and after his first years of studies, this tutoring helped to improve his financial circumstances. His special interest at that time, and for the rest of his life, was anatomy and pathology. In spite of Reich's statement that Gruby came to Vienna in 1828 (64) and the assertion of the biographer in the *Wiener Blätter* (79) that he had completed his five years of medical studies in 1834, the documents of the archive of Vienna's University prove that he finished the fifth year of studies only in 1836. His conduct is mentioned as good, his attitude as diligent, whereas each of the sixteen other students on the list got the mark "very diligent." His progress in studies is mentioned as "first rate" whereas eight of his sixteen colleagues on this list show "Eminenz" in progress. Gruby, therefore, was regarded as a very good but not as an unusually brilliant student. When finished with the official curriculum, he did not hurry to start his practice; instead he continued his academic work, and did not even apply for his doctor's degree until 1839, in spite of the fact that, though he was not yet a graduate doctor, his reputation already was attracting many patients. Whether it was financial difficulties or other obstacles that prevented him from obtaining his doctor's degree until 1839 cannot be determined; possibly he intended an academic and research career rather than that of a practitioner. Although he lacked funds and was a Jew and a Hungarian, both of which were handicaps at the University of Vienna at that time, and although he had to spend part of his time earning a living, Gruby's abilities and eagerness to work so impressed his teachers that he was made an assistant in surgery (Operations-Zoegling). The famous urologist and surgeon, Joseph Wattmann, appointed him assistant notwithstanding the fact that Jews were not eligible for such a position. We know also from his publication of 1840 that he did medical research under the direction of Berres and Rokitansky for several years, as a student and later.

The manner in which Wattmann's interest was drawn to the young Hungarian student is related by Gruby's first biographer in 1850 (79) as a story still remembered at that time among the physicians of Vienna General Hospital. When Gruby was in the last year of his medical studies, probably 1835 or 1836, he, along with other students, accompanied Wattmann's assistant on his rounds. When the latter presented to the students a patient with caries (corrosion) of the neck vertebrae, Gruby did not accept this diagnosis quietly, as students in Europe usually do in such a situation; he expressed the opinion that this diagnosis could not be correct because certain movements by the patient would not be possible, the muscles involved being attached precisely to the supposedly affected bones. The assistant Schuh, later Professor of Surgery in Vienna, was very indignant and reported the student for his disrespectful attitude toward the Chief. The following day, while on rounds, Wattmann called Gruby to the bedside of a patient and said to him: "Sir, as I hear, you know everything better than others; try here to make your diagnosis." Gruby, disregarding this subtle reprimand, examined the patient carefully and to everyone's astonishment presented a clear, logical, excellent diagnosis. Even Wattmann immediately changed his tone and was full of appreciation of Gruby's extraordinary anatomical knowledge and logical judgment. From that day on he became Gruby's friend and protector.

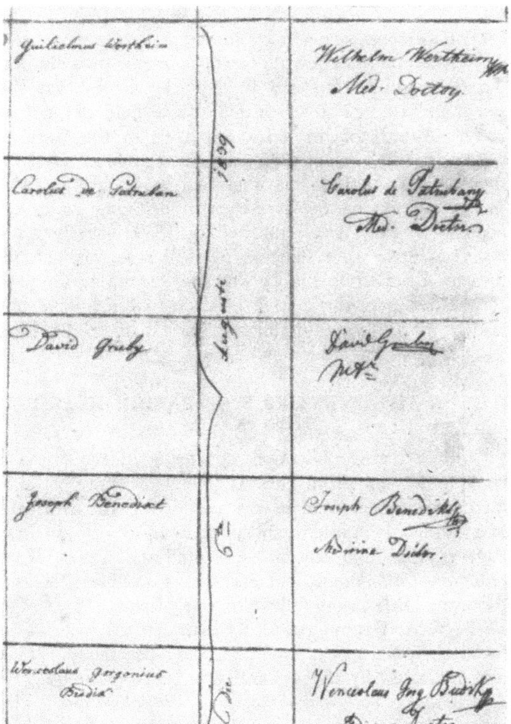

FIG. 23. One page of the "Reversalien-Protokoll," a register of those doctors of medicine and surgery who were graduated by the University of Vienna since 1818, with date of the graduation and the signature of the graduates. Notice how Gruby abbreviates or misspells his first name at such an important occasion.

In Austria at that time it was possible to be a practicing physician without having acquired the degree of doctor of medicine, but Gruby decided to take the official final step in his medical education by acquiring the degrees of doctor of medicine and master of ophthalmology. According to a list of the medical doctors graduating on August 6, 1839, still in the archives of the University of Vienna, Gruby passed his first medical examination on February 13, 1838 with excellent results (valde bene); the second examination followed on March 18, 1839, and he passed it with good results (bene). The day of his doctoral disputation was August 5, 1839; his medical diploma was dated August 6, 1839. The acting promoter was Professor Fischer. The entry in the register of the Vienna faculty concerning Gruby reads as follows (6): "Grubi [*sic*] David, n. Kis-Ker in Hung.an.1813, r.isrl, colleg. phil. Pesth. med.V. frequ: subiit examen prim. d. 13. Febr. 1838 valde bene. Idem secund. d. 18. mart. 1839. Bene. (Dipl. 6/8 1839)." [2] In the above mentioned list of graduating doctors of Vienna University his name is written Gruby.

It is possible that Gruby's name in Hungary was originally written Grubi; this is attested to by Bamberger, the German politician (1) who knew Gruby well in Paris. However, Bamberger's recollection, forty years later, that Gruby wrote his name Grouby is surely a mistake. As early as his Viennese publications and later in his French ones, on the medal struck in his honor in 1851 and in the title of his biography written by his own secretary Le Leu, his name is always written Gruby, and this is the way his name appears on his tombstone.

Gruby studied in Vienna's medical school for more than eight years. This was an unusually long time for the early nineteenth century, and there is no satisfactory explanation for this delay in the career of a diligent and brilliant student such as Gruby was. During this period he made his living by teaching, conducting courses for physicians, and by lecturing privately on anatomy and physiology. From the testimony of contemporary students we know that he, too, readily enjoyed the gay life of Vienna (57). According to the testimony of his friends, Gruby was one of the best waltzers in Vienna, and this may also have contributed to the delay in his graduation. A great part of his

[2] This writer was not able to check this document personally. In all the other documents known to him in the archives of Vienna University concerning Gruby the name is spelled Gruby.

time, however, was devoted to research and anatomical preparations. He became a very skilled anatomist, and many of his preparations were preserved in the anatomical museum in Vienna. In this activity he surely was influenced by the anatomist Hyrtl, master of injection technique and in Gruby's time assistant to Berres, Gruby's teacher. Even later in Paris Gruby continued with this type of scientific activity. Blanchard reports (46) that in Paris the Musée Anatomique de la Faculté de Medecine, called Musée Orfila, contained not less than 155 specimens prepared personally by Gruby. They were still in this collection in 1881 (6: 60).

One field of science that never lost its attraction for Gruby was microscopy. In the early thirties of the nineteenth century medical microscopy was still in its infancy. Ernst Abbe had not yet laid the scientific and mathematical foundation for microscope building, and the importance of this method for medical research was by no means yet generally agreed upon. Berres and Rokitansky in Vienna were among the first to realize the value of the microscope for medicine, and Gruby, full of enthusiasm joined these masters of anatomy in the employment of the new technique.

As a pupil of both, he was permitted to use an ex-

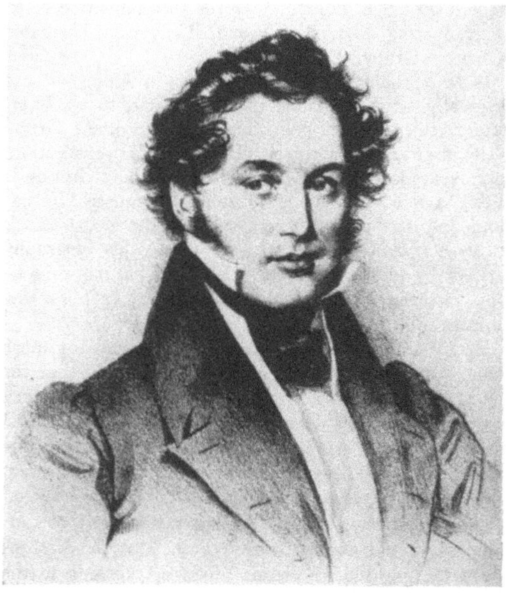

FIG. 24. Joseph Berres (1796–1844), Professor of Anatomy at the University of Vienna. He was Gruby's teacher in anatomy at the same time that the anatomist, Josef Hyrtl, was pupil and assistant of Berres. Hyrtl was famous for his improvement of the injection technique of vessels and, in this art, he was apparently Gruby's master. Courtesy of the Rare Book Department, Library of the Academy of Medicine, New York.

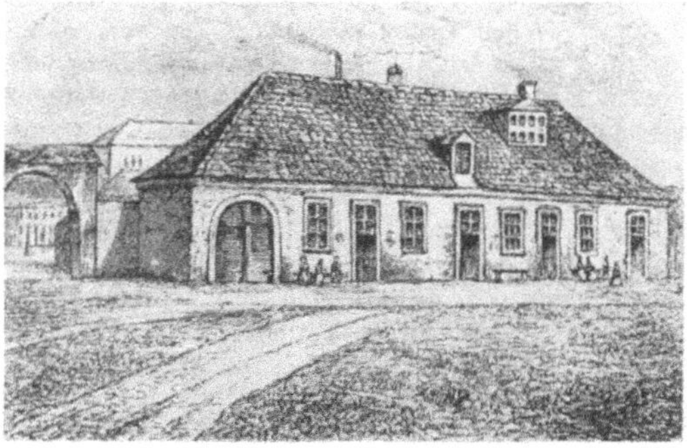

FIG. 25. The Morgue and "Pathological Institution" of the General Hospital in Vienna at the time when Rokitansky was working there and Gruby was his collaborating student. In these modest quarters modern pathological anatomy was created. From W. Kisch, *Die ältesten Strassen und Plätze von Wien's Vorstädten* **2**, Wien, Oscar Frank 1895.

cellent microscope made by the Ploessl Company, and he himself made simple microscopes for his own studies. The first publication that we have by Gruby was the result of years of investigation in the field of microscopy. A part of his work appeared in the German language (25), a greater part in Latin as Gruby's thesis (20). What was supposed to be his doctoral thesis, written on the influence of drinking water on health (6, 51), was published in 1839, shortly after his graduation; but that, as we will see, was not his thesis. Le Leu mentions that in Vienna Gruby received not only the degree of doctor of medicine but also of master of ophthalmology, and that he, Le Leu, had seen both the diplomas (57).

THE FIRST TEXTBOOK OF PATHOLOGICAL MICROSCOPY

Gruby's main publication, appearing in 1839, was a book interesting from various points of view. It was his doctoral thesis and it was intended as the first part of a handbook on microscopical pathology. On the first page of the 1840 edition is printed the words *Morphologia Pathologica,* but it bears a double title and two other title pages follow, as our picture shows (fig. 28). What Gruby apparently intended to write was a comprehensive work on microscopic pathology. This was indicated by the general title, *Observationes Microscopicae ad Morphologiam Pathologicam.* The other title of the book, apparently meant as a subtitle, is *Morphologia Fluidorum Pathologicorum,* "Tomi primi pars prima" (*Morphology of pathological fluids.* First part of the first volume). That was the first and the last installment of this exhaustive projected textbook. The title indicates that the work was planned to begin with a comparison between the microscopy of pathological fluids of the body and the normal findings. All observations were made in daylight with the Ploessl

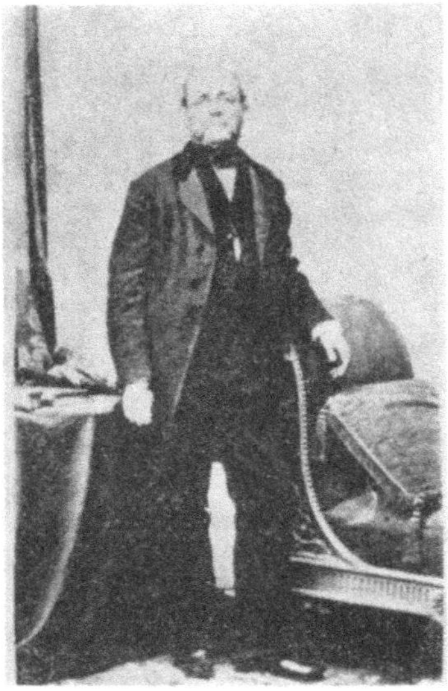

FIG. 26. Rokitansky. Courtesy of Rare Book Department, Library of the Academy of Medicine, New York.

microscope. The drawings in 40 × magnification were made by Gruby himself. On pages 12 and 13 Gruby gives an outline of the entire work. The first part was to contain the microscopic pathology of the body fluids: (1) mucus, (2) pus, (3) pseudomembranes, including coagulations (lympha plastica), (4) urine, under abnormal conditions, (5) milk, (6) tears, and (7) saliva. Of this plan only a part was executed, for the urine, milk, and tears were omitted from the book. In the second part Gruby intended to present the pathological morphology of vessels, nerves, cellular structures, membranes, muscle, fascias and ligaments, glands, and what he calls "telea corneae." The first installment appeared in 1839, that is, three years before Rokitansky's famous *Handbook of Pathological Anatomy*. Gruby's outline is that of a textbook on microscopical pathology, and the question arises, why he stopped after the publication of the first part of the first volume (20).

Gruby dedicated his doctoral thesis, his first publication in bookform, to his two outstanding teachers, Joseph Berres and Carl Rokitansky; in his dedication he calls Berres "fautori et literarum Maecenati." This appellation of patron and Maecenas gave Le Leu the idea that Berres may even have supported this publication financially. Perhaps he paid Gruby only during his years as student a salary for being his private assistant, for Gruby mentions in his autobiographical sketch (p. 209) his collaboration in the anatomical work of Berres. However his relationship to Berres must have been one of mutual sympathy. In a footnote of Gruby's paper on the venous system of the frog, published in 1842 in Paris (29: 212), he mentions Berres as his excellent teacher and friend. The dedication to Rokitansky is followed by the remark, "tam ingenii perspicuitate quam morum suavitate laudatissimo," which means that the book is dedicated to a man, outstanding not only for his excellent talents, but also for his extremely kind behavior toward others. From such dedications it can only be concluded that both leaders in anatomy in Vienna were well disposed toward the author as well as his work. This being the case, what was the reason for Gruby's stopping so suddenly and leaving Vienna just when the book was coming off the press? Looking through Rokitansky's famous *Handbuch,* which was published between 1842 and 1846, there is no question that the arrangement of the material shows many similarities to Gruby's plan, indicating Rokitansky's influence on Gruby. On the other hand, Gruby's work was probably intended as the

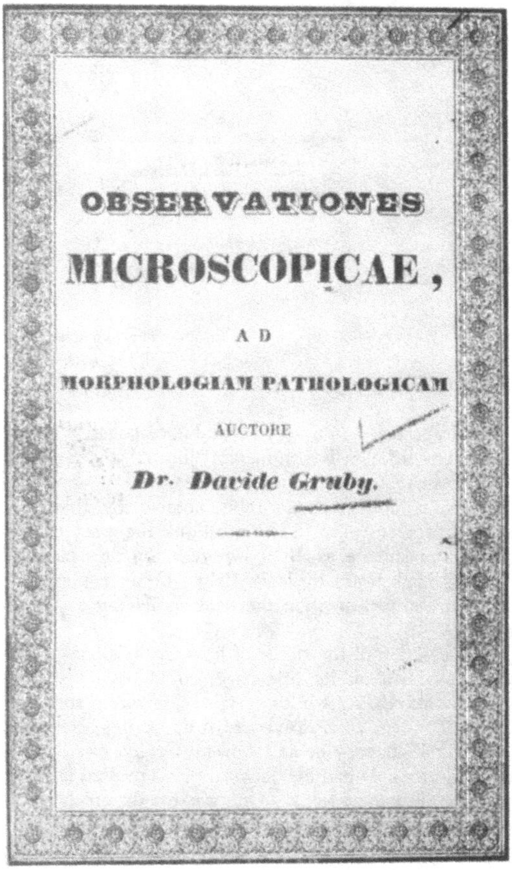

FIG. 27. Outside (brown) cover of Gruby's book on pathological microscopy.

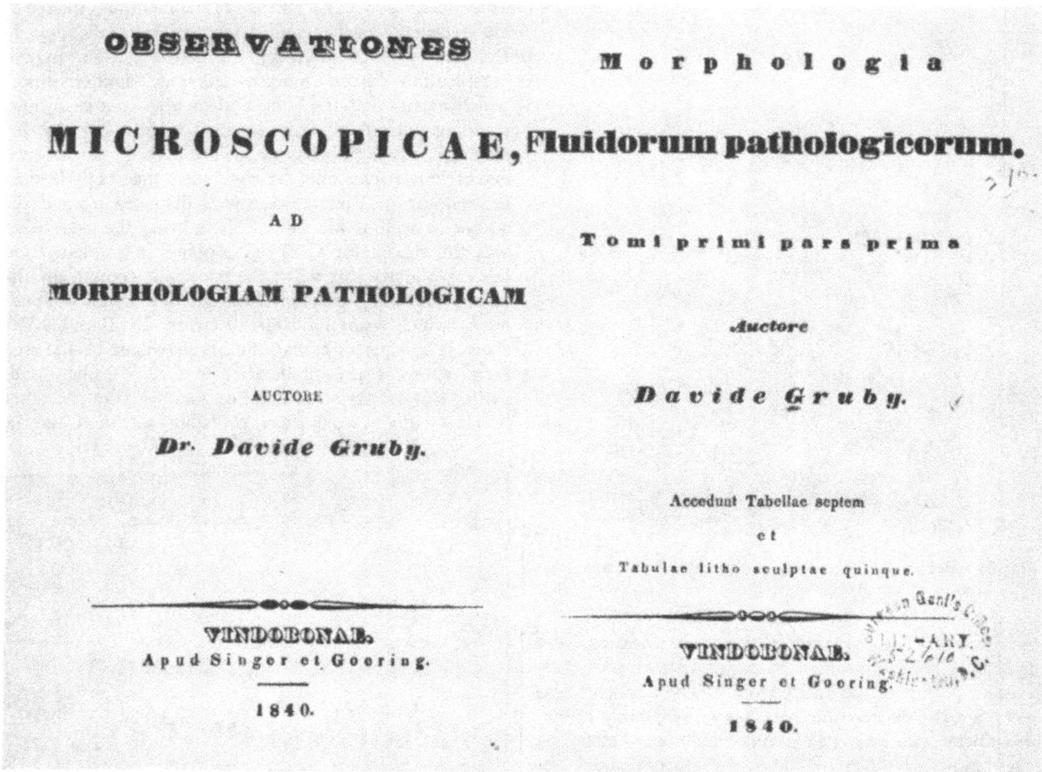

OBSERVATIONES
MICROSCOPICAE,
AD
MORPHOLOGIAM PATHOLOGICAM
AUCTORE
Dr. Davide Gruby.
VINDOBONAE.
Apud Singer et Goering.
1840.

Morphologia
Fluidorum pathologicorum.
Tomi primi pars prima
Auctore
Davide Gruby.
Accedunt Tabellae septem
et
Tabulae litho sculptae quinque.
VINDOBONAE.
Apud Singer et Goering.
1840.

FIG. 28. The two inner title pages of Gruby's book of 1840.

pathological counterpart to Berres's microscopical anatomy.

Gruby's book had a very favorable response. In the same year, 1839, a Berlin medical journal, the *Berliner Medizinische Centralzeitung,* carried a very appreciative two-column report. It is noteworthy that this review of October 5, 1839 mentions the year of the book's appearance as 1839, whereas the title page of Gruby's book bears the date 1840. Other contemporary sources also mention the book as having appeared in 1839 (48).

The solution of the riddle of how Gruby's book, with the year 1840 on its title page, could have been reviewed in 1839, while certain journals, such as *Schmidt's Year Book,* reviewed it as having been published in 1840, may be as follows. Gruby, like Robert Remak, probably had his doctoral thesis printed in 1839 and 1840 in two editions. One was for the official purpose of his degree, in accordance with the rules and requirements, with the title page in the prescribed form, of which no copy seems to be extant; the other had a different title page, like that of our illustration. This idea finds support in a remark in the review of Gruby's *Observationes* in *Schmidt's Jahrbücher.*[8] There the reviewer expresses the opinion that the book probably is a doctoral thesis, for at its conclusion was added the usual group of short statements (theses), which had to be defended publicly at the doctor's disputation and which would have no meaning at the end of a regular publication. He is surprised that the title page bears no statement that it is a doctoral thesis.

Le Leu (57) as well as Blanchard (6) asserted that Gruby's doctoral thesis was a since lost paper on medical effects of water. That Gruby's thesis was indeed his book of 1839 is proven beyond doubt by the entry in the list of "Doctores Medicinae" in the Archives of Vienna's University, where the "Thema disputatum" is mentioned as: "Observationes microscopicas" (*sic*). In the official *Taschenbuch der Wiener K. K. Universität für das jahr 1840,* edited by the office of the University beadles (78) we find a list of the past year's graduates where on page 156 it reads: "Herr David Gruby. Diss. sistens: *Observationes microscopicas ad morphologiam pathologicam.*" His supposedly lost

[8] 30: 100, 1841.

treatise on the medical effect of water is by no means lost, and was not only an unprinted manuscript as Blanchard thought (6). It was published in 1839 but not as Gruby's doctoral thesis. We will refer to it later (see p. 207). In the copy of this rare book of 1839 in the Library of the Surgeon General's Office in Washington, D. C. (see fig. 27) unfortunately no theses are included. It consists of a sixty-four page text (1–64), twenty-one pages devoted to explanations of 5 plates (pages 1–21), two pages of index, only four of these plates of lithographed figures, and seven large tables in the text summarizing Gruby's results. According to the *Archives* of the Vienna Faculty, Gruby was given his doctor's diploma on August 6, 1839, so his thesis, publicly defended on August 5, must have been approved in 1839, which is consistent with its having been reviewed in a Berlin medical journal in the same year. It was then republished in 1840 with a different title page as a new publication.

The contents of this book, though it does not strike us today as a fundamental revelation, were highly regarded in medical circles in Vienna and abroad as well. Canstatt, a very critical reviewer who wrote a lengthy report of five columns on it in *Schmidt's Year Book*,[4] was, in spite of his objections to a few weak spots, very much impressed by the work. He emphasized that such a doctoral thesis was by far outstanding among publications of this sort, and in this he was quite correct. Canstatt also mentions the contents of Gruby's doctoral thesis in his well known textbook *Die Spezielle Pathologie und Therapie*.[4a] There, in the first volume, he emphasizes how the different discrasias (the abnormal mixture of the body fluids which is supposed to be the basis of the different diseases) reflect in the pathological secretions of the body. After having mentioned the studies of Vogel, Henle, and Mandl on pus he quotes on page 84 especially the doctoral thesis of David Gruby, commending it highly as the first attempt to differentiate scientifically by means of the microscope the different kinds of pus in different diseases.

The level of work accepted at that time in Vienna for a doctoral thesis may be illustrated by one in the collection of this writer, which was approved and printed in Vienna a half-year before Gruby's thesis, at the end of 1838. The author was a Bohemian physician by the name of Josephus Seidlitz. This eighteen-page paper bears the title, "Concerning the main physical and psychological differences between men and women." That such a brief work can be no more than several short excerpts from a few textbooks is obvious. It is, therefore, not surprising that Canstatt was astonished to find a book of careful original investigation in a new field of medicine among those valueless manuscripts, so valueless in fact that some time later the farce of printing doctoral theses was abolished in Austria.

[4] *Ibid.*

[4a] Erlangen, F. Enke, 1841.

Canstatt concluded his review with the following words: "We finally leave the author with high respect, and we expect soon from his diligence, which is demonstrated in this book, further enrichment of our knowledge in pathological microscopy."

It is no wonder that if, in Germany, in these years of critical objective and scientific reform of medicine, Gruby's book was so much appreciated, it was still more highly valued in Vienna. As recognition the University of Vienna offered Gruby a professorship, but only on the condition that he embrace the Catholic faith (64, 57). We know that many an outstanding Jewish merchant and factory owner in Vienna at that time received baptism in order to escape the humiliating conditions of life a Jew had to endure there. But Gruby's logical mind did not understand what conversion to Catholicism had to do with the teaching of anatomy and microscopy. His pride and his character forbade him to use conversion as a tool to create a career, and so he refused the offer, remaining faithful to the Jewish religion. Probably this experience was so disappointing and revolting to Gruby that he decided to leave the work he had begun and the country where he saw no opportunity of continuing his beloved research successfully except by being baptized (57).

No doubt his book of 1839 (1840) contained many good observations, but for the modern physician it is disappointing as far as its practical results or the advancement of medicine are concerned. We do not agree with the very critical point of view of Blanchard that its contents are, so to speak, valueless. We should never forget that it was pioneer work in microscopical pathology, especially with respect to the fluids of the body. The 103 illustrations drawn by Gruby and contained in five plates show very distinctly the various media investigated, the easily recognizable cells in the fluids, their form, their size, nuclei, and so forth. Even though it must be agreed that this book presents no fundamental revelations to medicine, the following facts concerning the contents are proof of the outstanding talent of its author.

Gruby found and emphasized that none of the body fluids were simple liquids, but each of them contained what we would term today leucocytes and epithelial cells, though he called the leucocytes globuli (he also spoke of the red blood cells in the historic way as globuli sanguinis). In seven tables he compares the amount of these globules in different body fluids. For instance, he shows how, after an infection takes place, the microscopical appearance of the blenoroic secretion of the urethra changes from day to day. He observed (p. 29, table 5, figs. 87, 88, 96) that the sputum of tubercular patients may contain fragments of lung tissue. Of course Valentin thought that the striated muscle fibers found there too must have been of extraneous origin (72). Gruby contends that the cells in pus are formed originally in the parenchym of the sick organ. Gruby also states—correctly—that organs like the kidney and the liver become abnormally yellowish and fragile and an abscess forms when the tissue finally decays (fibrilae laceratae). He asserts that parts of blood corpuscles (moleculi minimi) may leave dilated capillaries with a stream of fluid, form cells in pathological secretions, and re-enter the bloodstream (p. 55 ff.) as cells and their disintegration products. These important though still vague statements about the penetration of particles and cells through the wall of capillaries first attracted general attention in 1877, when Cohnheim established that whole blood cells can penetrate the walls of capillaries. Gruby, likewise mentions the possibility of the creation of new capillaries, and he makes sound observations on the reabsorption of pus and metastatic suppurative abscesses. Under the microscope he saw how distilled water makes the white blood cells (globuli) swell and finally burst. In modern terminology he observed the effect of hypotonic solutions on cells. He watched the movement of granulated substances within the cells (the protoplasmic current) and also outside the cells and confirmed that nuclei treated with acetic acid became more easily visible. He made many excellent observations (p. 39 ff.) on blood coagulation and the crusta inflammatoria (phlogistica). He also saw that in typhoid fever not only is the spleen enlarged but a swelling of the regional lymph glands is visible if ulcers of the intestines are present.

Gruby sent out complimentary copies of his doctoral thesis not merely for the purpose of acquainting the medical world with its contents and making himself known among the leading physicians of his time, but because he really was anxious for criticism and to learn how outstanding medical men judged his work. A letter is extant which, after he moved to Paris, he sent with a copy of his book to Valentin, leading physiologist and anatomist in Bern, famous for his own microscopical work, asking him for his opinion. From this letter, which asked for Valentin's opinion of the book, we learn that the latter had previously received an injected zoological preparation from Gruby (a tapeworm). This letter reads in translation:

Hochwohlgeborener Herr Professor:

Before my departure from Vienna I had the honor to send you a Taenia soleum cera injecta. I have not yet any message whether this preparation was turned over to you in good condition.

The high esteem I cherish for Euer Hochwohlgeboren (your excellency) is the reason why I am sending you through Herr Dr. Lohner from Graz the first part of my morphologia pathologica for your judgment. Your veracity and your generally known keen interest in microscopical investigations gives me hope that you soon will confirm the difference I have found between pus and mucus and the presence of little living objects (animalcula conoidea) in the pus of small pox. Should these investigations not displease your excellency, I would be glad to have the pleasure of having pleased in some way the desire of a scholar whom I esteem and admire for various reasons.

I hope to be honored by an answer from your excellency and am with high esteem,

Dr. David Gruby

Paris. 13th of August 1840
My addresse: Rue Git-le-Cœur No. 5

This letter sounds, indeed, as though Gruby, when he came to Paris, intended to continue his work. The final remark that he esteems and admires Valentin for various reasons, probably is an allusion to Valentin's steadfast rejection of every offer of a chair at a university for which baptism was a prerequisite. Valentin's stand in this matter was well known to European Jewry, and Gruby, being in the same position in Vienna, had the highest appreciation for Valentin's exemplary behavior.

It is not clear whether the injected tapeworm mentioned in this letter was only a gift sent to an admired leader in medicine or whether Gruby made part of his living by selling anatomical preparations to other institutions. We know that Hyrtl, from whom he probably learned this technique in Vienna, sold many of his famous injected preparations to the most varied laboratories of the old and new world. This time-consuming activity may possibly explain why it took Gruby such a long time to finish his medical studies.

Valentin, like everyone, was indeed very much interested in this publication of Gruby's; announcing it in his *Repertorium,* he emphasized the assiduity and diligence expended by the author and wrote a report of no less than four pages (72). He very kindly pointed out all the valuable contributions of the book, but he also called attention to two main shortcomings: (1) Gruby did not compare all his findings with the pertinent findings of other authors. (2) Gruby did not adequately take into consideration Schwann's new cell theory. Indeed, no comparison is made even with Henle's pamphlet on mucus and pus (Berlin, 1838) (47).

Gruby may have felt the justification of this criticism, and this, too, may have contributed to his not continuing with the plan of the entire work. It may not be incorrect to put the criticism of Gruby's doctoral thesis in this way: The book is the product of extremely diligent work of a young student who unfortunately did not have for his guidance a teacher imbued with new ideas in modern medicine. Exactness and reliability he learned well from his teachers, but the revolutionary free spirit that created a new medicine had as yet no echo in Austria. Gruby soon did much better in his new environment.

Part of the content of Gruby's book, written in Latin, was published in the German language in the first volume of the *Proceedings* of the Viennese K. K. Gesellschaft der Aerzte zu Wien, where he presented it as a paper at the meeting of January, 1840. This Society of Physicians at Vienna was founded and chartered by

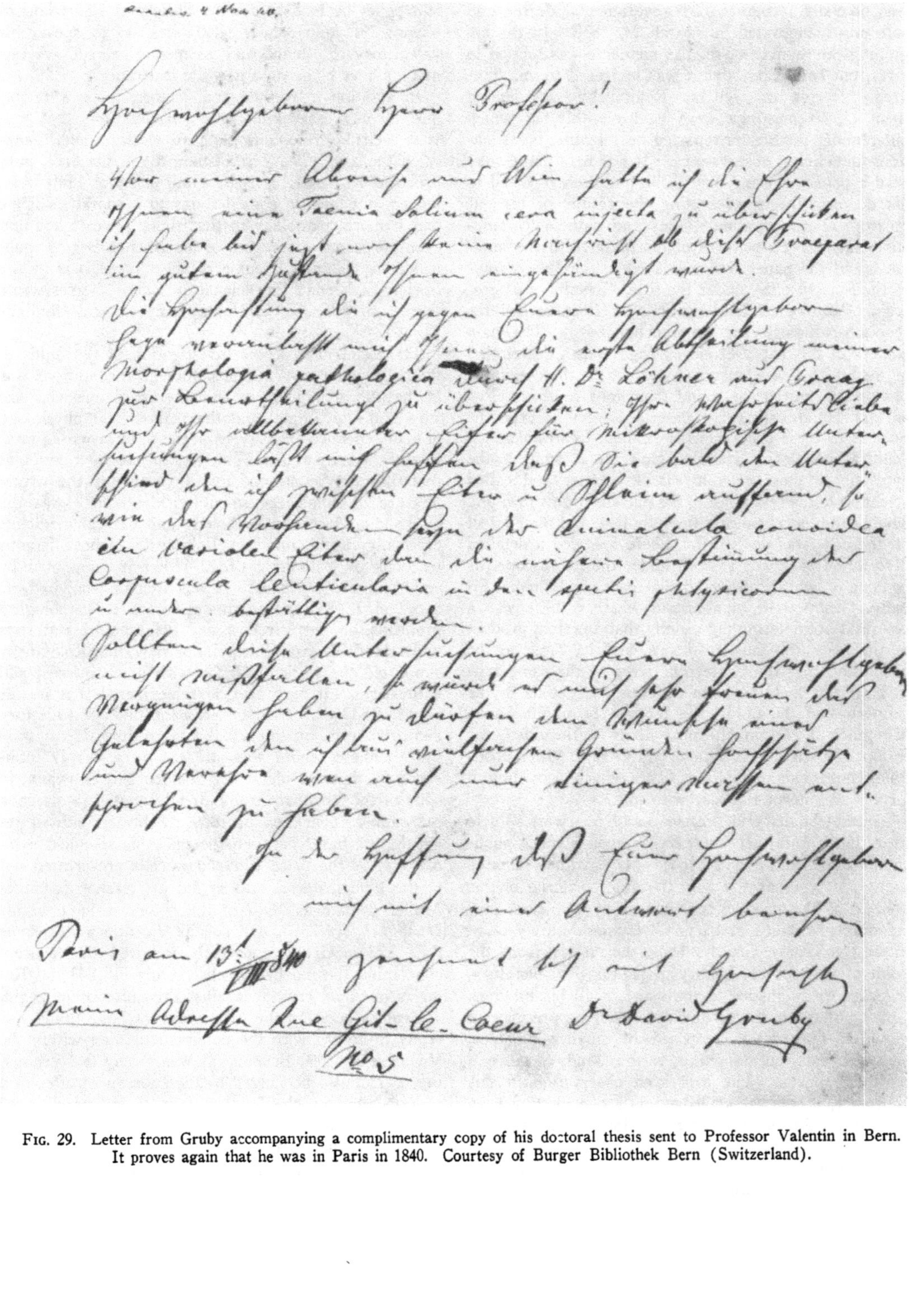

[illegible] 4 Nov 40.

Hochwohlgeborner Herr Professor!

Vor meiner Abreise aus Wien hatte ich die Ehre Ihnen eine Taenia Solium cera injecta zu überschicken ich habe bis jetzt noch keine Nachricht ob dieses Praeparat im gutem Zustande Ihnen eingehändigt wurde.

Die Hochachtung die ich gegen Euer Hochwohlgeboren hege veranlasst mich Ihnen die erste Abtheilung meiner Morphologia pathologica durch H. Dr. Löhner aus Praag zur Beurtheilung zu überschicken. Ihre Wahrheitsliebe und Ihr allbekannter Eifer für mikroskopische Untersuchungen lässt mich hoffen dass Sie bald den Unterschied den ich zwischen Eiter u. Schleim äussere, so wie das [illegible] der Animalcula conoidea im Variolen Eiter und die nähere Bestimmung der Corpuscula lenticularia in den sputis phtysicorum u. andere bestättigen werden.

Sollten diese Untersuchungen Euer Hochwohlgeboren nicht missfallen, so würde es mich sehr freuen das Vergnügen haben zu dürfen den Wünschen eines Gelehrten den ich aus vielfachen Gründen hochschätze und verehre wenn auch nur einiger Massen entsprochen zu haben.

In der Hoffnung dass Euer Hochwohlgeboren mich mit einer Antwort beehren

Paris am 13. VIII 840 zeichnet sich mit Hochachtung

Meine Adresse Rue Git-le-Coeur No 5 Dr David Gruby

FIG. 29. Letter from Gruby accompanying a complimentary copy of his doctoral thesis sent to Professor Valentin in Bern. It proves again that he was in Paris in 1840. Courtesy of Burger Bibliothek Bern (Switzerland).

the Emperor Ferdinand on November 17, 1837. It was officially recognized by governmental decree and solemnly inaugurated on March 24, 1838. In the beginning the number of regular members was limited to forty, but two years later it was increased to one hundred. Berres as well as Rokitansky was among them. Two meetings were held monthly, at which outstanding physicians reported on scientific investigations and clinical observations. It was here that Gruby read a paper covering part of his research reported in his doctoral thesis, presenting the results of his microscopical investigation of pus and pathological mucus. He showed pictures of his findings to the audience, and the paper was published in the *Proceedings* of the Society (25) under the title, "Results of Microscopic Pathological Investigations" ("Resultate mikroscopisch-pathologischer Untersuchungen"). The main content of this paper of eleven pages was a description of the white cells (leucocytes) which he discovered in pus and in mucus; he found them four times as large as red blood cells. He described very clearly the nucleus of these cells, which he called, *Centralbläschen* (central bubbles). He also gave an account of the cytolysis of these cells in distilled water and called attention to the resistance of the nucleus to this medium. Many different chemicals were applied, and their effect on the cells was described. There followed a detailed description of mucus as seen under the microscope, its content of white cells, epithelial cells, and fluid. Finally, Gruby tried to ascertain whether there was a possibility of determining exactly that a certain product of the body was pus or mucus, and he came to the conclusion that the white cells were of the same type in both and that the main difference might lie in the properties of the fluid. He thought he might find a difference if certain chemical fluids were added, for instance, hydrochloric acid or nitric acid. In mucous fluids these acids precipitated fibres, which, according to Gruby, was never the case with pus.

The objectivity and preciseness of this work which, in its biochemical aspects, exceeds even Henle's publication on pus and mucus (1838) (47) can be evaluated best if one compares it with the other material in this volume of the proceedings written by the most outstanding physicians in Vienna. It would surely be of interest to study Gruby's book thoroughly from the point of view of the history of pathological histology, in order to do justice to the value of all his findings. Among other things, Gruby described the presence of globules, apparently composed of smaller globules, similar to fatty substances, in various kinds of pus and puriform mucus. The first such observation in this substance, it was acknowledged as a contribution even in the critical *General Anatomy* of Jacob Henle in 1841 (p. 161).

However, Gruby's plan to continue the studies collected in his publications and to write a handbook on pathological morphology was interrupted. The excellent paper he read before the Society of Physicians of Vienna on January 31, 1840, was, so to speak, his valedictory to Vienna and its medical world. A few months later he began a new life in France.

In addition to the personal factors, there were unquestionably other important considerations that prevented Gruby from continuing his work on microscopical pathology. The first installment of his book published in 1839 and his lecture and paper of 1840 were, indeed, outstanding contributions to humoral medicine and humoral pathology of that time. It matched and even surpassed the report of his teacher Berres, published in the same volume of the *Proceedings* of the Society of Vienna Physicians (p. 195). Berres wrote there on contagia and his microscopical findings (1838).

The exact microscopic investigation of the fluids of the body under normal and pathological conditions was of the utmost importance and interest to one who was sure that the normal and the pathological physiology of man depended exclusively on the right or wrong mixture of the body fluids. This was the common notion at that time in Vienna, and the importance of the wrong mixture of fluids, the so-called "dyscrasia," was the outstanding factor in pathology and clinical medicine, especially in the mind of Rokitansky, whose famous textbook on pathology (1842–1846) is dominated by emphasis on dyscrasias. It was Remak who, in Germany in 1845, opposed this approach to pathological problems, as did Virchow and his school. But it is understandable, from this point of view, that Rokitansky supported the work of Gruby with much interest and enthusiasm. It may also be remembered that it was only in 1839 that Theodor Schwann published his fundamental work on the cell theory of animals; in 1839 the Viennese school was still not very deeply influenced by the new ideas of Schleiden and Schwann, in spite of the fact that Gruby already quoted in his book Schwann's publication of 1839. Schwann himself regarded the fluids between the cells, his so-called *cytoblastem,* as the place where new cells are created out of the fluid material, and so did his teacher Johannes Müller as late as 1840 in the second volume of his *Handbuch* (p. 759), and so did Valentin at the same time (73). Gruby apparently followed this concept concerning the red blood cells. Only in 1841 did Remak's one-man crusade against this misconcept begin.

Gruby's book on the microscopy of body fluids was really in accord with the dominant opinion within the Viennese Medical School. It was timely and promising, as can also be judged by the subsequent offer of a professorship on the medical faculty, but conditioned on Gruby's conversion.

If Gruby had planned to practice medicine in the Austrian capital, the chances for a gifted young doctor were not too bad there. In 1839 the *Kaiserstadt* had

350,000 inhabitants, not including the garrison. There were 341 civilian physicians and 158 civilian surgeons (48). With only one physician for each 1,100 persons, an already famous young doctor could surely assume the risk of establishing a practice. But Gruby's goal was very different, and his first and greatest desire was to continue his research work. To be able to do so he left Vienna.

Before he decided where to settle, he visited several German universities and English centers of research. In England he had a very prominent friend in the physician William Bowman, famous for his fundamental discoveries about the structure of the kidney (Bowman's Capsule) and the muscle. This friendship and Gruby's experimental approach to histological problems during his years in Vienna are attested to by a remark by Bowman which I found on page 509 in Volume 3 of Todd's *Cyclopedia of Anatomy and Physiology*. There Bowman writes (1847): "My friend Dr. Gruby in Vienna informed me that according to experiments with spiral rods of glass he conceives the fibrillae [of striated muscle] to be consequently spiral threads."

Bowman met Gruby in Vienna in 1838, while visiting the outstanding places of medical research and the most prominent clinics on the continent. The famous Sir Francis Galton, later on explorer, anthropologist, and meteorologist, was with him on this trip. At that time he was a young man of sixteen who, on his father's suggestion, accompanied Doctor Bowman for the purpose of getting in contact with the medical institutions of Europe. In this way he was to find out whether he really would like to become a physician and to follow in this profession his grandfather, Erasmus Darwin. Bowman was very much impressed by Gruby's work and personality. Years later in his article "Mucous Membranes" in *Todd's Encyclopedia* he mentioned with approval Gruby's doctoral thesis and his statement there that the mucous membranes do not produce viscous mucus under normal conditions. When at the end of this article Bowman enumerates the most outstanding scholars in modern microscopy in Germany, he mentions Gruby's name with those of Purkinje, Valentin, Henle, Schwann, Ehrenberg, R. Wagner, and other famous fathers of this new field of scientific medicine.

Gruby, therefore, had reason to see his friends in England and discuss with them his plans and personal problems. During his travel in Germany he, of course, became better acquainted with the still young Northern revolution, which, in opposition to the teaching of dyscrasia, emphasized Schwann's cellular concept of anatomy and physiology and admired Johannes Müller's organic and matter-of-fact approach to all problems of physiology and pathology. A bright mind like Gruby's must have been deeply impressed by these new revelations and that may have been a valid reason why, when he left Vienna disappointed, he also left Vienna's obsolete points of view in medicine. Kind hearted person that he was all his life, he may have hesitated to continue a work that, carried on in a new spirit, might have put him in opposition to his beloved teacher Rokitansky. But, when he arrived at the scene of his new activities in Paris, he went on in a new spirit with many of the investigations that had been started in this early period in Vienna. His textbook on microscopical pathology, however, remained a torso.

SUGGESTIONS IN HYDROTHERAPY

The microscopical and anatomical studies that Gruby reported in his doctoral thesis and in the first volume of the publications of the Society of Physicians in Vienna were not the only subjects that had attracted the interest of the young student. Besides microscopy, it was chiefly chemistry to which he devoted his efforts. Another subject to which Gruby was drawn from the chemical as well as the medical point of view was one of the highest importance for Vienna then and for many years to come. It was the problem of the water supply and the provision of safe drinking water for the population of Vienna (21) not solved until more than thirty years later by Eduard Suess' aqueduct. It was the time when an apparatus for filtering the water of rivers had been built and publicized by Doctor Grimaud de Caux, and in 1839 Gruby published an article on the dietetic and pharmaceutic use of spring water, well water, and purified Danube water in the twentieth volume of the Austrian *Medical Year Books,* an outstanding medical journal in Austria. Later, when Gruby came to live in Paris, he met again and worked together with Grimaud de Caux on the anatomy of *Murex brandaris,* the purple snail. They published the results of these investigations jointly in 1842 in the proceedings of the Paris Academy of Sciences (19). In his just mentioned paper of 1839 Gruby discussed from a chemical point of view, how water rich in organic salts may operate adversely on the body by the deposition of the salts at certain points and also through its effect on food as well as drugs of which decoctions are made. He praised purified Danube water highly and advised drinking it because of its low content of dissolved salts and minerals.

There is no question that Gruby overdid it by making the salt content of natural water responsible for gout and a great many other diseases, but it is a noteworthy fact that he was among the first to realize the role of drinking water and food on the health of people and that he saw here an important factor in popular hygiene, thus becoming one of the fathers of modern sitology or dietetics. Next to microscopy, dietetics remained a matter of major medical interest for him all through his life. Later a great deal of his success in his practice was based on his constant awareness of the fact that many diseases were due to wrong food—wrong either in quality or in quantity. His idea to use purified, mineral-free water as a treatment for concretions in the body was justified by the medical trend in the early twenties of this century. At that time, for example, the drinking of distilled water was recommended as a treatment for calculi by outstanding physicians like the late Professor Charles Glaessner of Vienna. The entire twentieth-century belief that transmineralization of the body was helpful in certain diseases was a confirmation of Gruby's early suggestions concerning the use of drinking water free of or low in minerals. According to Gruby, the use of purified water of the Danube River was indicated for the cleaning of teeth and skin. He found less need for soap because of the cleansing effect of mineral-free water. For hygiene of scalp and hair this kind of water was preferable to spring or well water. Gruby also suggested its use in gastrointestinal diseases and for the external and internal use for children and especially the newborn and infants.

The leading idea of this paper, the repeated appeal to the "rational physician," shows that Gruby at that time was already strongly influenced by the modern, rational and physiological approach in the study of medicine. In this respect he was surely in Vienna an exception to the average physician. It is also noteworthy that he stressed the general importance of his suggestions as a means of improving the hygiene and health of the people

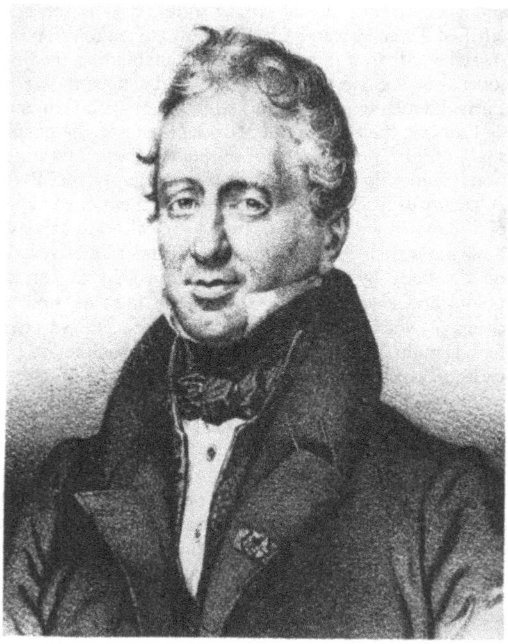

FIG. 30. The Paris surgeon, Roux, whose suggestion persuaded Gruby to settle in Paris. From a lithograph in the author's possession.

of Vienna. In the concluding sentence he asks that the poor be not excluded from the blessings of filtered Danube water. In a moving plea for the needy population, he asks the wealthy to pay the expenses of making the filtered river water available to the whole population.

Gruby presents himself in this publication, which appeared a few years after the terrible cholera epidemic of 1831–1832, as an enthusiastic advocate of small pox vaccination and of quarantine to prevent the spread of communicable diseases. In his later life he very definitely changed his opinion concerning vaccination.

The praise he bestows on preventive medicine in the introduction to this paper, the differentiation he makes between the money-making practitioner and the unrewarded idealist who, by his research work, helps to prevent plagues and diseases, is astonishing for a very young Viennese physician in 1839; moreover, what he says is true even in our day. This characterizes Gruby's mature mind and kind personality better than any biographer could do.

Gruby was very impressed by what he learned on his trip in Germany and England, but not so impressed by these countries and the life there as to decide to settle permanently in England or in any of Germany's reactionary places. His final decision was in favor of France.

While Gruby was still working in Vienna, he met many visiting foreign physicians. One of them, the French surgeon Philibert Joseph Roux, successor to the surgeon Dupuytren at the hospital Hôtel Dieu in Paris and a foreign member of the Society of Physicians in Vienna, suggested that he make his home in this famous center of medicine, for here microscopical studies were still a very new field and held promise for clinical investigations and for a talented young physician who might start to spread knowledge about them in Paris. Gruby decided to follow this suggestion of a famous and influential physician and settle in Paris. There he remained to the end of his long life.

START IN PARIS

At this time, in spite of Berlin's already growing reputation, Vienna and Paris were the two centers of medical studies in Europe to which interested students from all over the world flocked to learn new methods and become acquainted with new ideas. In this respect, Paris still outshone Vienna, where the second Viennese school of medicine was just beginning to flourish under the pathologist Rokitansky and the clinician Skoda. Paris was known for its many outstanding physicians and scientists, its scientific societies and collections, and its numerous large hospitals. Magendie, one of the founders of modern physiology, taught there, as did his pupil and already famous collaborator Claude Bernard, and Flourens and Orfila, all shining stars in the firmament of scientific medicine, and many famous clinicians. Among them were specialists in various fields, such as surgery, pediatrics, dermatology, syphilology, with knowledge and experience not to be found anywhere else. To mention only a few names still remembered in our day, there were, for instance, Lugol and Cazenave; Roux, the surgeon; and Lisfranc, Andral, and Piorry teaching clinical pathology. It is significant that just at the time when Gruby went to study in Paris, two books appeared in Germany on the faculty and medical studies in Paris. One of them was entitled *Vienna and Paris, a Contribution to the History and Evaluation of Present-day Medicine,* written by an outstanding pioneer in modern German medicine, Carl August Wunderlich, one of the fathers of clinical thermometry, at that time Privatdozent at the University of Tübingen (Germany) and later founder and editor of the journal, *Archives of Physiological Medicine.* This book was published in Stuttgart as a volume of 166 pages (76). The other, a book of 295 pages written by S. J. Otterburg, was entitled *The Medical Paris, a Contribution to the History of Medicine and a Guide for German Physicians* (63). There probably existed still more ephemeral literature on this subject than these two books. Paris at that time was the Mecca that attracted innumerable young European physicians. Gruby, therefore, showed good judgment by going from famous Vienna to the even more famous Paris to continue his medical studies, or, to use his own expression (57), for the purpose of his own information on medical problems.

The attractive power which France and especially Paris exerted on a young man was, of course, not limited to its medical institutions. Since the days of Louis XIV the reputation of France as the cultural center of Europe was well established. The glory of the Napoleonic era was still in everyone's memory. The political power and liberal tendencies of the common man in Paris compared with the despair and servitude of the common man in Germany, in Austria, and other European countries, attracted those who were suffering under political injustice in their own countries. Finally the fame of feminine charm and beauty in modern Paris, known, like its immorality and political corruption through the fascinating novels of Balzac and Stendal and of many second rate poets, may have attracted a gay young man who vividly enjoyed the happy life of Vienna in the days when Lanner and Johann Strauss senior created the Viennese waltz music.

We know too little about the weight of these different factors in Gruby's final decision to settle in the town which, according to the consensus of opinions, represented the best of all France and was regarded as its heart and center of life. On Gruby's last years in Vienna and his start in Paris Le Leu reports a few autobiographical notes dictated to him by Gruby in 1895, who, after more than half a century had passed, was still proud of the lasting contributions of his first publications, in which he demonstrated that every one of the investigated body fluids contained, besides the fluid, living cellular elements. It may be worth while to translate the passages in Le Leu's book which present these notes (57).

"If you wish to know details concerning my work in microscopy," said old Gruby,

> I should tell you that the first thing I published in Vienna was a paper on inflammation and pus read before the Medical Society of Vienna. That may have been about 1835 or 1836. The second work, entitled "Morphologia Pathologica," which I published in Vienna in 1840, was again a microscopic study. In these investigations I showed the presence of living units in the pus of small pox blisters and of other origin. There one finds the genesis and morphology of the globules of pus, their birth, development, and death, observed under the microscope. I demonstrated that cells were present in mucus and other material. At that time I worked at the side of my master Berres, Professor of Anatomy, and I collaborated with him for a period of several years on his own work. If you are interested in the work of Berres, unique from the anatomical point of view, I could let you see a copy which I possess.

At this point Gruby showed Le Leu the magnificent book and told him interesting details about Berres and their common work. But, unfortunately, Le Leu did not write down this part of the conversation, which would have been a valuable supplement to the anatomist's Hyrtl's report on his own collaboration on Berres's books (52).

> Later on, [Gruby continued,] I gave courses in descriptive anatomy in Vienna and in surgical anatomy to young applicants for the degree of medical doctor. At the same time, I was admitted to the surgical department under the direction of Professor Wattmann.
>
> After I received my diploma as medical doctor and master of ophthalmology, I undertook a scientific trip through Germany and visited various universities in Europe. Roux, the surgeon at the Hôtel Dieu in Paris, who, as a traveler in Vienna, saw the preparations I made for the museum, especially in the field of ophthalmology,[5] encouraged me to come to Paris. I took this trip with one of my colleagues from Vienna, and we arrived in Paris in the spring of 1841. I wanted to improve my knowledge in some field, in which I was not able to improve it in Vienna, especially concerning diseases of the newborn and diseases of the skin.
>
> I carried on the studies on the pathological anatomy of the newborn in the Foundlings Hospital. At that time, this branch of study was not much cultivated at this hospital.
>
> One of my colleagues, also interested in diseases of the newborn, assisted in the autopsies and tried to make this investigation more profound.
>
> When he came to study the diseases of the kidneys of the newborn, he consulted me concerning the obstructions of the urinary channels. The various questions he put forward and which I hastened to answer, increased his curiosity to know the name of the one who answered so promptly, and after having learned my name, he exclaimed that he had been looking for me for a long time already.

[5] These preparations must have been indeed most remarkable. Still in 1844 W. Herzig mentions in a book on medical Vienna as outstanding treasure in the museum of the ophthalmological clinic injected preparations made by Prochaska, Hyrtl, Gruby, and Patruban (48: 90).

He came with his colleagues from Vienna, where he went to look for me to attend my course in pathological and microscopical anatomy, and nobody was able to tell him where he could find me.

He insisted on seeing my preparations pertaining to the diseases of the kidneys of newborns, which I had made in Paris for my own instruction. I did as he wished, and he asked me to give a course in microscopical anatomy for him and his friends, who were looking for an instructor. In spite of the fact that I was very little inclined to start a course as instructor, being on the way to instruct myself and little able to give lessons to others, I finally, after some months of reluctance and hesitation, started a course for these young physicians. They were Dr. Berg from Stockholm, Lilienwald and Glasser from Sweden, and some young Austrian, German, and Russian physicians. At the same time they attended a course given by Claude Bernard, who was still a young physician, but already renowned for his studies in comparative physiology. When he saw that I was teaching a new branch, he joined as a pupil with his group and attended my course on microscopic anatomy. He was at that time the pupil of Magendie at the Collège de France, and Magendie himself took part in my course on microscopic anatomy.

Here you have my debut in Paris.

After a few words on Gruby's studies on "cryptogams," Le Leu's notes suddenly come to an end and he mentions that at this point old Gruby suddenly stopped dictating, saying that at the moment he had no more time left. He disappeared quickly to do some other, more important work, as for instance, offering some nuts to a monkey or some sugar to a parrot, or watering his plants, and with that the interesting autobiography of his early days in Paris remained a fragment.

Gruby's statement on his first paper read before the Viennese Medical Society, as reported by Le Leu, is not exact. Gruby read the paper on the mentioned topics before the Society of Physicians at Vienna, but it was not in 1835 or 1836; it was on January 31, 1840 (52), after the publication of his Latin dissertation on the same topic in 1839. The date of his lecture shows that he was still living in Vienna early in 1840. His 1839 paper on the use of filtered Danube water (21) was signed "David Gruby, practical physician at Vienna," indicating that he probably practiced medicine even before being graduated as Doctor. From the fact that nobody in Vienna knew of Gruby's whereabouts when the Swedish scholars inquired, it may be concluded that no close relationship bound him to any of the young stars in Vienna's medical centers. There is, also, no proof of any friendly relationship between Gruby and the anatomist Hyrtl, who until 1837 was also a pupil, collaborator, and youthful friend of Berres. In 1837, at the age of twenty-seven, Hyrtl left Vienna for Prague, where he became Professor of Anatomy. In no place in his caustic autobiographical publication did he mention the name of Gruby (52).

In 1840, as mentioned before, Gruby left the beautiful city of Vienna, where he had studied and graduated, and where he had lived during the horrible years of the cholera of 1830–1831, and where he had attended

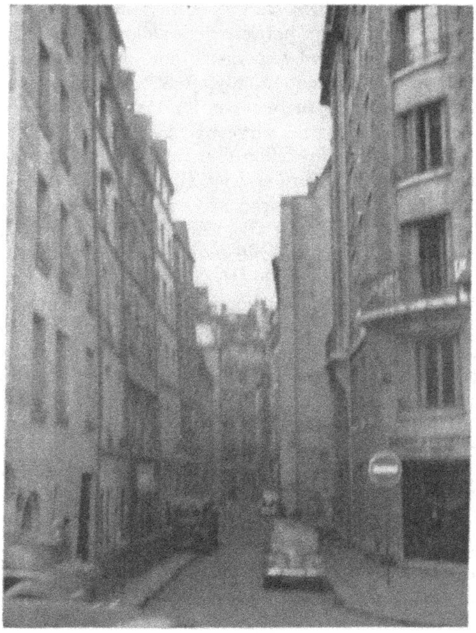

FIG. 31. Rue Git le Cœur seen from the shore of the Seine, the third house to the left is No. 5 where Gruby had his first apartment in Paris. Photo. taken by the author.

the great inspiring meeting of the 1832 convention of the Society of German Scientists and Physicians, which was postponed for a year because of the dangers of the cholera epidemic. Maybe this epidemic had an influence on Gruby's starting to study medicine in 1831. He left Vienna before the tornado of the "crazy" year 1848 produced so many changes in the lives of all Viennese citizens.

As indicated by his letter to Valentin, Gruby came to Paris in 1840. The political atmosphere there was tense. Louis Phillippe, the citizen-king, was ruling, but the Bonapartists were gaining in power. Paris was still flourishing as the medical center of Europe. At that time Gruby's reputation was great enough for his move from Vienna to France to be reported in the Berlin medical *Central-Zeitung* in the following way. It says, in the issue of May 15, 1840 (p. 396), reported from Vienna: "Dr. Gruby, a native of Hungary, who graduated from this [the Viennese] university and has already published excellent work on the subject of the microscopical pathological anatomy, departed for Paris to settle there as a practicing physician." This announcement also proves the spring of 1840 as the time of Gruby's settlement in Paris.

Gruby's start in Paris was a modest one. His first apartment was situated in the Rue Git le Cœur No. 5, where he gave his courses and lectures from 1841 until

1854 (6). He remained so fond of this apartment to the end of his life that he never failed to pay his rent to the former superintendent of the house, and after her death, even to her daughter (57), even though he no longer lived in this part of Paris.

Rue Git le Cœur, situated in the Sixth Arrondisment in the middle of Paris, still has today precisely the same appearance as at the time when Gruby came there in 1840. All the century-old houses on the narrow street are untouched. There are small exotic eating places such as may have existed already in Gruby's days and aroused his interest.

Of course, it is indicative of Gruby's esthetic sense and interests that this little street was located between the beautiful Quai des Grand Augustines, with a view over the Seine River, and the Rue St. André des Arts in the close vicinity of the historical building of the French Academy, the Institut de France, where Gruby was to present time and again in the following years his epoch-making medical research. He lived just between the centers of science and of art, next to the Louvre, the Jardin des Tuilleries, the church of Nôtre Dame, and the Royal Palace. As modest as this street and its old houses appear today to the visitor, Gruby displayed original and excellent taste in choosing Rue Git le Cœur No. 5 as his first headquarters in Paris.

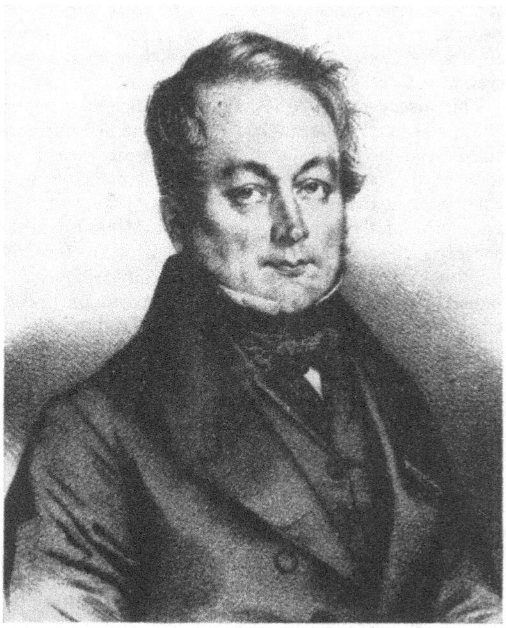

FIG. 32. François Magendie (1783–1855), the famous French physiologist. Strong opponent of the use of ether narcosis, regarding it as danger for morality. He was one of Gruby's students in microscopy.

His means were modest and limited, but it was not another start like the one in Pest or in Vienna. He came to Paris, with helpful letters of recommendation from Viennese friends, who also assisted him financially. Le Leu reprints a letter dated June, 1840 by a Mr. Sch . . . r, who sent Gruby a check for 500 Frcs. Le Leu emphasized the good relations which Gruby maintained with the Sch...r family until death. This chiffre may stand for his father's friend Schindler, who brought David from Kis-Kér to Pest and provided him with his first employment, as a waiter-bookkeeper.

In Paris Gruby submerged himself in his work, mainly in the Foundling Hospital under Jacques François Baron, one of the outstanding pediatricians and medical consultants in Paris (63). A former pupil of Berres and Rokitansky, he was soon entrusted with the work in pathological anatomy at this hospital. It was here that Frederic Berg, later Professor of Pediatrics in Stockholm, urged him to give courses for foreign students. Gruby did this for many years, in Paris, and at the veterinary school at Alfort, two hours away from Paris, where he introduced microscopical studies and found a faithful friend and collaborator in Professor O. Delafond. Delafond (also written De Lafond) was already professor at the veterinary school at Alfort when Gruby started his activities in Paris in 1840. In 1838 he had published a treatise on general veterinary pathology in two volumes (9) and also a book on the sanitary police of domestic animals (10). As author of two books on blood-diseases of animals which were subsequently published in 1843 and 1848 he was, of course, highly interested in Gruby's microscopical research. Both friends may have gained by their collaboration and may have mutually inspired their respective research.

In 1841 Gruby started a private research laboratory, teaching there microscopy of normal and pathological specimens. Besides Magendie, and Claude Bernard, Flourens, Milne-Edwards, and other outstanding figures were among his pupils (5, 6, 57), despite the fact that medical microscopy was already represented on the faculty by a compatriot of Gruby. Professor Delafond too attended Gruby's lectures and that started the friendship and collaboration of the two scholars in Alfort (6). Gruby's lectures were also attended by foreign physicians, coming to Paris from England, Sweden, and other countries (6) to study modern medicine.

At that time microscopical anatomy was taught in the medical faculty of Paris by Louis Mandl, a Hungarian who had the title of *Professeur Particulier d'Anatomie Microscopic.* Mandl gave courses exclusively for medical students of the *École Pratique de la Faculté de Médicine,* whereas Gruby's courses, in no connection with the medical school of Paris, were given for post-graduates, and therefore probably were on a higher level (6).

There is no evidence that Gruby was ever on friendly

terms with Mandl. Mandl did not mention Gruby's studies in his great work, *Anatomie Microscopique,* nor even in the chapter on microscopy of body fluids. It may be that this great work of Mandl with its many plates also helped to discourage Gruby from continuing with his own book, especially since he saw that it took Mandl not less than twenty years to complete and publish his two volumes. That Gruby at that time gave lectures and demonstrations on microscopy and on parasites of animals at the veterinary school at Alfort too is witnessed by his biographer Blanchard (5, 6) who knew it from Gruby himself and from Professor M. Weber, his colleague at the Academy of Medicine who attended these lectures as an assistant.

Gruby's reputation and his fame as author of the book published in 1840 was growing rapidly. That can be judged from a letter of his father, who in 1841 proudly writes of newspaper items concerning his son (57). Gruby's financial condition at that time may also have improved considerably, for in the above-mentioned letter telling of the death of David's stepmother the elder Gruby asks his son for 200 florins and Gruby's brother requests 100 florins for himself as a subsidy, at that time a considerable amount of money.

THE FOUNDING OF DERMATOMYCOLOGY

The year 1841 and those immediately following were the years of Gruby's greatest contributions to medicine. During this time he published in quick sequence in the *Proceedings* of the Paris Académie des Sciences his fundamental discoveries on the various molds that produce affections of the skin, the scalp and mucous membranes especially in children. The etiology of the several types of ringworm diseases was clarified by him in those years, and for the first time microscopy was introduced into clinical dermatology as an indispensable tool for the right diagnosis.

I omit a bibliography of Gruby's work, because, except for his above-mentioned papers published in the German language, Blanchard (5), Le Leu (57), and Salaün (68), each published one. Only his outstanding contributions will be mentioned. On July 12, 1841 he described clearly the causative fungus of Favus, a skin disease, establishing that Favus was a contagious disease produced by a fungus (22), announcing experiments to produce this disease in man and animals by inoculation of the specific molds. It was within the very short period of three years that he discovered the fungus of Favus, the microsporum (the cause of a scalp disease), and the fungi today called trichophyton tonsurans and oidium albicans, the latter the cause of thrush. Though his clinical descriptions of the different diseases produced by the various fungi he discovered may be inadequate for the modern clinician (66) his microscopical descriptions were so excellent that decades later, when his discoveries were rediscovered and confirmed, not much remained to be added to his original microscopical reports (70).

Gruby's enthused devotion to microscopy never waned. He even used the newly-invented (1839) procedure, photography, to make pictures of the microscopic objects which he discussed, and he and his Hungarian compatriot Mandl may justly be regarded as the outstanding pioneers in modern micrography in France (5, 6, 11).

Zakon and Benedek (77) are also right in calling Gruby the father of modern medical mycology. He is definitely the founder of a scientific approach to all the dermatomycotic diseases, i.e., diseases of the skin produced by parasitic fungi.

DISCOVERIES AND STUDIES IN PARASITOLOGY

Dermatomycology was by no means the only field of human and animal parasitology which received outstanding contributions from Gruby. In the same period of his highest scientific fecundity belongs the discovery of a corkscrew-shaped living parasite in the blood of frogs, similar to one reported two years before (1841) by G. Valentin (74), the physiologist of Bern University. Valentin found it in the blood of a fish. In 1842 Gluge had found such parasites in the hearts of frogs (17). Gruby attached to this discovery such importance that he published his findings in the *Proceedings* of the Paris Académie des Sciences (30) and in the *Annales des Sciences Naturelles* (31), naming this type of parasite Trypanosoma (1843), which name has been used ever since.

This discovery by Gruby, like his entire mycological work, was fated to be laughed at and remained unrecognized by most of his outstanding contemporaries. In spite of the fact that his report was accompanied by what were at that time good drawings of trypanosoma, the editor of the *Annals,* the famous Milne-Edwards, one of Gruby's audience in his courses on microscopy, could not refrain from adding an editorial footnote (31) signed (R) emphasizing that not only was he unconvinced that the trypanosoma was a special zoological type, but he did not regard these bodies as real animals at all but as products of the host animal's body, surviving for a time like ciliaries. He thought that they should be compared with spermatozoids rather than with helminths. R. Remak, who in 1842 saw similar parasites in the blood of freshwater fish and very commonly in the blood of pike was doubtful whether they are parasites or a kind of spermatozoa, which opinion [6] may have influenced Milne-Edwards.

Today nobody will doubt that in this controversy Doctor Gruby was right and his famous critical opponent Milne-Edwards was wrong. However there is no question that such public criticism without personal checking of the facts reported by Gruby dis-

[6] Canstatt's *Jahresberichte* 1842: 10.

credited the discovery and must have hurt the author, whose name never again appeared among the contributors to the *Annales des Sciences Naturelles.*

Gruby, however, was not discouraged nor did he waste his time on polemics. He rarely did. He continued his research on animals in Paris, studying the anatomy of the venous system of the frog. He probably had discovered the trypanosoma in the frog's blood during similar prior investigations. Apparently he had already engaged in this type of research in Vienna or he started on it immediately after coming to Paris, for the thirteenth volume of the *Proceedings* of the Paris Académie des Sciences, published in 1841, already contains a paper presented by Gruby in which he reports on his anatomical and physiological research on the venous system of frogs (24, 29).

In the same year that Gruby published his discovery of the trypanosoma in frogs, he made a discovery of equal importance in dogs. In the sixteenth volume of the *Proceedings* of the Académie des Sciences, together with his friend Delafond, he presented (40) the discovery of parasites in the blood of an apparently healthy dog; small threadlike living organisms, 3–5μ in length were found in the bloodstream, but not in the urine of dogs. This was the first discovery of microfilaria in the blood of a mammal, microfilaria being the larval form of filaria, a roundworm living in the blood. It was only in 1872 that T. R. Lewis in India discovered a microfilaria (the larva of filaria sanguinis hominis) in human blood. Gruby gives in this paper the size of the red blood cells in the dog as from 7–8μ which agrees fairly well with our knowledge today.

The discovery of filaria in the bloodstream of dogs by Gruby and Delafond was also reported in the Viennese *Oesterreichische Medizinische Wochenschrift*[7] and in Germany in Froriep's *Notizen.*[8] Finally, it should be mentioned that Gruby was the first to discover a fungus mycelium as basis and nucleus of a concretion extracted by Hirschler, Chief of the Clinique de Desmarres in Paris, from the lacrimal duct of a human being. This was in 1848 and Blanchard witnesses (6) to possess Gruby's own dated drawings of this microscopical observation. Molds producing such concretions in the lacrimal duct were later repeatedly reported, for instance by A. von Gräfe (1855), by W. Goldzieher (18, 1844) and others, but Gruby was again the first to recognize the real nature of this pathological condition in man. Gruby gave the entire group of diseases produced by molds the name "maladies parasitique végetales ou phyto-parasitiques." He was the master who conquered this entire field of human and animal pathology for medical understanding and modern treatment.

[7] 1844: 772.
[8] No. 645: 106.

ANATOMICAL AND PHYSIOLOGICAL DISCOVERIES

The investigations on the venous system of the frog, published in the reports of the Paris Académie des Sciences in 1841, on which he reported extensively in 1842 in the *Annales de Science Naturelle* (29) were evaluated by the greatest contemporary expert, Johannes Müller, in his annual report on the progress in anatomy in his *Archiv,*[9] as a very exact and meritorious work. Gruby reported his discovery of various, as yet unknown, veins in the head of the frog and also an unknown communication of the anterior abdominal vein and the umbilical vein with the heart before their entry into the liver.

Not only does this short paper testify to the fact that Gruby continued his anatomical research in the meticulous Viennese spirit, but it is the first indication of his interest in problems of experimental physiology, and this new trend appears time and again in his subsequent work.

It was, apparently, through his contact with and under the influence of Magendie and Claude Bernard, both of whom attended Gruby's lectures in microscopy, of Delafond and others that the young doctor came to realize the importance of physiological observation and experimentation. He corroborated, for instance, in the mentioned paper of 1841 (29), Flourens' finding (1832) that the great abdominal veins have an autonomous kind of pulsation independent of the auricles, a fact which, in 1839, was confirmed in America by M. Allison with respect to the vena cava and the veins of the lungs of different vertebrates. This fact was still doubted by Johannes Müller in the fourth edition of the first volume of his *Handbuch,*[10] where he only mentions Flourens' observations. Müller was of the opinion that the pulmonic veins and the venae cavae show a pulsation only where they are sheathed by muscle bundles originating in the heart muscle itself.

Gruby was so impressed by the rich vascular supply of the kidney that he also considered undertaking much needed research on the function of the kidneys in frogs.

"INFECTED BLOOD"—TRANSFUSION EXPERIMENTS

The new physiological direction of Gruby's research is revealed by his statement that the parasites he discovered in the blood of dogs may survive in preserved blood at a temperature of 15° Celsius. Gruby and Delafond repeatedly came back to the subject of these parasites. In 1843 and 1844 (40, 45) and as late as 1852 they published a second and third report on the parasites that may be found in the blood of dogs (46). A paper on the same topic was published by them in the *Edinburgh Philosophical Journal* (1852) and in the *Quarterly Journal of Microscopic Science* (1854).

[9] 1842: 233.
[10] 1844: 169.

They mention mainly two apparently different types of parasites. One is the microfilaria, reported in 1843 and 1844, which is described as "des entozoaires de genre filarie vivants dans le sang de certain chiens domestiques et circulant avec les globules de ce fluid dans tous les vaisseux." In the meantime these discoveries were confirmed by other authors on other mammals, for instance, in 1845 by Hyrtl, Gros, and Ecker. Gruby and Delafond gave their parasites the name *filaria papilosa haematica canis domestici*. In addition to this type, present only in the bloodstream, they found long, thin, mature parasites, male and female, 14–20 cm. in length and 1 mm. in width in the heart of certain dogs. According to Fülleborn (15), the species found by Gruby and Delafond was probably, what today is called *microfilaria repens*.

The research that Gruby and Delafond published as early as 1844 and, in detail, in 1852 shows an amazing modern experimental approach. They gave blood transfusions from infected dogs to healthy ones and were able to produce, in 1844, in one dog and in 1852 in two healthy dogs the same type of microfilariosis by transfusion of 200–800 cc. of defibrinated blood of an infected dog. This is an outstanding experiment in the history of communicable diseases as well as in the field of blood transfusion. It is also a definite advance beyond Valentin's concept of 1840 of a kind of spontaneous generation of parasites in the body liquids of mammals. A new era in parasitology opens with this approach to its problems. In the blood of healthy dogs that had been given a transfusion of infected blood, Gruby found the parasites for over three years up to the death of the animals. Thus, for the first time, it was established that a communicable disease could be induced in a healthy animal by intravenous transfusion of defibrinated blood of an infected animal.

Gruby and Delafond also gave transfusions of the infected blood of dogs to two rabbits and found surviving parasites in the blood of the rabbits eighty-nine days afterwards but not later. The autopsy performed after that time revealed no parasites, either in the blood or in the tissues of these animals.

Extremely interesting was the result obtained, already in 1844, by injecting the blood of infected dogs into the bloodstream of frogs. For a week the dog-erythrocytes could be found in the bloodstream of the frog and also the microfilarias. On the ninth and tenth days the red blood cells of the dog disintegrated, and the parasites disappeared, and all the frogs died of a scurvy-like disease.

From these first systematic efforts to produce, by hetero-transfusion of infected blood, an experimental haematogenous infection the authors came to the conclusion that the parasites investigated can exist only in the blood of dogs or of such animals that have a special suitable and not yet understood constitution.

No less important was their conclusion that the transmission of the parasites, even in dogs, is possible only if the infected blood is intravenously injected, but not if it is injected into tissues or into the serous cavities. Most surprising are their experiments in which the authors mated male and female dogs, one of them infected, the other not, and both of different breeds. They ascertained that only those puppies were infected that were of the same breed as the infected parent.

According to modern knowledge these experiments are not proof of inherited microfilariasis, for the puppies could have been infected later in the usual way. Nevertheless, there was sufficient ground to suspect an immunity based on breed. The first evidence of infection was found in the blood of the puppies at the age of five to six months, and could be traced for many years. Some of the dogs suffered epileptiform attacks. Gruby and Delafond submitted this outstanding piece of experimental work to the Paris *Académie* in competition for the *Prix du Physiologie Experimental*. It would be of special interest to know whether all these extraordinary facts, published by such a distinguished institution, ever came to the knowledge of young Pasteur and whether they impressed this father of pathogenic microbiology.

ODDS AND ENDS IN RESEARCH

The working capacity and the enthusiasm Gruby exhibited during these years must have been unlimited and his collaboration with Delafond a very close one. In the same year, 1843, both of them published other papers on very different topics in the same *Proceedings* of the Academy of Paris. It is easy to recognize that the work Gruby performed at the veterinary school at Alfort was partly a continuation of his Viennese microscopical studies, but with a more modern approach. In the sixteenth volume of the *Comptes Rendus* of the Paris Academy (41, 42, 44) he returned to the topic of his doctoral thesis, the investigation of the microscopical appearance of body fluids and, together with Delafond, published microscopical studies on the lymph and chylus of horse, dog, and rabbit. There they described granulated cells in the lymph. They studied the histology of the villi of the intestines and found a ciliary movement of the intestinal epithelium of dogs. They also made the statement that in horse and dog the content of the stomach is sour, whereas beyond the pylorus it is sour in the horse, but neutral or alkaline in the dog. Gruby and Delafond devoted careful research (41, 42, 44) to the anatomy, function, and movement of the intestinal villi as well as to the study of the chyme, the viscid fluid contents of the stomach before it passes into the duodenum. The cells found in the lymph are described as round and oval granulated cells with a diameter of 5–10μ already differentiated as leucocytes ("globul blanc") and another different type of white cell. Gruby and Delafond also describe the presence of many droplets of fat in the lymph, each supposed to be surrounded by a protein membrane. It is observed likewise that lymph coagulates when separated from the lymph vessels. The progress evidenced in this work, as compared with Gruby's 1840 book, is so apparent that his advanced insight and experience, too, may have prevented him from continuing the publication of the promised subsequent installments of *Morphologia Pathologica*. He had definitely outgrown, at that time, the type of his first publication. On the other hand, he may not have found the time needed for continuing such a venture, being busy with new fascinating discoveries.

Still in the same year both friends reported (43) on the abundance of living parasites in the stomach of higher animals, a new fact in mammal parasitology, which Froriep in Germany found important enough to review in his *Journal*[11] and of which an English translation appeared in the *Annals of Natural History* in 1844. In the same year (45) they described their investigations on the blood of 250 dogs, finding microfilariasis in only five of the animals. There were no parasites in the urine, bile, saliva, humor aqueus, and cerebrospinal fluid even when they were present in the blood. To accomplish all that, Gruby must have worked with all his energy, and consequently he may have had no time to write books.

However, there was other work done too by Gruby in the first years of his stay in Paris. In 1842 he continued to study various parasites of frogs (26, 27). He found little filaria-like parasites in peritoneal cysts of these animals, a discovery made independently in the same year by C. Vogt. Gruby, since his Viennese days skilled in injecting into vessels, describes a method for intravenous injections into living frogs. He injected some eggs of diastoma, a parasite flatworm of the frog, into other healthy animals and carefully observed their reactions with the microscope. He reports emboli produced in this way, and as their consequence, inflammation, adhesions, and suppuration. In the case of suppuration, the leucocytes were found to be larger than those of mammals, less opaque, and perfectly spherical. In these experiments Gruby found uratic concrements in the bladder and observed their formation microscopically. Gallstones of cholesterol up to 3 mm. in diameter were found in these frogs and tubercle-like formations in the lungs and the gastrointestinal tract.

It should be remembered that these investigations were very early efforts in experimental pathology, in which field Gruby was really an outstanding and unjustly forgotten pioneer. In the same paper he mentions experiments to produce necrosis in frogs by freezing with solid carbon dioxide the skin or the eyeball until stiff, and he is surprised that these organs recover entirely. His mind continuously returns to problems of parasitology. The son of the little farmer remembers the devastating epidemics of potato-sickness and we find Gruby in these busy years interested in animal and vegetable parasites producing this kind of potato-sickness (33). His differentiating of three kinds of potato-sickness shows the same keen and brilliant approach to problems of plant pathology which he presented in research in human pathology. At the same time he was also occupied with clinical studies in parasitology as presented in a paper submitted to the Paris Académie des Sciences in 1844 (32), when he reported on the introduction of a tube 8 mm. in diameter into the stomach of a sick woman to ascertain whether vomited particles consisting of "sporules" 4–9 μ in diameter came from the stomach or from the gullet. Finally, to show his versatility, a paper may be mentioned which he published in 1842 in the *Comptes Rendus* on the anatomy of *Murex,* the purple snail (19).

With each one of his discoveries during the years 1841 through 1845, Gruby proved to be not only a worthy offspring of the second medical school of Vienna, but also an excellent scholar in the field of anatomy, physiology, and pathology, original in his thoughts and his methods and reliable in his observations.

In the interest of fairness in the history of modern parasitology, it must be mentioned that the fungus which causes Favus had been discovered and, in a letter to Johannes Müller, described briefly by the Berlin Clinician Professor Schönlein, and this letter was published by Müller in his *Archiv* in 1839. But the mold had already been discovered by Schönlein's pupil, Remak, in 1837, though he did not recognize its nature as a fungus. Gruby, however, made his discovery (22) independently of Schönlein, whose publication apparently neither he nor any physiologist in France knew of at that time (23). Gruby himself admitted expressively Schönlein's priority when made aware of the latter's paper (53) in 1841 (23) and in 1842 when he published his studies concerning the skin disease *tinea favosa* in German in Müller's *Archiv,* however doubtful whether the fungi of Schönlein were identical with his own. There he also mentioned his first attempts (22, 23) to inoculate with the disease man, rabbits, amphibians, worms, and plants(!!), and he emphasized the superiority of his own observations and experiments over those of Schönlein (23). Gruby's original report was made with such thoroughness and exactness that Rille, himself an expert in modern microscopy, found it difficult to understand how such an accurate observation of so many details could have been made at that early stage in the development of microscopical technique. The name of the fungus producing the Favus disease of the skin is now the one given it by Remak in honor of his teacher and protector, Schönlein (in 1845), *Achorion Schoenleinii.*

The thrush-producing fungus was discovered at the same time by Gruby and by his pupil, Berg, and pub-

[11] No. 609: 233, 1843.

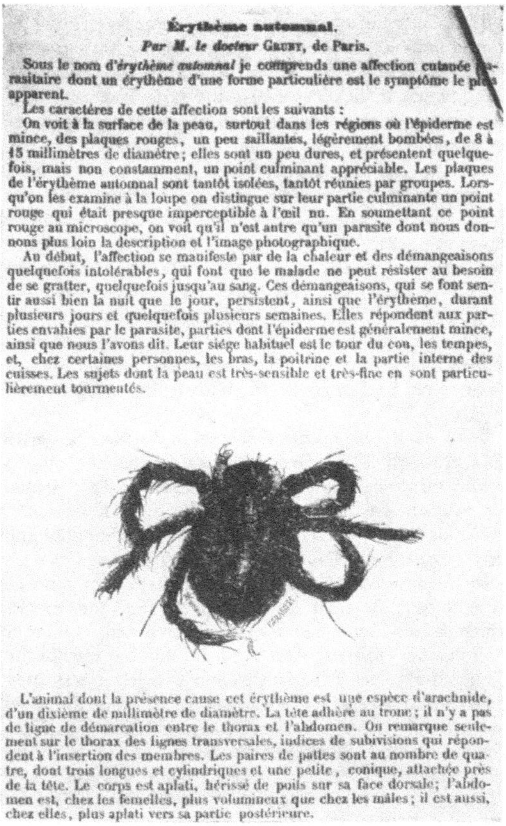

Érythème automnal.

Par M. le docteur GRUBY, de Paris.

Sous le nom d'*érythème automnal* je comprends une affection cutanée parasitaire dont un érythème d'une forme particulière est le symptôme le plus apparent.

Les caractères de cette affection sont les suivants :

On voit à la surface de la peau, surtout dans les régions où l'épiderme est mince, des plaques rouges, un peu saillantes, légèrement bombées, de 8 à 15 millimètres de diamètre; elles sont un peu dures, et présentent quelquefois, mais non constamment, un point culminant appréciable. Les plaques de l'érythème automnal sont tantôt isolées, tantôt réunies par groupes. Lorsqu'on les examine à la loupe on distingue sur leur partie culminante un point rouge qui était presque imperceptible à l'œil nu. En soumettant ce point rouge au microscope, on voit qu'il n'est autre qu'un parasite dont nous donnons plus loin la description et l'image photographique.

Au début, l'affection se manifeste par de la chaleur et des démangeaisons quelquefois intolérables, qui font que le malade ne peut résister au besoin de se gratter, quelquefois jusqu'au sang. Ces démangeaisons, qui se font sentir aussi bien la nuit que le jour, persistent, ainsi que l'érythème, durant plusieurs jours et quelquefois plusieurs semaines. Elles répondent aux parties envahies par le parasite, parties dont l'épiderme est généralement mince, ainsi que nous l'avons dit. Leur siége habituel est le tour du cou, les tempes, et, chez certaines personnes, les bras, la poitrine et la partie interne des cuisses. Les sujets dont la peau est très-sensible et très-fine en sont particulièrement tourmentés.

L'animal dont la présence cause cet érythème est une espèce d'arachnide, d'un dixième de millimètre de diamètre. La tête adhère au tronc; il n'y a pas de ligne de démarcation entre le thorax et l'abdomen. On remarque seulement sur le thorax des lignes transversales, indices de subivisions qui répondent à l'insertion des membres. Les paires de pattes sont au nombre de quatre, dont trois longues et cylindriques et une petite, conique, attachée près de la tête. Le corps est aplati, hérissé de poils sur sa face dorsale; l'abdomen est, chez les femelles, plus volumineux que chez les mâles; il est aussi, chez elles, plus aplati vers sa partie postérieure.

FIG. 33. Gruby's first publication on the discovery of the mite producing *Erythema autumnale*. *La Clinique European* 1: 171, 1859.

lished by both in 1842 in the same journal and in friendly cooperation (4).

Gruby's fundamental discoveries and his justifiable demand for a fundamental change in the treatment of Favus (22, 23), and his discovery of *Trypanosoma* (31), met with suspicion and sarcasm, especially in France. They were ridiculed in scientific journals and newspapers. Even Bazin writes in his textbook on dermatomycoses in 1858 (2: 144 and 196): "malheureusement, la plus grande partie du memoire de M. Gruby n'est qu'un roman," and even in 1873 the dermatologist Cazenave declared in his textbook that Gruby's fungi were the illusions of a microscopist and "rêveries allemands." Modern research has proven how right Gruby, the excellent observer, was and how wrong those who had criticized his discoveries. Rokitansky, in his famous *Handbuch der Pathologischen Anatomie*,[12] gave credit to his pupil Gruby for his discoveries, and so did Bazin, the first in France, officially in 1853 and 1854, and Sabauraud, who in 1892 rediscovered the microsporon (69). In Germany, Gruby's discoveries were published by Froriep in his *Journal* in 1842,[13] who referred to a confirmation of Gruby's findings through microphotograms by Rayer and Montagne in Paris. Gruby also published some of his findings in the *Österreichische Medizinische Wochenschrift*, a medical Archive in Vienna, in 1843, and he and his work were highly regarded in Sweden by P. H. Malmsten, who gave to one of the pathogenic molds discovered by Gruby the name used until the present, *Trichophyton tonsurans*.

Finally, Gruby's interest turned also to diseases caused by parasitic mites, and in this field, too, he did remarkable pioneer work. He was the first to describe the scab produced in dogs by an acarus-mite, and in 1859 in the *Clinic European*,[14] and in German in the *Allgemeine Wiener Medizinische Zeitung* [15] reported on "the parasite, producing *erythema autumnale*" with an excellent microscopic picture of it.

NEW DISAPPOINTMENTS

Aware of the value of his contributions in the field of clinical microscopy, micrography, and mycology, and of the success of his courses, Gruby tried to become associated with the Paris University or at least with the Veterinary School in Alfort (82) and to acquire French citizenship. We do not know the details of this endeavor—I was not able to find any traces of it in the archives of the Paris medical faculty. Whether here, too, at a time and in a country ruled by bias and discrimination, his Jewish faith lost him the well-deserved teaching position cannot be established. Perhaps the fact that all his life Gruby spoke French poorly and with a pronounced accent had something to do with it. We know only that he did not succeed in resuming a university career in Paris. According to Blanchard he did not even obtain French citizenship, but received only permission to stay in France (December 1, 1846). He became a French citizen in May 1848 (61).

At that time, the political situation in France was still more tense than in the year 1840 when Gruby settled in Paris. In 1848, the February revolution finally ended the kingdom of France, and the Second Republic was created. Adolphe Cremieux as Minister of Justice became the most prominent figure in the Cabinet and under him his friend and physician, Gruby, was naturalized on May 6, 1848, as a French citizen (6). He received the Grande Naturalization. However, he did not obtain his license to practice medicine until six years later (1854).

It was Gruby's fate for a second time to be denied a position entitling him to study and teach in connection

[12] 1: 469, 1846.

[13] Nos. 504 and 524.

[14] 1: 171, 1859.

[15] 6: 19, 1861.

with a university when he had just started brilliant research work. When this happened to him the first time, he had left Vienna in 1840; now, in 1845, he apparently slowed down his research work, lost interest in the laboratory he had built and in his courses, and turned mainly to practicing medicine. His publications in the *Proceedings* of the Académie des Sciences became scarcer after 1845, and he devoted his time and interest, without a legal license, to his steadily growing practice. This soon brought him into serious trouble.

START OF MEDICAL PRACTICE

One night Gruby received an urgent call to see a person in the house where he was living, who apparently was dying. He found the patient in critical condition, owing principally to improper treatment by the French physician. Gruby stopped the treatment and the patient was well after three days. The French physician, however, filed a lawsuit against the doctor from abroad who had dared to interfere with his medical work, effectively, it is true, but nevertheless illegally. This was a serious offense, especially since a Medical Congress at its Paris session in 1845 had decided on the strict prevention of the practice of medicine by physicians not licensed in France. Such violation could indeed result in the gravest legal consequences for the offender. Gruby had only received his permit of steady residence as foreigner in Paris on December 1, 1846 (6). Gruby's patients felt deeply with their beloved and now threatened physician. They flocked to his home to express their sympathy, and some of them presented him with a beautiful medal struck in his honor as a token of their affection.

Renowned and friendly physicians, such as the surgeon Denonvillier, knowing Gruby as physician of members of his own family, and the dean of the medical faculty, Bérard, tried energetically to help their eminent colleague, and some of his prominent patients intervened in Gruby's behalf. Finally, he received his license to practice medicine in 1854.

In these days of his youth in Paris the young doctor

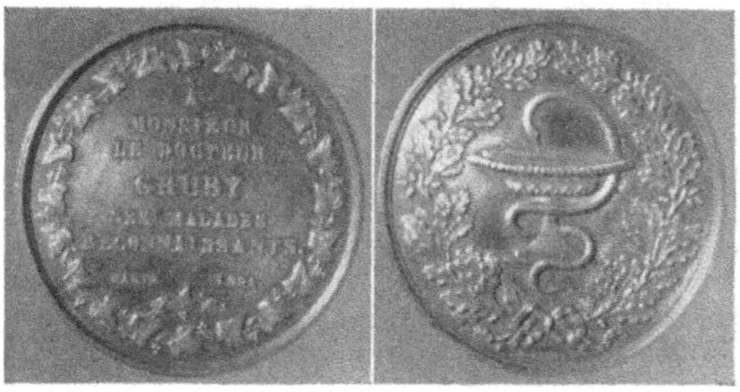

FIG. 34. Medal (by B. Marrel) dedicated to Dr. Gruby by thankful patients when he was endangered in 1851. Courtesy of the Welsh Medical Library, Johns Hopkins University, Baltimore, Md.

delighted in having company at his house, and gay, animated symposia with friends. A student who visited him in 1848 described two such evenings he spent with Dr. Gruby (64), and we have similar reports of visitors who saw Gruby at the end of the 1850's (80). A vivid picture is given of the group that gathered at that time, evening after evening around Dr. Gruby in his home, where he gave goulash parties and served the excellent Hungarian wine from Tokay, enjoying philosophical and other discussions with his guests. Attending these gatherings were old friends, patients of his, politicians, artists, musicians, and poets, a salon of interesting personalities, and among them some poor, Jewish students from Hungary (64), who came to see their famous compatriot and found him even on his busiest days always with an ear willing to listen to their worries and a hand open to help them with their financial problems.

Such a Jewish student reports that when he saw Gruby at his home in Paris in 1848 and spoke to him about his own difficulties in that city, Gruby took him immediately into another room where, in the sight of no more than their own four eyes he gave the young man a large sum in such a manner as though he had been indebted to him and was glad to be able now to pay back what he owed. As a visitor in 1859 reports, never was a certain dignity lacking in Gruby's congenial gatherings after the day's work was finished, and never did Gruby indulge in frivolities during them (80), but each aspect of human life and psychology drew his deepest interest and evoked a lively discussion. This same admirer emphasizes (80) that Gruby as a physician always had at the bedside the approach of the researcher and physiologist to clinical problems, and unlike the ordinary physician, emphasized the influence of food, clothing and daily habits of life on health and disease. In France in those days this was a most unusual procedure for a practitioner and it was one more factor in Gruby's great success as a physician. He personally went to the markets to study the quality and the condition of the food, and as this witness confirms (80):

> There was no housewife who would have had a better knowledge of the quality of milk and butter in every place in the center of Paris than he. Nobody knew the secret of the large and small restaurants, of the large and small empoisoneurs better, and he could teach a butcher the special qualities of the various kinds of mutton. He investigated the several markets and was at home in the different slaughter houses.

These types of knowledge were extraordinary in a physician in those days and so were his interest and talent for all mechanical work.

The same visitor writes:

> It is extremely amusing to see how Gruby with a practical eye tries to reform everything that surrounds man from morning till evening, from the cradle to the grave, and how his knowledge of physics helps him in this work. On

clothing and bedding, on stoves and lamps, on everything he puts his improving hand, and his apartment is a peculiar kind of museum of objects which everyone wants to own, too, but which, indeed, can be found nowhere except in his home.

There is no question that a physician of such original character with a good background of knowledge and experience and a sound judgment of human qualities and shortcomings, and above all being an excellent psychologist, must have attracted many patients, especially among the intellectual, higher classes of Paris, and indeed Gruby soon developed a most lucrative practice. Among the celebrities of the Second Empire many—such as Dumas Père and Dumas Fils, Chopin, Lamartine, Alphonse Daudet, Adolphe Cremieux, George Sand, Moritz Hartmann, Heinrich Heine—were his patients. Ludwig Bamberger (1) was a close friend of the poet, Moritz Hartmann, who during a protracted illness (periostitis or osteomyelitis) was attended by Gruby in Paris. Bamberger in his autobiography gives an eye-witness report on Gruby's activities. He praises not only Gruby's high qualities as physician, but also his devotion to Hartmann, who, as the beloved center of the foreign intelligentsia, always had in his room a coterie of famous foreigners to keep him company.

We learn from Bamberger not only how absorbed Gruby was in his animal experiments still in the early fifties of the nineteenth century, but also the names of the celebrities who in those years were friends and close acquaintances of the famous patient and his famous doctor. Among them were the Hungarian, Frederic Szarvady, stanch follower of the revolutionary Kossuth who introduced Gruby as a physician to Hartmann. There was the Comtesse d'Agoult, future mother-in-law of the composer Richard Wagner, and Cosima, daughter of the Comtesse and Franz Liszt. The Austrian poet Alfred Meissner and the Russian poet Ivan Turgenev were members of this illustrious coterie. Gruby's reputation among these personalities was well deserved. He had a critical mind, was a fine understanding psychologist and never prescribed more of strong drugs than he thought necessary. His use of cotton for the most diverse purposes in medicine since the 1840's—when no colleague of his in Paris did so—may also have contributed to his success as a practitioner. The aged Professor Charles Laubry in Paris told this writer that he remembers how in his youth he watched on the street respectfully from a distance the still legendary as well as famous Dr. Gruby.

Innumerable were the tales regarding his psychosomatic method of treating patients and his miraculous success with allegedly incurable diseases (6, 57, 82). One such case may be mentioned, reported by Ludwig Bamberger, who was living in Paris at the time and was an acquaintance of the patient in question (1). This lady was suffering from a supposedly incurable chronic pain in the throat. Gruby's prescription was: You will buy daily in a certain shop a bag full of Spanish grapes; you will carry them to the garden of the Palais Royal, where you will arrive daily before twelve noon. At noon at each single stroke of the clock you will swallow one single grape without crushing it. The lady did so and was soon entirely cured.

Gruby's kindness was known to everyone in Paris. His fees were moderate (as a rule 10 francs) and he seldom sent out bills. If urged by his patients, he would send them only a statement of the services rendered but never bills. Sundays were devoted to charity patients. Nevertheless, Gruby made a fortune as a practicing physician, as can be seen from his patriotic expenditures during the Franco-Prussian War and the estate he left when he died in 1898 (57).

As mentioned previously, from 1846 on Gruby's research fell off substantially in favor of his activities as a general practitioner.

It happens, though rarely, that a young scientist, after an extremely promising start in research and fundamental discoveries, suddenly turns away from science and never again returns to the field of his early success. That was, as is well known, the case with the Italian Marchese Corti who, after having discovered Cortis' organ in the ear in his thirties, and after having made important discoveries relating to the histology of the retina of the eye, took up the life of an Italian country nobleman, forsaking medicine forever (49). Most of Gruby's biographers see him in this same light. But that is incorrect; Gruby was not only a fine psychologist, he was also a philosopher who would not change the entire trend of his life because of a discouraging experience. We have one small booklet of his, published in the field of philosophy. It is entitled *De l'Homme et de la Machine* (Paris, 1866), and was reprinted by Le Leu.

Even though Gruby may have felt hurt by his double experience with universities and the disregard for his discoveries displayed by his colleagues of the faculty, he never during his life really stopped being the ardent student and independent research worker he had been as a young man. He never was unfaithful to the ideal activities of a research physician, which he praised in his publication of 1839 (21). The courses he gave so successfully were conducted up to 1854 even though he had no connection with the teaching of the medical faculty.

Evidence that his interest in research remained very much alive even later can be found, for instance, in his presentation in September 1855 of the kidney of a cow at a meeting of the Biological Society in Paris (37). This cow had a hydronephrosis containing sixty-six pounds of fluid; neither stones nor ureteral obstruction was found. The fluid was analyzed by Berthelot.

PHYSIOLOGICAL STUDIES ON NARCOSIS

Gruby's interest and working hours, as far as they were not devoted to his medical practice, soon turned to new fields of research, and here again he did important work whose value medicine never recognized and for which it gave him no credit.

In 1847 and 1848 Gruby performed animal experiments on the effects of the new sensational anesthetics, ether and chloroform. It was on October 16, 1846, that Morton performed his first successful ether narcosis in the Massachusetts General Hospital in Boston. The news was published in November, 1846, and only two months later the surgeon Velpeau reported at the January 1847 meeting of the Paris Académie des Sciences (75), when priority of this great discovery was claimed by Ducros and by Jackson, on his first clinical experiences with the new anesthetic. He continued his reports at the following meetings (January 25 and February 1) and so did Roux, the surgeon. Only at the February 1 meeting did a physiologist take the floor in the Académie to express his opinion. It was Magendie, sixty-three years of age, world-renowned and the outstanding representative of physiology in France (58).

In extremely strong words he discouraged the use of the new anesthetic. He did not offer any constructive comment or experimental explanation. He objected to the use of ether because he doubted its advantage to the clinic and, besides, he regarded it as a danger to the public morale. He said "For my part, and I believe that every man with self-respect will join my sentiments, I would not agree for any reason to be put in a situation where my entirely defenseless body is given into the hands of a surgeon who may be unskilled, not capable, and inattentive."

A vehement discussion between Velpeau, Magendie, Roux, and others followed this onslaught of destructive criticism from the master physiologist of France and was continued in some of the following meetings. However, by the following week at the meeting of February 8, the Académie already received the valuable report of two other physiologists. Flourens described experiments performed on the spinal cord of a narcotized dog and rabbit (14) and Serres reported on experiments on the direct influence of ether on exposed nerves (71). But it was Gruby who at the same meeting presented an elaborate discussion of his physiological experiments on the effect of ether anesthesia on various animals (34).

Gruby's experiments on ether and chloroform narcosis were published in the *Comptes Rendus des Séances de l'Académie des Sciences* of Paris (34, 35, 36). In a short time he had conducted comparative studies on frog, mouse, rabbit, young and old dogs, with respect to the time required to narcotize these animals, the duration of the narcosis and the time it takes to kill them by narcosis. He summarized his findings in thirty-four precise statements. Gruby emphasized a point which neither Magendie nor Flourens had mentioned, to wit, the wonderful opportunity of using narcotized animals for physiological experiments, for instance to study microscopically the circulation in the capillaries of the liver, kidney, lungs, and transparent membranes of frogs, in the mesenterium of rabbit and dog, and the circulation in lymph vessels. It is further proof of Gruby's fine personality that he was the first to advocate that in the future animal experiments should be performed on narcotized animals. For this suggestion alone Gruby deserved that a monument be erected to him by an organization to prevent cruelty to animals.

Gruby described the progredient decrease after an initial increase in the rate of respiration as a consequence of ether inhalation, and the decrease in the heart rate when the animal is narcotized to death, and the increase in both these functions as soon as the narcosis is interrupted before it is too late. In frogs the beginning of the narcotized stage is delayed after loss of blood, severe wounds, and decerebration. In young dogs the state of narcosis is reached more quickly than in old dogs, but the narcosis wears off more quickly, too. Circulation in the capillaries is maintained even in deep narcosis, but there may be a partial stasis in the capillaries in protracted narcosis. Gruby observed that muscles retain their contractibility for a time in dogs narcotized so deeply that no spontaneous movement of the extremities occurs, and when they do not react to pinching or pricking with a needle. Even if narcosis is protracted to a standstill in breathing, the dog may be resuscitated by a phlebotomy. Gruby also described the initial state of excitation in dogs when ether narcosis is performed and compared it to the effect of alcohol.

As an effect of chloroform narcosis, Gruby especially called attention, in 1847 (35) and 1848, (36) to the brighter color of the venous blood of dogs during narcosis than before narcosis. He also emphasized the higher toxicity of chloroform, and its quicker action compared with ether narcosis.

His practical approach to biological problems becomes evident in his reference to the fact that the meat of animals, even after it is boiled, is not edible if they were narcotized with ether, but chloroform narcosis does not spoil its taste.

Gruby's studies, in animal experiments, on the pharmacology of ether narcosis were indeed the very first of their kind. Yet when the centenary year of 1946 brought us books and papers on the history of ether narcosis, these books had nothing special to say about Gruby's pioneer work, not even noting his emphasis on the need for a sufficient oxygen supply in inhalation narcosis (36: 176). This neglect and ignorance of Gruby's contribution to the early studies in this field may be due to the fact that early writers on this subject, such as the American Buckminster Brown (7), the Frenchman Henry Chambert (8), and the German surgeon J. F. Dieffenbach (12), writing in 1847 and

1848, cited the discussions of Professors Velpeau, Roux, Magendie, and Flourens in the Paris Academy early in 1847, but they did not mention the statements of one Doctor Gruby, who was not even an *agrée* at one of the big Paris hospitals.[16] Later authors probably did not take the trouble to check the original sources for themselves. Shortly afterwards Gruby gave up this type of research, presenting the familiar tragic figure in the history of medicine: the able scientist, denied the privilege of having his own laboratory and adequate help; the brilliant teacher denied the opportunity of teaching in a school; the outsider whose very valuable contributions were ignored by those of the inner circle.

WAR MEDICINE AND THE MEDICAL USE OF COTTON

Soon, however, other important and demanding problems were on Gruby's mind. It was the time of the empire of Napoleon III when wars in and outside of Europe absorbed the interest of everyone in France.

During the period between Gruby's settlement in Paris and the catastrophe of 1870 there was the Revolution of 1848 and the war in the Crimean Peninsula (1854–1856), in which France was involved, and the war of Austria in 1859. France took part in the war in China in 1860; she observed the war between Prussia and Austria in 1866, and finally in 1870 the Franco-Prussian War ended the Second Empire.

Gruby, who had gradually discontinued his anatomical and microscopical research work for an extensive practice, was on the other hand, through his practical activities as a physician, becoming increasingly interested in clinical problems and in the problems of military medicine and surgery, at this time a new field for modern medical consideration.

It is hard to understand how it was that Gruby, who found fungi to be the cause of varied skin diseases and who was the first to observe microfilaria in mammals and trypanosomas in frogs, was not aware of the tremendous importance of the new discoveries in the field of clinical bacteriology. However, we know that even a man like the surgeon Billroth was for a long time very hesitant in accepting this new gospel. Gruby stubbornly refused to recognize the importance of germs in different diseases, and in his later years he no longer believed in the value of vaccination. Indeed, he was an active member in the anti-vaccination societies of England and Germany, though in his first German paper in 1839 he praised vaccination and its blessings. During the last years of his life he suffered from a purulent infection of the bladder, but when his physician, Delefosse, suggested disinfectant bladder irrigations, Gruby rejected the treatment; so far did his disapproval of the germ-theory of infectious diseases go (11).

Despite this incomprehensible attitude, Gruby contributed a most important suggestion and valuable clinical experience to the progress of asepsis in medicine, especially in surgery and war medicine. In 1859, through various publications, he effectively urged the wide use of cotton in medicine, surgery, gynecology, and, above all, for wound dressings. It was mainly through his influence that the use of lint (charpie) and similar material in surgery was eliminated in France.

This fundamental contribution was first published in 1859 in *Clinique Européen,* an international medical journal published weekly in Paris by Dr. Kraus of Vienna and Dr. Pichler of Paris. A long article by Gruby on this subject appeared in the January 29 and February 5, 1859 issues [17] on pages 36 and 45 of this journal. A short time later the article was reprinted in the German language in the *Allgemeine Wiener Medizinische Zeitung,*[18] a journal edited by the same two physicians, Dr. Kraus and Dr. Pichler. In these articles Gruby revealed that for many years he had used cotton exclusively in his practice instead of lint, and he assailed the dangerous and disagreeable use of lint (charpie). Modestly he disclaims any priority for this suggestion. According to Gruby, Hebra in the Department of Dermatology of the Vienna Hospital often used cotton in the treatment of skin diseases. It may be concluded from this remark that Gruby personally knew Hebra, who once was also a pupil of Gruby's teacher, the surgeon Wattmann. As a matter of fact, a short note on the use of cotton on wounds produced by blister plasters was also published in 1838 by a Dr. Koch in Laichingen, a little village in South Germany (55). But these few lines had no lasting effect and were apparently not known to Gruby.

In his enthusiasm for the clinical use of cotton Gruby followed Mathias Mayor, a physician in Lausanne, Switzerland, who devoted a pamphlet and two chapters of a surgical book to this topic (60). However, even in the third edition of this book (1838), Mayor still complained (p. 60) that nobody followed his advice and that all the outstanding surgeons of his time abhorred the use of cotton and preferred the dirtiest lint to clean cotton. Gruby now indicated many new medical uses for cotton, which today are a matter of course. It is doubtful whether Gruby knew of Mayor's book. He does not mention it, as he mentions Hebra, but he became one of the first to use and to preach the use of cotton as an indispensable material of widespread application in medicine. He suggested cotton for the following purposes: to dress every kind of wound, not only skin lesions, to prepare tampons of cotton for the nose, and to use cotton as a carrier for medications to be applied in cavities of the body. He emphasizes that cotton is less irritating and can be more easily removed than lint, and makes the keen observation that wounds heal

[16] Gruby's contributions are mentioned in the book by Fulton and Stanton (16).

[17] Nos. 5 and 6.

[18] 4: 71, 75, 91, 1859.

more quickly and more frequently *per primam intentionem* (without infectious complications) in cases where cotton is used in preference to lint (charpie). Like Hebra and Koch, he used it to cover the skin in cases of skin diseases (intertrigo, for instance) and skin lesions and in burns and frostbite, in rheumatic joint diseases to cover and protect the joints, and for cataplasms. He recommended the use of cotton by the surgeon many years prior to Guérin (1870), by the gynecologist, the ophthalmologist, and the dentist, and in the treatment of the ear, nose, and mouth. All Gruby's experiences with this material are today well known to every practitioner; they may account in part for the enormous success Gruby had as a physician.

This one achievement alone would entitle Gruby to be remembered in the history of medicine, especially in the history of surgery, as well as of military medicine.

Besides his publicizing the use of cotton, Gruby's sympathetic intellect was later occupied largely with the desire to alleviate and reduce the suffering of war victims on the battlefields. Nothing can give a more vivid picture of Gruby's mind and character than a paragraph from his report on the World's Fair in Paris in 1867 (38). There he describes the apparatus and instruments used in first aid in wartime. He outlines the purpose of war medicine on the battlefields in classic form, saying (in literal translation): "Because the science of war devotes all its genius to the problem of finding the best means of destroying as much of the world as possible in the shortest time possible, the genius of beneficial charity ought to find the means of providing for each victim the most immediate help he needs."

Gruby, who since childhood and youth had known what it meant to suffer helplessly, and who also knew from his later years what it meant to be defenseless against bias and prejudice, had a compassionate heart for every weak creature. That led him in 1847 to sponsor the idea of using narcotized animals for experiments. He did not even permit horseshoes to be put on the hoofs of his three horses (6, 57), lovingly tended all the plants and pet animals in his home, and always took good care of his old horses until their death.

For many years his mind was occupied with the problem of how best and most quickly to help the wounded on the battlefields. He is supposed to have been the first in France to design a stretcher on wheels. One of his last publications contains pictures of various stretchers and portable chairs for wounded soldiers that he had constructed for use in wartime and also a collapsible hospital tent to be set up at the place where it was most needed in war (39). Such a mobile hospital-tent was to provide the wounded with all the necessary comforts, an adequate heating system and supply of fresh air. He did not abandon this excellent idea when the war of 1870 was over. Such a hospital, of iron and canvas, movable and well-furnished, aired and heated, was actually constructed according to his plan and at his expense. It was set up in Paris and received the Grand Prix at the Paris exhibition of 1889.

When, in the same year, an epidemic of grippe (influenza) swept France, and all the hospitals were overcrowded with the sick and dying, Gruby's great hospital tent served very well the charitable purpose for which it was created. This may also have been one of the reasons why in the following year, 1890, the Octagenarian Gruby was made a Knight of the French Legion of Honor. In view of his patriotic and selfless activities during the War of 1870, he well deserved this public recognition twenty years earlier, but in 1871 he was awarded only the *Croix de bronze* by the French Committee of the Red Cross.

Among his other contributions during the Franco-Prussian War were the following: In his house in Montmartre he maintained at his own expense a hospital of forty beds acting as head physician and surgeon. He also donated many thousands of francs for equipment for soldiers, and he generously supported the Italian hospital in the Rue Taitbout.

MEDICAL METEOROLOGY

During the years when Gruby took care of many patients daily, beloved and adored by them and denounced as a charlatan by many of his colleagues, everyone in Paris was familiar with the peculiar carriage of the stout and eccentric little doctor—the carriage having its only window on top. At this time Doctor Gruby not only devoted himself to the problems of war medicine, but spent a great deal of time and money on another scientific hobby—astronomy and meteorology. This interest of his was even mentioned on his tombstone. In his house on Montmartre he set up in 1860 an observatory with good telescopes which he placed at the disposal of the French Government during the Franco-Prussian War. Another laboratory for meteorological observations was established in his house, 100 Rue Lepic, with the interesting purpose of establishing a laboratory for medical meteorology. Here again Gruby exhibited his extraordinary vision for problems related to modern medicine. Even now, this field opened by Gruby is still very unsatisfactorily studied. Gruby's interest in medical meteorology was so great that he published a monthly bulletin under the name: *Bulletin Météorologique de L'Observatoire Gruby, Rue Lepic 100.* He personally constructed various astronomical instruments, and Blanchard (6) had a clock designed and made by Gruby himself. This clock had to be wound only once in three months and worked perfectly.

In the War of 1870, Gruby's observatory at Montmartre was directed by Colonel Sozdat, the Director of the Musée des Arts et Metiers, and proved to be very helpful during the siege of Paris. Up to the time of

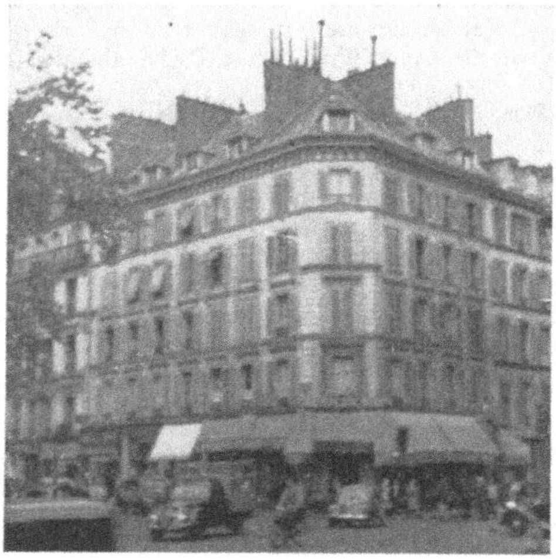

FIG. 35. Gruby's great corner building, Rue St. Lazare 66, where he lived for a long time and where he died in his big duplex apartment. Photo. taken by the author.

Gruby's death his meteorological station was still working under Casse and the aeronaut Jovis.

FINALE

During the years when Gruby was not publishing medical research in the *Proceedings* of the Paris Academy of Sciences, he did not refrain, as we have seen, from all scientific investigation. Further evidence of this is the fact that after his death, Blanchard and Le Leu found in his house on Montmartre a veritable museum of hundreds of preparations, especially carefully injected ones, skeletons and mulages and, in addition, about 15,000 microscopical slides and 2,000 photomicrograms. In the field of photomicrography Gruby, next to Mandl, was one of the outstanding pioneers in France. It is a great pity and loss that in later years he did not publish any of his findings, and that all this material, except for what was acquired by Blanchard, was destroyed or lost after his death just because nobody took a real interest in it.

With advancing age Gruby gradually lost interest in all these pursuits. The elderly bachelor became a lonely and odd personality, confining his activities to his patients, his pet animals, and his plants that crowded his rooms. It was a secluded life he led in his beautiful spacious house at Rue St. Lazare 66. He still maintained two more apartments in his houses at Montmartre and Rue Lepic, but during the last years of his life he probably never visited them. Like his first apartment in Paris at Git le Cœur No. 5, this last one in his own house on the Rue St. Lazare was typical of his taste and personality. It is still there, a large corner house facing the plaza in front of the big Trinity Church, close to the great boulevards. In the foyer of the house, in a niche, still stands the bust of the son of Napeleon III, a reminder that the second empire was the time of Gruby's greatest success as a well-to-do practitioner, in a happy and successful Paris and France.

In 1885 Gruby hired as a librarian for his collection of about 8,000 volumes housed in his duplex apartment on Rue St. Lazare, a Mr. Le Leu, who soon became his private secretary, and in this capacity remained with him until 1898. Gruby's popularity, even in his old age, is confirmed by Le Leu who, ten years after his employer's death, found a publisher and sponsors for a 285-page book on Gruby's last years, entitled *Le Dr. Gruby. Notes et Souvenirs.*

When Le Leu entered the service of Doctor Gruby, the latter was already seventy-five years old and apparently retired from all medical research work. There were still many patients coming to see him. What

L. LE LEU

LE

Dr GRUBY

NOTES ET SOUVENIRS

PARIS — 1er
P.-V. STOCK, EDITEUR
(Ancienne Librairie TRESSE & STOCK)
155, RUE SAINT-HONORÉ, 155
DEVANT LE THÉATRE-FRANÇAIS
—
1908

FIG. 36. Title page of Le Leu's biography of Gruby.

Le Leu witnessed, however, was more or less the final chapter in the book of life of a once very efficient, busy, and up to his death, most interesting personality. He met in Gruby a stout, lively little gentleman with blue eyes and a bald head, extremely meticulous in his appearance, eccentric in his behavior and manner of living. Patients came to see him in the morning from ten until twelve. At noontime, for lunch, and afterwards he retired to the inner sanctuary of his apartment, to a room that even Le Leu almost never entered. Gruby's physician was not admitted into this room, even during Gruby's last sickness (11). From two o'clock on patients came again or he went to see them. Being very much interested in gastro-intestinal diseases and dietetic treatment, he continued, even in his old age, to go to the food market to purchase all that was needed for the kitchen: fowl, fish, fruit, potatoes. He selected them himself. According to Reich's biography (64), already as a young doctor he was known as an expert, not only on gastronomic problems, but on all questions pertaining to what we today call "hygiene of food and alimentation." His personal food requirements were very simple. When the gay time of his younger years was over, he entertained with food and philosophical discussions a small group of his closest remaining friends twice a month, on Friday evenings, in his house. He was especially pleased whenever he received from his home country, Hungary, any kind of cake or fruit, which he enjoyed more than anything else, even though Le Leu was very often not able to share this patriotic enthusiasm. In the evenings after dinner, he dictated letters to his secretary, who would then work until 11 o'clock or later. Upon retiring at bedtime, Gruby would daily grease his entire body carefully and cover it with a kind of tissue paper.

Gruby was a heavy smoker of cigars and pipes, but that did not prevent him from becoming a member of the French society against the misuse of tobacco, and he even sponsored a hundred franc prize of the society for the best paper against tobacco smoking. The man who won this award with a learned paper was his secretary, Le Leu, himself a very heavy smoker. Gruby's membership in this society was chiefly an act of friendship toward its founder, his old friend M. Decroix, a military veterinarian whom he knew from the time of his research activities at the veterinary school in Alfort. Decroix was also known for his sponsorship of hypophagy, which means persuading people to eat horse meat. On this subject, however, we have no proof that Gruby ever followed his advice.

Gruby, who was admired by all his patients, male and female, never wore any kind of jewelry, not even a watch chain; his only personal luxury, an excellent gold pocket watch, was buried from sight in his vest pocket.

In contrast to Gruby's meticulously clean and proper appearance was his apartment. The room with the extensive library looked like a storage room, with books in tall heaps all over the floor and those on the shelves scarcely accessible. New magazines and books came in daily, most of them never read; at least during the last years of his life, Gruby, who never stopped buying books, did not have the time to read them. He liked to buy other things, too, whenever he saw anything interesting, and he never threw anything away, so that his entire apartment, including the rooms to which patients were admitted, was overcrowded, filled with bric-a-brac like an old curiosity shop. Often, when patients came, it was a problem to make chairs available for them, every piece of furniture carrying its cargo.

In the late 80's and in the 90's the rooms in Gruby's apartment not meant for visitors were even worse. Le Leu had only a small table on which to do his secretarial work, part of the writing material and documents having to lie on the floor. The rooms of the house were filled with an inconceivable chaos of objects that were never used. Gruby also kept always a number of pet animals and flowers; the latter he watered regularly and so abundantly that the tenants of the apartment below his were continually getting watered along with them. Food that he bought or that came from Hungary was stored there also; even when it began to rot,

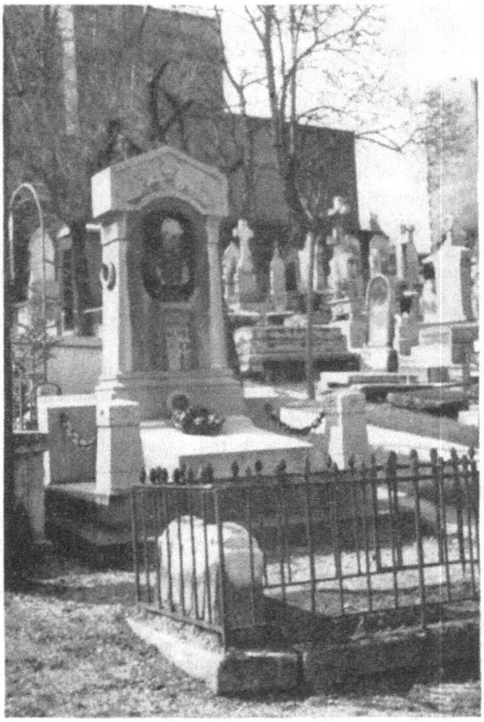

FIG. 37. Gruby's tombstone in the cemetery of St. Vincente in Paris. Photo. taken by the author in 1952.

it was rarely removed. When, after his death, Le Leu and Blanchard went through his two other apartments, they found still worse chaos. Scientific preparations heaped together with putrefying legs of horses, broken containers not checked by anyone for many years and smelling terribly, filled this private museum of comparative zoology. The description Le Leu gives of Gruby's home reminds us very much of Goethe's account in his day and year diaries of the state in which he found the apartment of his friend, the physicist, Professor Büttner in Jena, when the latter died.

Up to his eighty-eighth year, the last year of his life, Gruby was in fairly good physical health, seeing patients, receiving and writing letters, interested in everything that happened in the world. Only in his last year did his health decline. Patients dropped away, and finally there were none left. When he felt that the end of his life was near, he retired to his bedroom and nobody was permitted to enter. This room, of course, did not deserve the name of bedroom. When, after his death, the police, Le Leu, and the servants entered it, they found no bed, and it was evident that for many years Gruby had not slept in a bed, but either in his chair or on the floor. There his body was found on November 14, 1898, after he had not answered his servants' calls for two days. The police were summoned, the room was opened, and there he was, dead on the floor, lonely in death as he had been in life.

Gruby left no last will, and no wife or children. His various relatives fell heir to about 300,000 francs. His belongings, including his library and real estate, brought this sum. At the public auction where everything was sold, some of his instruments were bought by a German bookdealer from the Librairie H. Welter (5); most of his scientific manuscripts and preparations, especially the photomicrographs, were purchased by his biographer, Blanchard, who kept part of them for his own laboratory and donated the others to various public collections such as the Bibliothèque du Musée d'Histoire Naturelle in Paris, the Laboratoire d'Histoire Naturelle des Ecoles Veterinaires d'Alfort and to that of Toulouse, and a part to the Bureau of Animal Industry of the American Department of Agriculture (5) in Washington, D. C., where they are probably hidden away in some drawer, but I was not able to trace them there.

Gruby is buried in the cemetery of Saint Vincent near Montmartre. First buried in the Cimetière du Nord (Montmartre), his body was transferred on January 14, 1899, to his last resting place in Cimetière de St. Vincent nearby (13 Division, 1 Ligne), where a beautiful tombstone marks the place. In a niche of the monument made of artificial stone is a fine life size bronze bust by Georges Lemaire, showing the ribbon of the Légion d'Honneur in his lapel. The stone bears the inscription, "Au Docteur Gruby 1810–1898." Among leaves, flowers, and stars can be seen a cup,

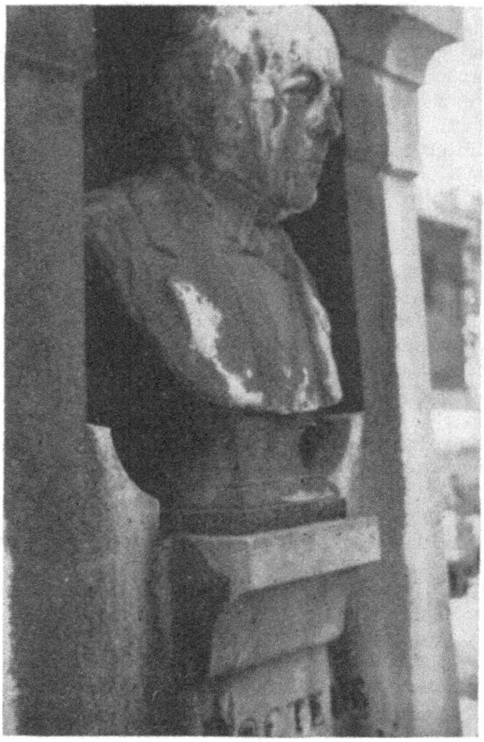

FIG. 38. Bust of Gruby at his tombstone in Paris. Photo. taken by the author.

two serpents, and two telescopes, and a ribbon with the inscription: "Médicine, Science, Astronomie."

The grave is kept clean and in good order, but none of the employees of the cemetery was able to tell me who takes care of it. Gruby left no descendants or close relatives in Paris, only a group of thankful patients and admirers. When I visited Gruby's burial place fifty-four years after his death, it was conspicuous among the other generally very neglected graves by its clean, dignified, and tasteful appearance. In a small wreath of artificial material I found a fresh branch of a tree placed there by someone apparently a short time before.

REFERENCES

1. BAMBERGER, L. 1899. Erinnerungen. Berlin, G. Reimer.
2. BAZIN, ANTOINE P. E. 1858. Leçons théoriques et cliniques sur les affections cutanées parasitaires. Paris, F. Chamerot.
3. BEESON, B. B. 1931. David Gruby, M.D., 1810–1898. *Archiv. of Dermat. and Syph.* **23**: 141–144.
4. BERG, F. F. 1842. De la structure anatomico-microscopique du muguet. Lettre a M. le Dr. Gruby. *Clinique des hôpiteaux des enfants* **2**: 143 and 191.
5. BLANCHARD, RAPHAEL. 1899, 1900. David Gruby. *Chronique Médical* **6**: 96 and **7**: 42.

6. ——. 1899. David Gruby (1810–1898). *Arch. de Parasitol.* 2: 43–74.

7. Brown, Buckminster. 1847. On the pathological and physiological effects of ethereal inhalation. Boston, D. Clapp.

8. Chambert, H. 1848. Des effects physiologiques thérapeutiques des éthers. Paris, J. B. Baillière.

9. Delafond, O. 1838. Traité de la Pathologie General Vétérinaire. Paris, Dupont.

10. ——. 1838. Traité sur la police sanitaire des animaux domestiques. Paris, Dupont.

11. Delefosse, D. 1900. Chronique Médical 7: 125.

12. Dieffenbach, J. F. 1847. Der Aether gegen den Schmerz. Berlin, A. Hirschwald.

13. Ebstein, E. 1929. David Gruby (1810–1898) als Forscher und Arzt Heinrich Heine's. *Dermat. Wochenschr.* **88**: 507–510.

14. Flourens, Marie P. 1847. Note touchant les effets de l'inhalation éthérée sur la moelle épinière. *C. R. Acad. Sci. Paris.* **24**: 161–162.

15. Fülleborn, F. 1929. *Filariosen des Menschen.* In *Hand buch d. pathog. Microorg.* 6/2: 1097–1224. Jena and Berlin. G. Fischer and Urban & Schwarzenberg.

16. Fulton, J. F., and M. E. Stanton. 1946. The centenial of surgical anesthesia. New York, G. Schumann.

17. Gluge, G. 1842. Ueber ein eigentumliches Entozoon im Blute des Frosches. *Müller's Archiv* 1842: 148.

18. Goldzieher, W. 1884. Streptothrix Försteri im unteren Thränenröhrchen. *Cbl. f. Augenheilkunde* **8**: 33–35.

19. Grimaud de Caux and David Gruby. 1842. Description anatomique d l'organe qui fournit la liqueur purpurigène dans le Murex brandaris et analyse microscopique de cette liqueur. *C. R. Acad. Sci. Paris* **15**: 1007–1008.

20. Gruby, David. 1893. Observationes Microscopicae. Vienna, Singer & Goering.

21. ——. 1839. Ueber den diätetischen und pharmazeutischen Gebrauch des Quell-Brunnen-, und gereinigten Donauwassers. *Med. Jahrb. d. K. K. Oesterr. Staates.* **20**: 567–586.

22. ——. 1841. Mémoire sur une végétation qui constitue la vraie teigne. *C. R. Acad. Sci., Paris* **13**: 72–75.

23. ——. 1841. Sur les mycodermes qui constituent la teigne faveuse. *C. R. Acad. Sci. Paris* **13**: 309–311.

24. ——. 1941. Recherches anatomiques concernant le sysème veineux de la grenouille. *C. R. Acad. Sci. Paris* **13**: 923–926.

25. ——. 1842. Resultate microscopisch-pathologischer Untersuchungen. *Verh. d. K. K. Ges. D. Aerzte zu Wien* **1**: 184–194.

26. ——. 1842. Note sur les entozoaires de la grenouille et sur quelques points de la pathologie de ce Batracien. *C. R. Acad. Sci. Paris* **15**: 33–35.

27. ——. 1842. Note. *C. R. Acad. Sci. Paris* **15**: 71–72.

28. ——. 1842. Ueber Tinea favosa (aus brieflicher Mitteilung). *Müller's Archiv.* 1842: 22–24.

29. —— [misspelled Gruy]. 1842. Recherches anatomiques sur le système veineux de la grenouille. *Ann. des Sci. Nat.*, 2nd Ser., **17**: 209-230.

30. ——. 1843. Recherches et observations sur une nouvelle espèce d'hématozoaire, Trypanosoma sanguinis. *C. R. Acad. Sci. Paris* **17**: 1134–1136.

31. ——. 1844. Sur une nouvelle espèce de Haemotozoaire, Trypanosoma Sanguinis. *Ann. Sci. Nat.*, 3rd Ser., **1**: 104–107.

32. ——. 1844. Note sur des plants cryptogamiques se développant en grand masse dans l'estomac d'une malade atteinte, depuis huit ans, de difficulté dans la déglutition des aliments, soit liquides, soit solides. *C. R. Acad. Sci. Paris* **18**: 586–588.

33. ——. 1845. Recherches sur les Acarus, les Annélides, les cryptogames et la coloration noire qui constituent la maladie epidémiques des pommes de terre. *C. R. Acad. Sci. Paris* **21**: 696–697.

34. ——. 1847. Tableaux et conclusions des expériences faites sur l'inspiration des vapeurs d'éther chez les animaux. (Extrait par l'auteur.) *C. R. Acad. Sci. Paris* **24**: 192–194.

35. ——. 1847. Effets du chloroforme sur les animaux, comparés a ceux de l'éther. *C. R. Acad. Sci. Paris* **25**: 901–903.

36. ——. 1848. Action du chloroforme. *C. R. Acad. Sci. Paris* **26**: 175–176.

37. ——. 1855. Cas d'hydronephrose chez une vache. *C. R. Sci. Biol. Paris* **7**: 119–120.

38. ——. 1867. Appareils et instruments de l'art médical, materiel de secours a donner aux blessés sur les champs de bataille a l'exposition universelle de Paris. Paris, Lacroix.

39. ——. 1878. Rapports sur l'exposition universelle de 1878. Paris, Lacroix.

40. Gruby, David, and A. Delafond. 1843. Note sur une altération vermineuse du sang d'un chien, déterminée par un grand nombre d'hématozoaires du genre filaire. *C. R. Acad. Sci. Paris* **16**: 325–326.

41. Gruby, David, and O. Delafond. 1843. Résultats des recherches faites sur l'anatomie et les fonctions des villosités intestinales, l'absorption, la preparation et la composition organique du chyle dans les animaux. *C. R. Acad. Sci. Paris* **16**: 1194–1196.

42. Gruby, David, and O. Delafond. 1843. Note, contenue dans le paquet cacheté deposé. *C. R. Acad. Sci. Paris* **16**: 1197–1200.

43. Gruby, David, and O. Delafond. 1843. Recherches sur des animalcules se développant en grand nombre dans l'estomac et dans les intestins, pendant la digestion des animaux herbivores et carnivores. *C. R. Acad. Soc. Paris* **17**: 1304–1308.

44. Gruby, David, and O. Delafond. 1843. Résultats des recherches faites sur la composition organique de la lymphe chez les animaux. *C. R. Acad. Sci. Paris* **16**: 1369–1372.

45. Gruby, David, and O. Delafond. 1844. Deuxième note sur l'altération vermineuse du sang des chiens par l'hématozoaire du genre filaire. *C. R. Acad. Sci. Paris* **18**: 687–688.

46. Gruby, David, and O. Delafond. 1852. Troisième Mémoire sur le ver filaire qui vit dans le sang du chien domestique. *C. R. Acad. Sci. Paris* **34**: 9–14.

47. Henle, J. 1838. Ueber Schleim- und Eiterbildung und ihr Verhältnis zur Oberhaut. Berlin, Reimer.

48. Herzig, W. 1844. Das Medizinische Wien. Wien, Braumüller & Seidel.

49. Hintzsche, E. 1944. Alfonso Corti (1822–1876). Bern, P. Haupt.

50. Houben, H. H. 1926. Gespräche mit Heine. Frankfurt a.M., Rütten & Loening.

51. Houel, C. N. 1881. Catalogue du Musée Orfila. Paris, Dupont.

52. Hyrtl, Jos. 1869. Vergangenheit und Gegenwart des Museums für menschliche Anatomie an der Wiener Universität, Wien. W. Braumüller.

53. Kettner, 1841. Note. *C. R. Acad. Sci. Paris* **13**: 147.

54. Kisch, Wilhelm. 1883. Die alten Strassen und Plätze Wiens. Wien, M. Gottlieb.

55. Koch, D. 1838. *Monatsschr. f. med. Augenheilkunde und Chirurgie* **1**: 653–654.

56. Le Leu, L. 1898. La Mort du Docteur Gruby. *Le Figaro.* Nov. 16.

57. ——. 1908. Le Dr. Gruby. Notes et Souvenirs. Paris, P. V. Stock.
58. MAGENDIE, F. 1847. *Remarques. C. R. Acad. Sci. Paris* **24**: 134–138 and 142–144.
59. MAYOR, M. 1834. Sur le cotton et la charpie. Lausanne.
60. ——. 1838. Bandages et appareils à pansement. 3rd ed. Paris, Baillière.
61. MONTEMERLI, C. 1875. Biographie du Docteur Gruby offerte par les membres de la Companie humanitaire italienne à ses amis. Paris.
62. NEUBURGER, M. 1918. Entwicklung der Medizin in Oesterreich. Wien & Leipzig, C. Fromme.
63. OTTERBURG, S. J. 1841. Das medizinische Paris. Karlsruhe & Paris, A. Bielefeld.
64. REICH, IGNAZ. 1859. David Gruby. *Beth El.* **2**: 162–168.
65. REMAK, ROBERT. 1840. Zur Kenntnis von der pflanzlichen Natur der Porrigo Lupinosa. *Med. Ztg.* **9**: 73–74.
66. RILLE, J. H. 1926. David Gruby. *Dermat. Wochnschr.* **82**: 512–526.
67. ROSENTHAL, TH. 1932. David Gruby. (1810–1898.) *Ann. of Med. Hist.* **4**: 339–346.
68. SALAÜN, A. P. M. 1935. La Vie et l'œuvre de David Gruby. Doctoral Thesis, Bordeaux, J. Bière.
69. SABAURAUD, RAYMOND. 1894. Ta Teigne trichophytique et la Teigne spécial de Gruby. Paris, Rueff & Cie.
70. SABAURAUD, RAYMOND. 1910. Les maladies cryptogamic. Les Teignes. Paris, Masson & Cie (see p. 25).
71. SERRES, E. 1847. De l'action de l'éther liquide sur le tissu nerveux. *C. R. Acad. Sci. Paris* **24**: 162–168.
72. VALENTIN, G. 1840. Note. *Repertorium* **5**: 23 and 279–282.
73. ——. 1840. Zur Entwicklung der Gewebe des Muskel-des Blut-und des Nervensystems. *Müller's Archiv* 1840: 194–235.
74. ——. 1841. Ueber ein Entozoon im Blute von Salmo fario. *Müller's Archiv* 1841: 435–436.
75. VELPEAU, A. 1847. Remarques. *C. R. Acad. Sci. Paris* **24**: 76–78.
76. WUNDERLICH, C. A. 1841. Wien und Paris. Stuttgart, Ebner & Seubert.
77. ZAKON, S. J., and T. BENEDEK. 1944. David Gruby. *Bull. Histor. of Med.* **16**: 155–168.
78. 1840. Taschenbuch der Wiener K. K. Universitaet für das Jahr 1840. Wien, P. E. Mechitaristen.
79. 1850. Der Arzt Gruby in Paris. *Wiener Blätter* zu No. 4. Aug. 4, 1850: 31–32.
80. 1859. Dr. Gruby. *Orvosi Hetilap.* No. 47.
81. (No year. *ca.* 1860.) Médecins et Chirurgiens célèbres. Paris, Rosselin.
82. 1900. Ein Heilkünstlerleben. *Deutsche Med. Wchnschr.* **26**: 118–120.

III. ROBERT REMAK

1815–1865

INTRODUCTION

In 1815, the year when the town of Posen was turned over to the Prussian government after the final downfall of the empire of Napoleon I, Robert Remak was born to Jewish parents in the Ghetto of this town.

Except for anatomists, hardly anybody nowadays knows, even by name, this man whose discoveries are landmarks in the development of modern medicine. No bibliography of the work of this outstanding scholar existed up to the present. Even today not a great deal is known about Remak's personal life. A few lines here and there in the writings of his contemporaries, such as the pathologist Rudolf Virchow and the anatomist Waldeyer, furnish meager though important hints. A paper by Adam Wrzosek, who in 1925 published a short study on Remak's relationship to Poland (85), is valuable, and so is A. Kronthal's publication (45).[1] Besides these, there are a few biographical data, for instance, in the *Allgemeine Deutsche Biographie* by Pagel (55), some eulogies after Remak's death (3, 14, 92), and, last but not least, his *Vita* submitted with his doctoral thesis in 1838. This autobiographical outline is omitted in copies of this work, which were printed in the same year, 1838, not as a doctoral thesis, but as an independent publication.

Much valuable information supplementing these scanty data is available from Remak's own publications. These contain instructive personal details about the sort of work he did, his travels, and his acquaintances. In spite of all these sources of information, which were extensively used for the present sketch, his biography is still incomplete, owing partly to the inaccessibility of many archives in Germany at the present time and partly to their destruction in wartime. Probably a good deal of the pertinent material in private possession was also destroyed during the Nazi terror in Germany and in the course of military operations. A biographical sketch, published in 1915 by Professor Ludwig Geiger in the Jewish journal, *Allgemeine Zeitung des Judentums,* commemorated the centenary of Remak's birth. A compilation of excerpts from some of the previously mentioned eulogies, it does not add any new details, except for a photograph of Remak from the later years of his life (20). Remak's family gave Geiger not only this picture, but also the remaining fifteen letters Remak received between 1839 and 1855 from Alexander von Humboldt. These letters, deciphered and published by Geiger (21), represent an extremely valuable source of biographical material, especially for the years of Remak's struggle for a teaching position at the University of Berlin. They are at the same time valuable testimony to Humboldt's splendid character.

Two other very important and forgotten sources concerning the life of Remak exist and were consulted. One is the two-column eulogy of a student of philosophy, Adolf Ehrlich (14), published shortly after Remak's death in the Jewish journal, *Allgemeine Zeitung des Judentums,* in Leipzig on October 3, 1865. The value of this much-too-short outline of Remak's life lies in the fact that the data given were obtained from Remak's family, and consequently have a high degree of reliability. The other source is a book by M. Kalisch (40), published in Leipzig in 1860, which contains copies of all the documents in Governmental Archives pertaining to Remak's university career and other material of the greatest value dealing with the history and cultural life of the Jews in Germany in the first half of the nineteenth century, especially their relationship with the Prussian universities at that time. Nowhere in this book does Kalisch mention Remak's name or a title of his quoted publications, but if there

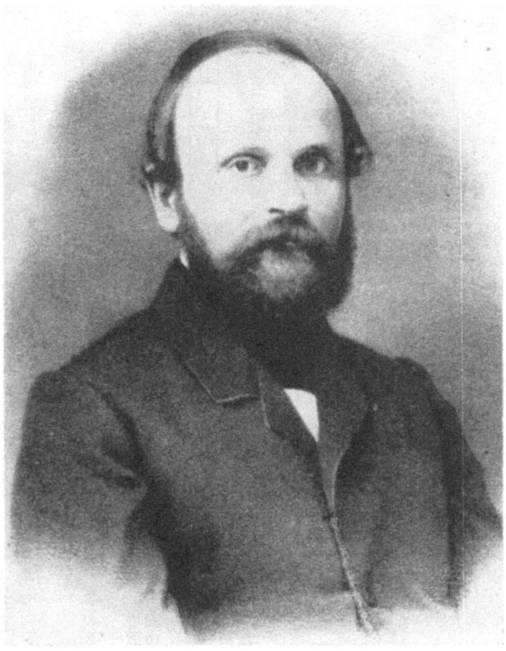

FIG. 39. Robert Remak. Courtesy of the Rare Book Department, Library of the Academy of Medicine, New York. Picture taken after 1859.

[1] Numbers in parentheses indicate references at end of chapter, p. 294.

REMAK'S FAMILY TREE

(*Courtesy Mrs. F. Litthauer*)

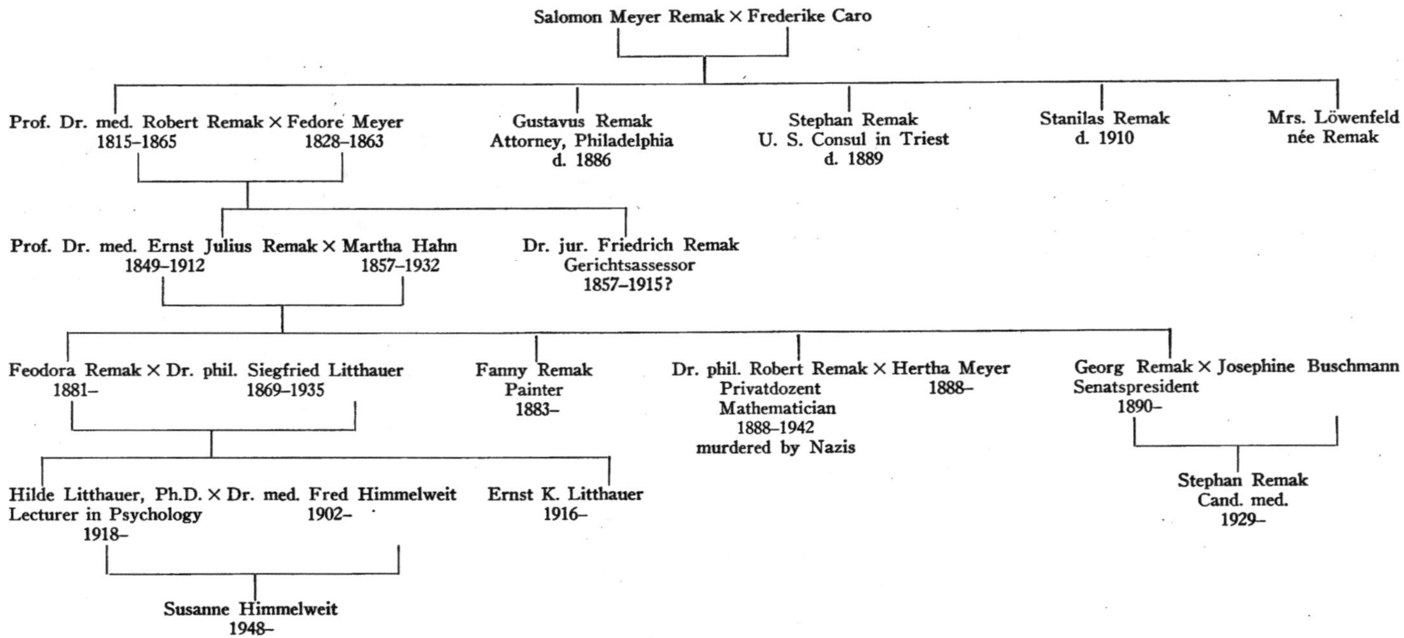

exists any doubt as to whether the "Dr. R," who is the subject of Kalisch's report, should be identified with Dr. Remak, it is dispelled by an express statement in Ehrlich's eulogy referring to Kalisch's book as a source of information.

Finally, I was fortunate to be beneficiary of the most friendly and valuable cooperation of Mrs. Feodora Litthauer and Miss Fanny Remak, both granddaughters of Robert Remak, who supplied valuable data and family traditions and the family tree that appears on p. 228. My sincerest thanks go to both these ladies, to whom Kalisch's publication concerning their grandfather was also well known.

YOUTH

Robert Remak was born (64) on July 30, 1815 in Posnan (Posen). He was the son of a Jewish merchant, Salomon Meier Remak, who, according to the recollection of Remak's classmate, Motty (85), was a well-to-do man. Humboldt, however, mentions Remak's parents in 1847 as orthodox and poor Jews. Remak's mother was Frederica Caro. Family tradition has it that the name Remak is taken from the most famous ancestor of this family, Rabbi Mose ben Jakob Cordovero (1522–1570), who, as usual in Hebrew literature, was called by the initials of his name, Rabbi Mose Cordovero, "ReMaK." This rabbi was one of the most famous authorities in Cabbalistics; his principal book (*Pardes rimmonim*) was often reprinted and repeatedly translated into Latin, and is supposed to have had an important influence on the teachings of Spinoza.

Concerning Robert Remak's father, Mrs. Litthauer, Remak's granddaughter, informed me that, from what her father said, he was the owner of a cigar store and ran a lottery office. That would not be a contradiction of Motty's recollections, but father Remak's finances may have been different later on, when he was further along in years. Arthur Kronthal's assertion [1a] that Robert Remak was the son of a physician, Dr. Julius Siegfried Remack in Posen, is definitely erroneous according to the statement of Remak's granddaughters. But Kronthal (*loc. cit.*) found in the documents of the Staatsarchiv in Posen (No. C. XVIII 67) the names of not less than nine well-to-do Jews of this town by the name of Remak who received Prussian naturalization as citizens between 1834 and 1837. They all were related to each other and among them was the physician, Dr. Julius Siegfried Remack, and one Salomon Meyer Remak, keeper of a lottery office. The latter was indeed Robert Remak's father. Kronthal remembers having heard from his grandfather, a contemporary of Robert Remak's father, how both the keeper of the lottery office and the physician Julius Remak used to boast about their famous ancestors in Spain and tell of their fate after the expulsion of Jews from Spain in the fifteenth century. These recollections of Kronthal seem to prove the family relations between Remak's father and Dr. Julius Remak in Posen.

The first instruction Remak received was in the parental home and in a private school of one named Apstein (64). He then entered a higher public school in his home town, which he attended for two years. Then he fell sick, and because of his poor health was compelled to abstain from all studies for more than a year.

Stadtrat Arthur Kronthal, a German-Jewish historian, found in the records of the Marien-Gymnasium in Posen a certified copy of Remak's school record from 1829, which reads in translation as follows:

> Robert Remak, fourteen years of age, attended from October, 1828 up to now the III grade of the German Bürgerschule. Diligence, attendance, and conduct must be regarded as exemplary. Progress in all subjects was excellent so that I am able to certify with good conscience: I never before had such an excellent pupil in my class.

The exact agreement of this school record with the classbook original was certified in Posen on September 30, 1829 by the pastor and school principal, J. G. Friedrich. This certificate was probably needed later when Remak entered the Polish Royal Gymnasium in Posen after his recovery. He attended this school for two and a half years and graduated at the age of eighteen with the *Testimonium Maturitatis,* which entitled him to attend any university in Germany.

Remak's education in this Polish Gymnasium gave the young student a nationalistic bent for the rest of his life. That a strong political attitude prevailed in this school we may judge from a remark in a letter from Kronthal to Remak's granddaughter. According to him the school that Remak attended was dissolved after the Polish revolt of 1830–1831. This was probably in 1833, because in its stead in 1834 two similar schools, a Catholic and a Protestant Gymnasium, were established. That Remak's sympathies were with the Poles and not with the Prussians is evident from the fact that his university studies in Berlin were, according to his granddaughter, subsidized by some Polish aristocrats. This seems to contradict Motty's statement that Remak's father was a well-to-do man. Time and again in the following years we find Remak joined in friendship for the most part with Polish personalities and helping the cause of the suppressed Polish people. Also he published scientific papers in the Polish language, which is indebted to him for various new expressions in the field of medical technology (85).

Remak's Polish patriotism was well known among his Berlin compatriots. When he was recognized as a research scholar in medicine and was admitted as a teacher at Berlin University, he was chosen, during the most dangerous days of the Berlin revolution in 1848, with two other Polish delegates (Dr. Adalbert Cybulski and Marceli Motty) to appear at an audience before

[1a] *Jüd. Familienforschung* 3: 872, 1937.

King Friedrich Wilhelm IV of Prussia to ask for the release of some Polish patriots imprisoned in Moabit because of their supposed connection with the Polish conspiracy of 1846 (35).

In 1833, when Remak left his home town to enroll as a student at Berlin, the Jewish proportion of Posnan's inhabitants was quite high. It was still 20 per cent of the entire population in 1849, and this in spite of a continuous migration of Jews to other German towns, such as Breslau and Berlin. In the first half of the nineteenth century many Jews left the religious and cultural center that had long bloomed in Posnan. It was precisely in the early years of the nineteenth century that Jewish life in that city was under the leadership of one of the most famous rabbinical scholars and authorities, Rabbi Akiba Eger (1761–1837). Nevertheless, the migration of the Jews and their settlement in other Prussian towns was very understandable. A famous governmental decree of 1812 had brought to the Jews of Prussia a high degree of emancipation from medieval injustice. Actually they were not yet full-fledged citizens, but the decree opened the gates to a more dignified existence and cultural development as compared with pre-Napoleonic times and with other countries.

When, in 1815, Posnan was ceded to Prussia as the grand duchy of Posen (since 1850 the province of Posen), the Jews living there did not automatically receive the rights and status of the other Jews in Prussia. It was only on June 1, 1833, when Remak had to decide on his future education at one of Germany's universities, that a new decree was promulgated concerning the Polish Jews in Prussia. This Preliminary Decree, the *vorläufige Verordnung wegen des Judentums im Grossherzogtum Posen,* represented by no means a generous, democratic change in the status of the Jews in this region, but still it was good enough to excite an overexaggerated feeling of enthusiasm, gratitude, and patriotism among this segment of the population. It speaks well for Remak's character that, neither by this meager gesture on the part of the Prussian Government towards the Jews of Posnan nor by any later events was he influenced to change his attitude towards the Poles generally or toward his Polish friends.

A STUDENT IN BERLIN

Like so many young Jews from the East who were eager to acquire modern knowledge and Western culture, Remak was attracted to the new radiant center of research, study, and modest luxury that began to grow up in Berlin, the capital of Prussia, where the new University, only a few decades old, had since 1810 attracted to its teaching staff and especially to the medical and science faculty some of the most renowned celebrities of Europe. It is his granddaughter's recollection that Remak's parents did not go to Berlin at the same time, but remained in Posnan.

Berlin was famous among European Jews as a center of culture that had many advantages to offer from the special point of view of a Jewish student. There were, of course, all the generally known scientific opportunities to study. There was also a well-known Jewish community in Berlin. The name of Moses Mendelssohn, the philosopher, who was a friend of the German poet Lessing and whose German writing was admired by the young Goethe, was connected with the city. Here his struggle to further the emancipation of the Jews had started. Jews, who were the first among their brothers to become graduates of universities and who had settled in Berlin long before the founding of its University, were still well known and admired as pioneers of a new era. The renown of such men as Mendelssohn's teacher, Dr. Abraham Kisch, who as the first Jew of Prague in Bohemia was duly graduated as an M.D. from Halle (1749) and settled for some time in Berlin, and that of the Berlin physician, Professor Marcus Herz, pupil and friend of the philosopher Kant, friend of Mendelssohn and Lessing, who had a kind of legendary fame among contemporary Jews and non-Jews from the eighteenth century, lured the inhabitants of the dark Ghettos of the East. Rumors of an incredibly high standard of living and of real modern culture among Berlin Jews, anecdotes and stories about the splendor and riches of certain Jewish families in the Prussian capital, unquestionably figured in the dreams of many a poor Jewish student in the East and were a powerful magnet for the well-to-do ones. The fame of Jewish ladies, in whose homes the Jewish and non-Jewish intelligentsia of Berlin used to meet, was no less impressive to these young people than the reputation of the stars of the medical world. Among the latter Alexander von Humboldt was especially popular and famous. His fair and friendly attitude towards each scholar in the field of science, non-Jew and Jew alike, was world renowned.

The Baron Alexander von Humboldt and his brother, Wilhelm, were known to be very prominent at the Prussian court and in scientific Germany. They were among those who asked earnestly for the right of the Jew to be admitted as a full-fledged citizen of the state in which he lived. At the same time Alexander von Humboldt was most influential at the University of Berlin, despite the fact that he never was a regular member of it. Later Remak came in personal contact with Alexander von Humboldt and repeatedly expressed his gratitude to and admiration for this man.

It seems probable that Remak was not the first of his family to become a physician. The Berlin journal, *Allgemeine Medicinische Centralzeitung,* announced on May 19, 1849 the death of a physician, a Doctor Remack, in Posen. The name Remak being not too common and Posen being the birthplace of Robert Remak, it seems probable that these physicians were related to each other. Callisen's *Biographical Dictionary*

(9) mentions also as living in Berlin in 1833 a Doctor Julius Siegfried Remack, who was born in Posen in 1793 and studied in Breslau and Berlin, being graduated from the latter in 1818. He may have been identical with the one Kronthal (*loc. cit.*) states was naturalized between 1834 and 1837 in Posen, and who died there in 1849. The slightly different spelling of the name is not very significant for those days, but it seems noteworthy that Remak gave his oldest son the name Ernst Julius. Callisen's dictionary of scientific writers (9) cites Robert Remak's name [2] as Remack too, and on page 407 remarks expressly that the spelling of his name is neither Remak nor Remarck but Remack. Remak himself, however, always used the spelling Remak.

Remak came to central Germany with the desire to study medicine. We find him in 1833 on his way to Berlin, and there it was that he spent the remainder of his life in learning, in research, in teaching, and in fighting—unfortunately, very often in vain—for justice and recognition for his work and for himself.

The year Remak entered the University of Berlin as a student was a remarkable one for its medical faculty. In that year Johannes Müller, Professor at Bonn, was called, on his own application and suggestion, to the chair of anatomy and physiology at the Berlin University. Müller soon became the center around which the most promising and brilliant minds of the younger generation flocked, exactly as in the years before, during the period when he was professor at the University of Bonn in the Rhineland. Even students who never intended to study medicine or science, like the philosopher and founder of the science of racial psychology, Professor M. Lazarus, were enthusiastic auditors in Müller's classes (46), enjoying his fascinating personality. To mention the names of his most distinguished pupils would be to enumerate most of the outstanding physiologists, anatomists, and zoologists of the following generation in Germany. Among them were, for instance, Theodor Schwann, Jacob Henle, Robert Remak, Adolph Hannover, Emil Du Bois-Reymond, Ernst Brücke, Herman Helmholtz, Albert Koelliker, Rudolf Virchow, Ernst Haeckel, Georg Meissner, Leopold Auerbach.

Remak became one of the group of Müller's early pupils in Berlin. In his pre-medical program he attended classes in physics with Professor Ermann; he studied chemistry with Mitscherlich, botany with Schultz, zoology with Ehrenberg and Lichtenstein, and logic and metaphysics with Henning. The most important among his teachers, who had a lasting and intensive influence on his entire development, were Ehrenberg, the famous microscopist, and Johannes Müller, whose lectures on general and special anatomy, comparative anatomy, physiology and pathology he

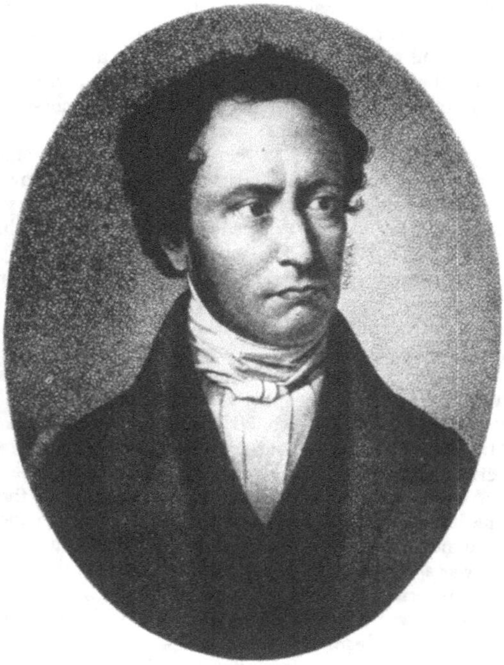

FIG. 40. Johannes Müller. Etching by L. Linsen. From the author's collection. A lithograph of this drawing by Werner from the original drawing by Rinck was published by Ebbecke (*Johannes Müller,* Hannover, Schmorl von Seefeld, 1951), from the collection of Müller's grandson.

attended in addition to Schlemm's anatomical courses (64).

We have a vivid description of Müller's personality drawn by his pupil, assistant, and later successor to the chair of physiology at Berlin, Emil Du Bois-Reymond (11). He described his professor in those early years as "not very friendly towards the average student of medicine." This is understandable, because Müller was taxed to the utmost by all his personal duties. The anatomical collections of the University had to be built up and developed. As a teacher he had to devote much time to his students in lectures and demonstrations, in spite of the fact that the Government had generously given him a free hand to decide for himself the extent of his teaching activities. Much time also had to be devoted to endless faculty meetings and to the obligatory examinations of prospective graduates. All that, however, was not his main occupation. Most of the time had to be spent in his own scientific research. Müller also had to study carefully all the published material on anatomy, physiology, and zoology for his own work and for the annual reports in his own journal, known as *Müller's Archiv,* which he founded in 1834, and in the

[2] 30: 416.

editing of the journal itself, although in this part of his work he was relieved by the managing editor, his young friend and pupil, Jacob Henle. It is easy, therefore, to comprehend that Müller had to be economical with his time and could not dissipate it in friendly discussions with the average student; consequently, as Du Bois-Reymond observed, it was very difficult for such a student to have any personal contact with Müller. However, it was quite another matter when he discovered in a pupil talent, eagerness, and ability to do research. Then Müller immediately became interested, friendly and generous with his time and material. This, for Müller, was the real life element up to his death. Such a fortunate student was Du Bois himself, who, like Müller's other collaborators, found him to be the personification of kindness, offering in the most courteous way his own experience, his wonderful library, and all the tools he had that would be useful in their work. His library was a unique collection of the literature pertaining to anatomy, physiology, and zoology.

Another picture of life in Müller's laboratory at the time Remak began to work there is given by the anatomist Jacob Henle in his eulogy for Theodor Schwann (32). In 1834 Jacob Henle became the second prosector in Müller's laboratory; at the same time Schwann was appointed to a position as *Gehülfe am anatomischen Institut,* with a salary of 10 Thalers a month. This was before Ernst Abbe initiated the fundamental reform in the building of microscopes and before he constructed his light condenser for illuminating microscopic specimens, which today is a part of every microscope. It was before the time even of the general use of gas illumination, which was introduced on Berlin's streets only in 1826. The students had, therefore, to be economical with their working time and utilize the daylight hours fully, especially in the winter. It is indicative of the times that Müller, writing to Professor Valentin in Bern on New Year's Eve, 1837, sends his best wishes for the New Year and "especially for good light in winter time" (see p. 174). Henle describes these early days of his collaboration with Schwann under Johannes Müller, the time when Remak began to work under Müller, too, as follows:

> I recollect the working place of what was called, euphemistically, the anatomical laboratory behind the Garnisonkirche, where we stayed with our kind chief Johannes Müller till late in the afternoon. So as not to miss the light hours, each of us took his main meal according to the English custom, and at noontime we used to gather in the director's room for a second breakfast. For this the janitor's wife supplied the food, and we, each outdoing the other, supplied the wine and the good sense of humor. Those were happy days for which the generation of today may envy us (32).

We have no real proof that in those years or later Remak had any close personal relationship either with Henle or with Schwann or with any other of the famous circle in Müller's laboratory. The way in which he is mentioned in Henle's textbook on general anatomy (31), the way in which Henle, even in 1841 and 1844 rejects Remak's fundamental discoveries pertaining to the connection of the nerve fibre with the nerve cell and of the unmedulated nerve fibres of the sympathetic nervous system, and finally, Henle's published polemic against Remak [8] give no ground to suppose that he and Remak were ever on very close terms. In his early years at Berlin the circle of Remak's close friends seems mainly to have embraced students and physicians from his home town and its vicinity.

In those days Henle (49, 56) was Müller's influential friend and right-hand man. He was a friend of Müller's wife since his early youth, when they both grew up as neighbor children in Coblenz. There he also first met Müller, also a native of Coblenz, who was in love with his future wife, Nanny, while Henle fell seriously in love with Mrs. Müller's sister. Both these young men were soon attached to each other in close friendship. Henle later studied under Müller at Bonn and accompanied him on scientific trips to Paris in 1831 and to London in 1837.

From the start of his *Archiv* in 1834 Müller made Henle a kind of managing editor of the journal, with a salary of 200 Thalers a year (49).

This famous anatomist, Jacob Henle, was a Jew, too, but as a child had been baptized. Close friendship between him and Remak may well have been blocked by the fact that the latter emphasized his Polish nationality whereas Henle was, like Müller, a member of one of the very politically active fraternities that existed at German universities (*Burschenschaftler*). Furthermore, Remak, offspring of orthodox Jews, stuck to his Judaism, while Henle, like so many baptized Jews, occasionally professed an anti-Semitic feeling. We find various such expressions still in his letters, published and surely carefully selected by his son-in-law, the anatomist Merkel (49), where he makes derogatory remarks about Jews (pp. 89, 324), and in one letter to his father even speaks of "filthy Jews" (p. 173). It was impossible that two such different characters as the exoteric Henle and the esoteric Remak could ever have been bound by a really close friendship, especially after the little Polish Jew Remak, at twenty-one already famous for his microscopic discoveries, proved to be right in several important scientific controversies with Henle.

However that may have been, Remak was fortunate enough soon to attract the attention and friendly interest of his great teachers Ehrenberg and Müller. A picture of his personality in these early days is given by the anonymous writer of Remak's eulogy in *Deutsche Klinik* (94), who says: "This writer recalls the days in 1836 when he met Remak as a slender young man with vivid eyes and short dark hair, and with an outspoken enthusiasm for microscopical studies." At that

[8] *Müller's Archiv,* 1839.

time Remak was seen frequently at Froriep's autopsies, in Barez's Children's Clinic, and assisting in Jüngken's eye clinic. He was especially popular among the foreign physicians who at that time already flocked to the center of modern medicine in Berlin. They always found a friendly, understanding, and helpful soul in the young student who, himself a stranger in Berlin, had a sympathetic feeling for all the needs and difficulties of the foreign doctors visiting the institutions and clinics of this city (94).

Besides being a diligent and eager student in the different clinics, he spent most of his time in microscopic studies, then a new, promising and always fascinating field in medicine. Rudolf Virchow, six years younger than Remak, described in the first volume of his *Archiv* in 1847 the still prevailing disregard and the contempt with which the average physician in Germany used to look upon the microscopist and his revolutionizing achievements. In America the first compound microscope was built in 1838 by Spencer (78) and in 1847 there were not more than four or five achromatic microscopes in the city of New York (97). Remak, like Berres, Purkinje, Müller, Valentin, Gruby, Schwann, and Henle, was one of those investigators who early recognized the value of microscopical studies for medicine.

From the beginning of his medical studies until Müller's death in 1858, Remak remained in close contact with him, his most inspiring and, because of his enormous wealth of knowledge, his most admired teacher. He was permitted to use Müller's microscope as well as Ehrenberg's, which were excellent for those days, and the very limited laboratory space in Müller's anatomical department in Berlin. Indeed, there was so little working space that even the master's most prominent pupils, like Schwann and Henle, and all the younger students, like Remak, had to set up at least a part of their laboratory equipment at home in their own rooms (49), which surely gave no pleasure to their parents or landlords!

It was Johannes Müller's way (11) not actually to conduct in detail the research of his favorite pupils, but to give a hint or suggestion, and then it was up to the pupil to work on this suggestion adequately. Through his teacher Ehrenberg's recent studies on ganglionic cells of invertebrates, Remak became interested in the microscopical structure of the nervous system, but it was the inspiration he received from Müller that put him on the way to making his first fundamental discoveries. A remark Müller once made to him personally (62), and which Müller repeated later in one of his annual reports in his *Archiv,*[4] that "we surely are not yet acquainted with the most primitive fibrils of the nervous system" and that "the so-called primitive ones may contain still more primitive ones," started Remak on an intensive microscopic study of the nervous system. In 1836, when Remak was still a student, the first results of this investigation were published in *Müller's Archiv,* later (1837) in Froriep's journal (62, 63), and extensively, in his doctoral thesis in 1838 (64).

[4] 4: iii, 1837.

Remak's studies in the early years of his career were by no means restricted to this one problem. He delighted in every kind of microscopical research (94). As a young student he did not concentrate his work on the nervous system exclusively, neither did he do so later. In one of his early papers (1837) in Froriep's journal, where he reports on the histology of the nervous system, he mentions at the same time, for example, his studies on the fibrillatory movement and on the spermatozoa of the salamander (*salamandra*). Ehrenberg, whose classes on invertebrate zoology Remak attended, had published a paper in *Poggendorf's Annalen* in 1833 (13), in which he expressed the opinion that microscopical differences might exist between the elements of motor and sensory nerve fibres (13: 454). In this paper and unquestionably in discussions with his pupils also, Ehrenberg suggested that someone make a special microscopical study of this point.

Magendie's discoveries on the physiology of the anterior and posterior roots of the spinal nerves, the anterior being the motor, the posterior the sensory fibers, were published in 1822. Every physiologist and anatomist was deeply impressed. Johannes Müller contributed important experimental proof for the newly-discovered facts, and the Bell-Magendie controversy over the priority of this fundamental discovery was still going on in a heated spirit when Ehrenberg performed his investigations with the purpose of accumulating proof of a microscopic difference between both roots of the spinal nerves, as the missing link in the chain of investigations on this important problem. His conclusions were not shared by Müller, who, in spite of close personal contact with Ehrenberg and with due respect for the latter's skill and experience, expressed the view that an anatomical difference between anterior and posterior roots in Ehrenberg's sense did not exist and contradicted Ehrenberg's findings in reviewing his work in the first volume of *Müller's Archiv.* Müller's objections were without any personal bias. So it came about that Remak, a gifted young student eager to do research and a pupil of both Ehrenberg and Müller, started on this work. Both offered Remak their facilities and assistance, and in his first paper (61) he thankfully acknowledged how both his teachers had put their fine modern microscopes at his disposal, how Müller had checked his findings, and how he had demonstrated to his teacher Ehrenberg his recent observations on the *rami communicantes* of the frog (61).

FIRST DISCOVERIES IN NEUROHISTOLOGY

The results of the investigations that Remak carried out were interesting enough to be entered in a prize contest (61) conducted by the faculty in 1835. They were favorably regarded by the university (40: 123) and won second prize (21: 116). The results are included in the introductory part of Remak's first publication (1836). Originally, he intended to investigate the nervous plexus, but soon he was led to the microscopical study of the structure of the spinal nerves. Here he sided with his teacher Ehrenberg, asserting that as a confirmation of Bell's law, he expected to find a microscopical difference between motor and sensory nerves. Of greater importance than such a theoretical opinion was the young student's discovery, in the course of this research, of the axis cylinder, the most important central part of each nerve fibre, and the discovery of the connection of nerve fibers with nerve cells. Here he met with the doubts and incredulity of his teacher Müller. In the annual report in his *Archiv*,[5] when Müller announced the discovery of the axis cylinder by Remak, he asserted that in his view the anatomist Valentin at Bern was correct in maintaining that the nerve fibres with their terminal parts only surround the ganglionic cells, though Remak had already stated in this first paper that nerve fibres stem from the ganglionic cells. This is a fundamental difference, and Remak's excellent observation is to this day a basis for all neurology. It is a great credit to Müller's character and scientific integrity that he accepted his young pupil's findings for publication in his own *Archiv*, in spite of his doubts as to their validity.

In the same volume (1836) in which Remak's first paper appears, Müller also mentions his name on page 18 in his annual report in connection with Remak's observations of a ganglion connected with the accessory *nervus Villisii*. That may be the first time that Remak's name was mentioned in medical literature. The following year Remak was working diligently with the nervous system, and the next results which he published in Froriep's journal contain confirmation of his own previous findings and a deeper understanding of the anatomical structure of the nerves. Remak wrote those papers in a style that was as far as possible from the then usual romantic, so-called philosophical metaphysical kind of style. He was a pupil of Ehrenberg and of Müller who, with his *Handbook of Physiology*, put an end to the school of natural philosophy in medicine. Remak himself remarks that in his opinion a certain dryness in the presentation and the most simple and precise kind of description of results can only be of high merit in reporting microscopical observations (62).

The principal new discoveries that Remak made between 1835 and 1838 in neurohistology were as follows: (1) Remak found the sympathetic nerve fibers to be of a specific unique type, non-medulated, that is, not provided with a myelin sheath like other nerve fibers, as we know today. These most primitive fibers were later called Remak's fibers. (2) Still more important was his discovery of the real relationship between ganglionic cells and nerve fibers. He found that the nerve fibers stem from ganglionic cells—a fact which he established in cattle, sheep, and rabbits, in 1837. (3) He found a fine central band in the myelinated nerve fibers, which he called the primitive band, being the most primitive nerve fiber for which he had been looking.

All these facts, today familiar to every student of medicine, were by no means immediately accepted by the profession nor recognized as great discoveries. In the first place, it was the famous physiologist and anatomist Valentin at Bern, Switzerland, who tried to disprove Remak's findings and to support his own opinion that the relationship between ganglionic globules and nerve fibers is not that of an organic unit, but of a "juxta-position," that is, only a contact and not an organic connection. A heated argument arose on this problem. Johannes Müller himself, in the third edition of his *Handbook of Physiology*, confirmed his pupil's findings with respect to unmedullated nerve fibers, and so did Theodor Schwann.[6] Both were considered authorities in their time.

But Valentin, also an outstanding expert, regarded Remak's findings as wrong,[7] and other distinguished scientists, too, held opposing opinions. Henle, for instance, in his book on pathological investigations,[8] was first to favor recognizing Remak's organic fibers as real nerve fibers even against Valentin's opposition; but only a year later in his textbook *Allgemeine Anatomie* (1841) and subsequently, he decided against Remak, against his own previous, better judgment, and joined Valentin's destructive criticism. Henle, of course, was a close friend of Valentin, and Valentin was instrumental in Henle's becoming full professor at Zürich in 1840 (49). It was otherwise with Valentin's famous teacher, Purkinje. When this scholar was in Berlin in 1837 and visited Johannes Müller, he met the young and already famous student, Remak, and he became acquainted with his microscopical findings on the axis cylinder and with the unmedullated nerve fibers (40). Purkinje soon became convinced, unbiased as he was in scientific problems, that Remak's fibers were no artifacts, and that the primitive band, newly discovered by Remak in the center of medullated nerve fibers, really existed, and that these facts were important anatomical discoveries. To Remak's primitive band he gave the name, still used, of "Axencylinder" (axis cylinder).

Purkinje was more reluctant to accept Remak's still more important discovery of the origin of the nerve fibers from ganglionic globules. However, Remak had proved that fact for the spinal ganglia and also for the central nervous system (spinal cord), as he emphasized

[5] 4: III, 1837.

[6] *Microscop. Unters.*, Berlin, 179, 1839.

[7] *Repertorium* 3: 72, 1838; *Müller's Archiv* 1839: 137.

[8] Berlin, 1840, p. 87.

in a short excerpt from his doctoral thesis in *Froriep's Notizen.*[9]

Purkinje, Ehrenberg, and especially Valentin had been for years continuously busy with microscopical studies on the nervous system. Then a student of twenty-one years of age appeared on the scene with fundamental discoveries that had escaped the attention of the most famous workers in microscopical research of his time. To take this gracefully, without envy or resentment, one would have had to be a philosophical, wise scholar, especially since Remak presented his new discoveries in the youthful apodictic manner of one who is sure, without any doubt of what he has seen. Valentin, the famous twenty-eight-year-old professor, the one most interested in those problems, was neither the aloof philosopher nor the phlegmatic student to accept the new discoveries with equanimity. He reacted immediately and vehemently with emotion and prejudice. In his quarterly, *Repertorium,*[10] Valentin in 1838 called Remak's chef d'œuvre, *Observationes,* a presentation of partly very good, partly misinterpreted observations, "proferred with deplorable arrogance." Without taking the pains to repeat Remak's observations exactly before criticizing them, at least out of respect for Johannes Müller, from whose laboratory they were published, Valentin condemned Remak's unmedullated nerve fibers and his central primitive band (axis-cylinder) as wrongly interpreted artifacts,[11] not to speak of the imagined connection between ganglionic cells and nerve fibers. Valentin's reasoning culminated in the following statement: "Concerning the conception of organic nerve fibers, this reviewer has to confess that he regards this idea, a relic of bygone times, incompatable with the objective trend of our day." He regarded Remak's fibers merely as a word, a phrase to hide our ignorance of the influence of the nervous system on metabolic processes, and compared Remak's stupendous epoch-making discoveries with the attempts to conceal our ignorance about the nature of light and heat by such expressions as lightstuff, heatstuff (Lichtstoff, Wärmestoff), common in those days.

For years Valentin insisted on this stubborn point of view. He opposed his own teacher Purkinje (*Repertorium* **5**: 80, 1840), his "gratefully revered father in science," when the latter, like Adolph Hannover, Johannes Müller, and others, already agreed with Remak's discoveries. In September 1837, shortly before he met Remak in Berlin, Purkinje presented his findings on what he later called the axis-cylinder at the Conference of German Scientists and Physicians in Prague (59). However, his drawings are much less convincing than Remak's, and their interpretation by Purkinje was wrong. Only after meeting Remak and being shown the "primitive band" of the nerve fibers by the latter did Purkinje give up adherence to Ehrenberg's previous opinion (13). This wrong opinion he still expressed in Prague in 1837. At that time he regarded the central part of the nerve as a channel, a hollow tube filled with fluid. But after his visit in Berlin he accepted Remak's findings of a central structure in nerve fibers, only applying to it the new name, axis-cylinder. These facts are attested to by Henle, who personally attended the meeting between Purkinje and Remak, and who wrote four years later in his *General Anatomy* (p. 782):

> What Purkinje here explained [Proceedings of the Prague Meeting of German Scientists and Physicians in 1838, p. 177, Figs. 9 and 10] as a central channel was later on, when Remak's work and Valentin's and my objections to it were published, described by him as a solid cord in the axis of the fiber. He called it cylinder axis.

Henle, of course, tried to dissuade the honest Purkinje from his belief that Remak had priority in this discovery, which the sincere Purkinje never doubted. Henle, however, says on page 783: "Purkinje does injustice to himself and to me [Henle] by proclaiming the identity of his axis-cylinder with Remak's primitive band." Valentin found Henle's disagreement with Remak much to his liking. In 1838 he convinced himself of the existence of Remak's "organic nerve fibers," as is clear from a letter he wrote Remak (B.B.B.), but he gave them an incorrect interpretation, regarding them as processes of the sheath enclosing the ganglionic cells (see p. 170). He and Henle, who joined this fight against Remak, became close friends. Only in 1842[12] did Valentin reluctantly admit his mistake, at least with respect to Remak's fibers and the axis-cylinder, and so did Henle in 1849. Remak was the victor, but only after a hard, nerve-racking struggle at a time when he was suffering from a serious chest disease and fearful of imminent death (see p. 168). The Valentin-Remak controversy is an unfortunate blot on Valentin's brilliant career as a scientist.

Following Purkinje's visit to Müller's laboratory and his meeting with Remak, Purkinje's pupil, Rosenthal, wrote his doctoral thesis, published in 1839 in Breslau, under the title *De formatione granulosa.* Purkinje and Rosenthal were, as mentioned above, not entirely in accord with Remak's opinions. They confirmed the actual existence of Remak's unmedullated fibers in sympathetic nerves and their similarity to the embryonic nerve fibers was emphasized. However, Rosenthal, like Purkinje, did not agree with Remak on the question of the continuity of nerve cells and nerve fibers. A very similar point of view was presented still later (1842) by F. H. Bidder and A. W. Volkmann (16) in a special monograph on the sympathetic nervous system. They, too, recognized the existence of a specific unmedullated nervous system, but they also denied that its fibers had their origin in ganglionic cells and re-

[9] No. 132, 1838.
[10] **3**: 14, 1838.
[11] *Repertorium* **3**: 73, 74, 76 ff., 1838.
[12] *Repertorium* **7**: 113, 115, 1842.

OBSERVATIONES ANATOMICAE ET MICROSCOPICAE
DE SYSTEMATIS NERVOSI STRUCTURA.

DISSERTATIO INAUGURALIS
QUAM
CONSENSU ET AUCTORITATE
GRATIOSI MEDICORUM ORDINIS
IN
ALMA LITERARUM UNIVERSITATE FRIDERICA GUILELMA
UT SUMMI
IN MEDICINA ET CHIRURGIA HONORES
RITE SIBI CONCEDANTUR
DIE XXX. MENS. JANUARII A. MDCCCXXXVIII.
H. L. Q. S.
PUBLICE DEFENDET
AUCTOR
ROBERTUS REMAK
POSNANIENSIS.

OPPONENTIBUS:
J. DE MIANOWSKI, MED. ET CHIR. DR. PROF. ACAD. VILNENSIS
A. DE BENTKOWSKI, MED. ET CHIR. DR.
M. COMITE DE CZAPSKI, JURIS UTRIUSQUE CAND.

BEROLINI, FORMIS KRIMERIANIS.

FIG. 41. Remak's doctoral thesis. Rare original first edition as thesis. Courtesy of Berlin University.

garded them as not identical with Remak's fibers. So difficult was it for outstanding scholars to break with the traditions of their time and to realize the enormous progress in Remak's new concept and new findings.

It took years of controversy between the most prominent scientists of the period before Remak's statements were finally proved to be valid. The most important confirmation came from his younger colleague in Müller's laboratory, Hermann Helmholtz. What Remak proved in 1837 concerning the connection between the ganglionic cells and nerve fibers in vertebrates was corroborated for invertebrates in Helmholtz's doctoral thesis in 1842 (30). This work was dedicated to and approved by Johannes Müller, who must therefore in 1842 have already recognized the error of his own views on Remak's discovery.

Remak's doctoral thesis of forty-two pages with two plates of pictures, under the Latin title, *Observationes anatomicae et microscopicae de systematis nervosi structura* (Berlin, 1838) will remain for all time one of the classic publications of early modern medicine.

Leo Königsberger, the enthusiastic biographer of Helmholtz, in his three-volume work on the scientist, creates an erroneous impression of the main content of Helmholtz's doctoral thesis (44: 48), saying: "His microscopical discovery that the nerve fibers stem from the ganglionic cells, which Ehrenberg discovered in 1833, is, according to the unanimous opinion of the physiologists, the histological basis of the entire nerve physiology and pathology." Many later authors accepted this version, and indeed it is right to emphasize the importance of this discovery, but the credit for it should go to Remak; a genius like Helmholtz does not need any undeserved recognition.

It was Müller who suggested these investigations to Helmholtz. As for Remak's findings, he still was reluctant to give up his own doubts. When Helmholtz was able to confirm Remak's discovery of the origin of nerve fibers in nerve cells and Müller approved, he nevertheless put it in this way, that Helmholtz's discovery with respect to invertebrates "was already assumed, but not yet proven for vertebrates." Without mentioning Remak's name Helmholtz reports these remarks by Müller in a letter to his father dated August 1, 1842 (31: 46). It was surely difficult for Müller to admit that his pupil Remak in 1837 was right, while he himself still wrote in 1839: "Concerning the direct connection of the ganglionic globuls with the gray fibers, I never was convinced of that."

We feel Müller's influence when Helmholtz, writing in his thesis of gray fibers, fails to mention Remak's priority, and when, at the end of this thesis (30: 28), without citing Remak's paper, he mentions only the

VITA.

Ego Robertus Remak, Posnaniensis, natus sum d. XXX. m. Julii a. MDCCCXV. patre Salomone, mercatore, et matre Friderica e gente Caro. Fidei judaicae addictus sum. Primis litterarum elementis postquam tum in parentum domo, tum in schola privata Cl. *Apsteini* imbutus sum, scholam publicam civium altiorem, quae etiam nunc viro humanissimo et summopere de me merito Cl. *Friedrich* rectore floret, per duos fere annos frequentavi. Tum anno et quod excurrit praeterlapso, quo propter improsperam corporis valetudinem litteris fere omnino abstinere coactus eram, in Gymnasio Posnaniensi, directoribus Cl. *Stoc* et Cl. *Jocob* quem mox Cl. *Wendt* excepit, per duos annos et dimidium versatus sum.

Testimonio maturitatis munitus auctumno anni MDCCCXXXIII Berolinum me contuli, ibique almae litterarum universitatis civibus ab Ill. *Strauss* t. t. rectore magnifico, atque medicinae studiosis ab Ill. *Busch*, t. t. decano, summe spectabili, adscriptus sum. Lectiones autem, quibus per quadriennium interfui, hae sunt: physicen generalem, atque de calore et luce Ill. *Ermann* me docuit, chemiam Ill. *Mitscherlich*, osteologiam, syndesmologiam et splanchnologiam Ill. *Schlemm*, anatomiam generalem et specialem, comparatam, pathologicam atque physiologiam Ill. *Mueller*, botanicen Ill. *Schultz*, zoologiam Ill. *Lichtenstein*, historiam naturalem animalium sceleto articulato destitutorum Ill. *Ehrenberg*, logicen et metaphysicen Ill. ab *Henning*, pathologiam et therapiam specialem Ill. *Hecker*, materiam medicam Ill. *Osann*, elementa artis obstetriciae Ill. *Busch*, akiurgiam et anatomiam chirurgicam Cel. *Froriep*, chirurgiam generalem et specialem Ill. *Juengken*, de fracturis et luxationibus Ill. *Kluge*.

Praeterea exercitationibus clinicis medicis, chirurgicis, ophthalmiatricis, obstetriciis virorum illustrissimorum *Bartels, Busch, de Graefe, Juengken, Osann, Truestedt, Wolff* tum auscultando tum practicando intra annum unum et dimidium usus sum, atque in morbis infantum curandis Cel. *Barez* per annum moderator benignus mihi fuit.

Quibus omnibus viris summe de me meritis gratias ago quas habeo maximas semperque habebo.

Tentaminibus tam philosophico, quam medico, nec non examine rigoroso rite absolutis, spero fore, ut dissertatione thesibusque defensis, summi in medicina et chirurgia honores mihi concedantur.

FIG. 42. Autobiography as printed in Remak's doctoral thesis (Vita). Courtesy of Berlin University.

latter's "conjecture" on the origin of nerve fibers in vertebrates and leaves it to the judgment "of more experienced physiologists whether his own findings may support Remak's opinion." This is literally what Müller had told Helmholtz on August 1, 1842.

The hesitancy of the great teacher to give credit to his great pupil was certainly not due to purely objective judgment. The proper thing for Müller as well as Helmholtz to have said would have been: "Remak was right in his observations, even though all the outstanding men of his time did not believe him, but now his findings are confirmed in a less difficult subject by Helmholtz and therefore credit should be given to the real discoverer of this important fact."

GRADUATION

On January 30, 1838 Remak received his degree of doctor of medicine and surgery *cum laude* from the medical faculty of the Friedrich Wilhelm University in Berlin. His attitude toward science and medicine is expressed in the motto which stands at the beginning of his doctoral thesis. It is a quotation from Francis Bacon: "Nec manus nuda neque intellectus sibi permissus multum valet," which means: Neither manual work alone nor imagination unchecked by facts is worth much.

Remak's doctoral thesis was published in the customary Latin. Printed by Reimer in Berlin it was also issued in another edition without the "theses" presented for solemn disputation and without the Vita. The title page, too, was changed, and in this form the work was presented as an independent publication. The doctoral thesis in its original form and the non-thesis edition were both dedicated to Remak's friend the physician De Bentkowsky.

This De Bentkowsky was one of Remak's three official opponents on the occassion of his graduation as a doctor, the two others also being gentlemen with Polish names. It is noteworthy that Remak, after

THESES.

1. *Hodierna morborum cutaneorum divisio multis in rebus cum systemate plantarum sexuali convenit, atque probe exculta ad divisionem illorum naturalem rectamque cognitionem perducet.*
2. *Non omnes eruptiones cutaneae ex causa venerea exortae luem universalem indicant.*
3. *Quo quis medicus junior, eo minus in morbis acutis pectoris curandis auscultationem sequatur.*
4. *Tuberculosis retardata plerumque phthisin floridam producit.*
5. *Sine medico judex nullus.*
6. *In plurimis aegrotis praestat, canalem lacrymalem imperveium destruere, quam tubulis impositis curare.*
7. *Diversa officia, diversa structura.*
8. *In hoc placito: — rerum virtutes rerum natura sunt, rerum autem natura res ipsae — unica physiologiae spes.*

FIG. 43. Theses of Remak to be publicly defended at the occasion of his graduation as M.D. Courtesy of Berlin University.

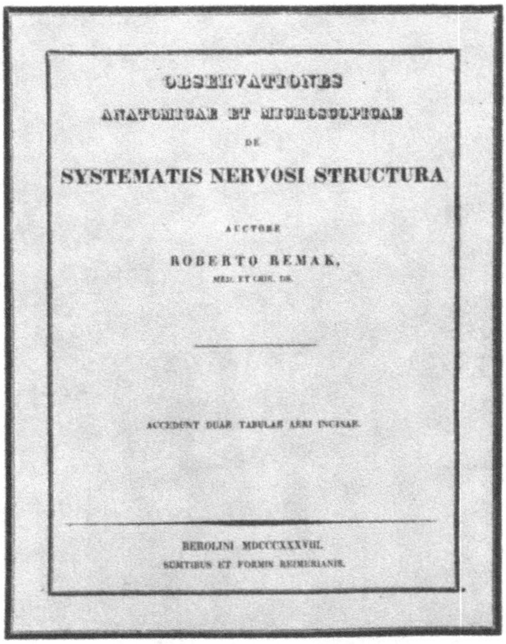
OBSERVATIONES
ANATOMICAE ET MICROSCOPICAE
DE
SYSTEMATIS NERVOSI STRUCTURA
AUCTORE
ROBERTO REMAK,
MED. ET CHIR. DR.
ACCEDUNT DUAE TABULAE AERI INCISAE.
BEROLINI MDCCCXXXVIII.
SUMTIBUS ET FORMIS REIMERIANIS.

FIG. 44. Remak's doctoral thesis. Second edition with changed title page. Size of the original 10½" × 8½". Courtesy of Historical Library, Yale University Medical School.

living for five years in Berlin and being a member of the inner circle of Johannes Müller's laboratory, when he had to select the friends to be his opponents, as was usual for this solemn occasion, did not choose even one of them from among his German colleagues in Berlin or from Müller's assistants. One of his opponents, a Count Czapski, was not even a medical man, rather strange in the case of the dissertation of a medical graduate. Perhaps among these Polish friends were some of his benefactors, who had subsidized his studies at Berlin.

Two years Remak's senior, De Bentkowsky, to whom this thesis is dedicated, was the son of a Polish university professor in Warsaw. He was a physician in Posen, Remak's home town, but later went to Rome to study theology and became a priest (85). Remak's choice of friends to participate in his solemn graduation demonstrates clearly that he did not have very close contact with German students and doctors in Berlin or in Müller's laboratory. This is easily understandable for one who knows the general ways of most German students at this time, their pleasures and amusements, and their attitude towards Jewish colleagues.

That Remak was not just one of the usual graduating flock is also apparent from the "theses" offered for

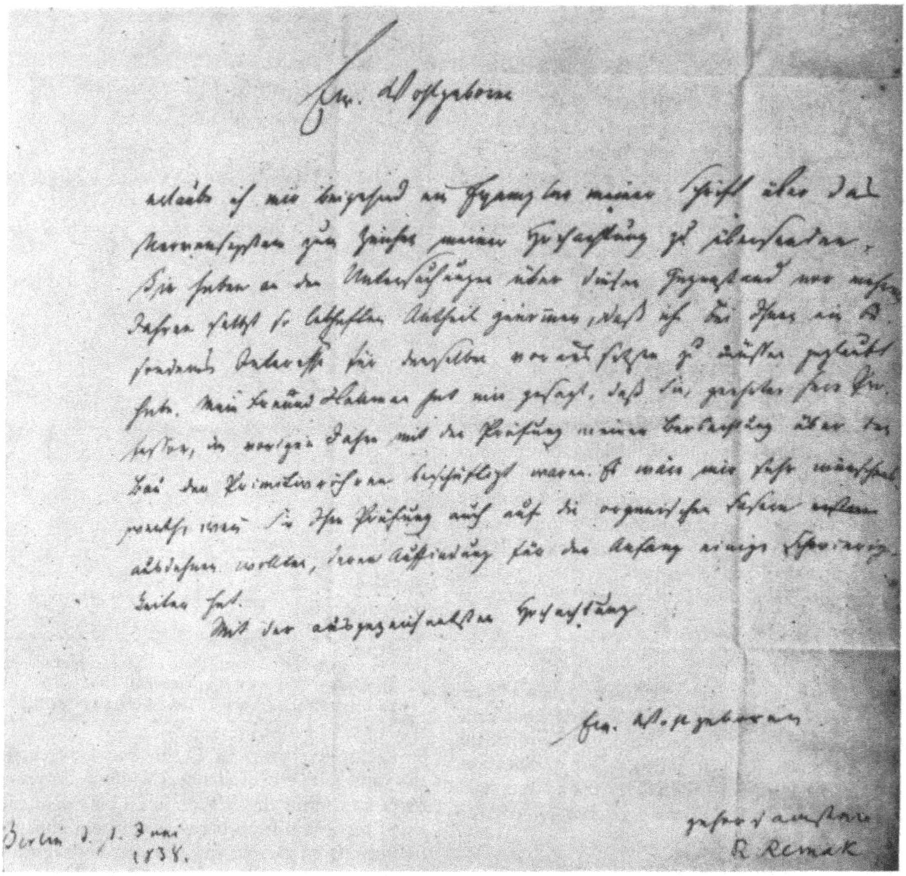
Berlin d. 1. Juni 1838.

R. Remak

FIG. 45. Letter of Remak accompanying the copy of the second edition of his doctoral thesis dedicated to Prof. Krause. Size 8″ × 6″. Courtesy of Historical Library, Yale University Medical School.

discussion at his graduation as a doctor. Some of these general statements which were selected by Remak and which had to be defended in public, sound peculiar, such as the statement "sine medico judex nullus" (without the physician no judgment is possible). Point 7 of these statements asserts that "a different function is connected with a different structure of tissues." This is unquestionably an extremely important statement, based on his own studies comparing the structure of spinal and sympathetic nerves. It also shows that Remak in 1838 had not yet abandoned the view held by Ehrenberg and him, and published in 1836, that microscopical differences may be found between motor and sensory nerve fibers. This question still awaits modern, especially electronmicroscopic, methods for a final decision. Revealing Remak's philosophical conceptions with respect to science is the last statement of the thesis, which emphasizes that the only hope for physiology is the fact that "the properties of things present their nature and the nature of things is the things themselves." There is no question that such a statement was based on his own careful study of Kant's philosophy. Such a statement and attitude may also explain why he included a non-medical man among his friends as an opponent.

The newly graduated doctor, too busy to translate his thesis into German, as he had originally intended, proudly sent it out to the distinguished men in the profession. Alexander von Humboldt was among those who received a complimentary copy.

Humboldt, the last universal genius among scientists, had a keen eye for outstanding contributions, and as Remak himself thankfully mentioned years later in 1855 in the introduction to his standard work on the *Embryology of Vertebrates,* he received the most favorable response from this much admired man (69). To quote

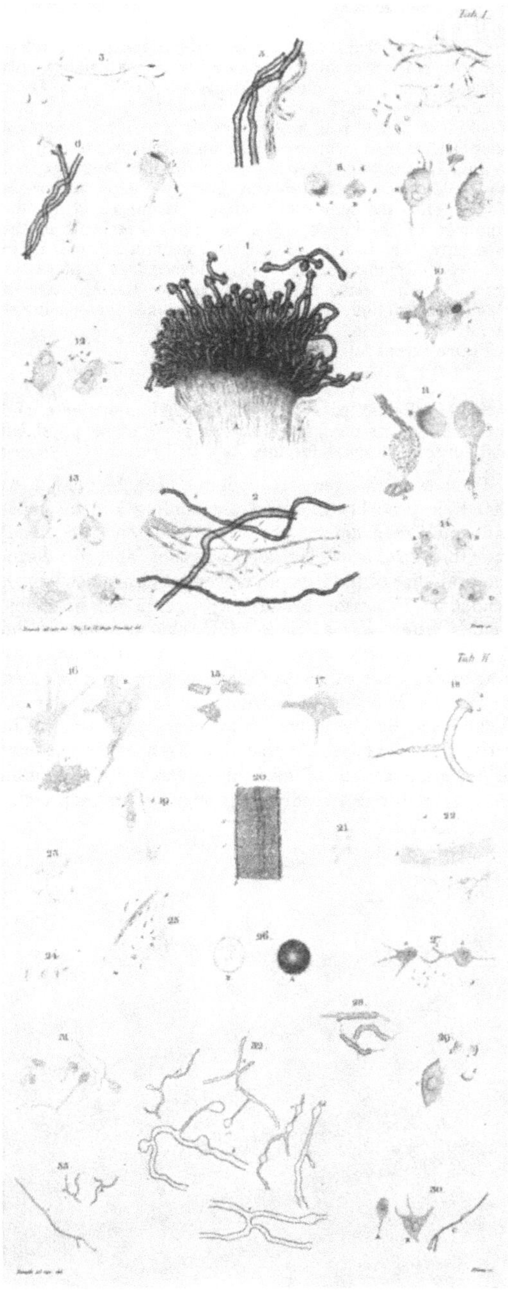

FIG. 46. The two tables from Remak's doctoral thesis showing: nerve fibers, axis-cylinder, unmyelinated fibers (organic—or Remak's fibers) and the origin of nerve fibers from ganglionic cells. Ganglionic cells with nuclei and nucleoli.

Remak's own words on Humboldt's reaction to the receipt of Remak's thesis: "I not only received encouraging words, but I gained untiring advice and help against religious and political intolerance which brought strife into my life, divided my energies, and denied my activities the necessary scope." "How little," says Remak, "is this dedication able to express the thankfulness that will accompany me to the end of my days" (69).

All the tragedy in Remak's later life, the bitterness and aggressive attitude, often marked by others, in his publications of later years, can to a great degree be explained by the fate he suffered owing to his steadfast adherence to his Jewish faith and Polish education. Indeed, his gratitude to Humboldt never waned, and another book (1858), which Remak regarded as one of his main contributions to practical medicine, was dedicated to Humboldt on the occasion of Humboldt's eighty-ninth birthday (73).

Here we present a picture of Remak's two tables, published in his doctoral thesis. Today they are so rare that even Stieda (80), when he wrote his history of our knowledge of the nerve cell, did not know them. Stieda, however, emphasizes that, as little as is known, it was Remak who first reported on and depicted in his early drawings those oblique partitions interrupting the myelin sheaths of each segment of a nerve fiber, which today are called Lantermann's incisures or Schmidt-Lantermann's clefts, but actually are Remak's discovery.

A glance at Remak's drawings shows better than any discussion how well he saw the axis-cylinder. The picture published by Purkinje in 1838 (59) demonstrates the superiority of Remak's observations and the exactness of his drawings, and the same holds for his pictures of nerve cells and their connections with nerve fibers, the multipolar ganglionic cells, and so on. Remak returned to the multipolar ganglionic cells in an important paper of 1855, which, as Deiters himself later admitted, was the start of his own work and of the modern neuron theory.

RELATIONSHIP TO POLAND

The main contents of Remak's thesis were soon published by him in the Polish language also. An extensive paper of fifty printed pages on nerves and the nervous system, it appeared in a medical journal in Warsaw (1838). As a footnote on the title page indicates, it was submitted on the condition that nothing should be altered in the language of the text. This shows how certain Remak was of his perfect knowledge of the Polish language (85) in the time of its modern development; and, indeed, many expressions used in this paper and later in the Polish medical literature were his own creations and a lasting contribution to Polish medical terminology. Later on he published several other papers in Polish and supervised the translation and edition of a Polish handbook for midwives in 1841. In 1843 a paper by the polyglot Remak in French was included in the *Memoirs* of the Society of Medicine in Warsaw, dealing with the indications of destruction of cancerous and non-cancerous tumors.

At the time of Remak's graduation, Jews were by the law not admitted to any teaching positions at a Prussian university. The young scholar, therefore, looked for another country where he might find a suitable position to safeguard his future research activities. His mastery of the Polish language, his education in the Gymnasium of Posen and his friendly connections with outstanding Polish personalities in Berlin as well as in Poland drew his interest to the Medical School in Wilna, where the vacancy of the chair of physiology in the medical faculty presented a timely opportunity. At that time Count Ouwaroff (1786–1855), an enlightened man eager to advance the standards of the Russian universities, was Minister of Education in Russia. Educated in Germany, he was an acquaintance of Goethe, to whom he dedicated a published paper. Remak secured Alexander von Humboldt's friendly support of his application. Humboldt's letter to Ouwaroff has been preserved in a copy written by Remak and published in the original French by Geiger (21). In English translation it reads:

To his Excellency Knight d'Ouwaroff, Minister of Public Instruction, President of the Imperial Academy, Grand Cordon, etc., at St. Peterburg.

Sir:

Your Excellency has been kind enough to permit me from time to time to introduce to you men, who by their talents and their work in the various fields of science have become in some way known to me and to call your attention to them. The kind benevolence with which you have continued to accept such communications evokes my most sincere appreciation. Here we have a young scholar, a native of Posen, Dr. Remak. After having received a second award of the Faculty of Medicine of the University of Berlin, he distinguished himself in anatomical and physiological investigations, which are very excellent and important, concerning the structure of nerves, their plexus, and the ganglions of nerves. I was able to follow the work of Dr. Remak together with my friend, Mr. Ehrenberg, by means of the microscope. It manifests great acuteness of observation, a laborious assiduousness, and the kind of general conception which characterizes modern physiology. I will not tire Your Excellency by enumerating the various papers that Dr. Remak has published in Latin, in German, and in Polish. I only mention that one of the most outstanding anatomists of Europe, our academician Johannes Müller, will be greatly pleased, if Your Excellency desires it, to confirm the commendation which I give to the talent, the diligence, and the moral character of Dr. Remak.

At the moment there is, as I believe, a vacant chair of physiology at the Medical Academy of Wilna. Mr. Mianovski, Professor at this institution, has given Mr. Remak some encouragement.

The young man belongs to the Mosaic religion, and his tender sentiments, for which you can hardly blame him, prevent him from becoming a Christian in order to serve his better interests. He immediately wrote to Wilna that he is a Jew, so that the Academy would not be ignorant of this fact.

Could I say that, regarding your legislation, very tolerant with respect to adherence to a certain nationality, this difficulty could be overcome in certain cases by a favor in accordance with the merits. I would like to hope that Your Excellency will bestow the favor of an exception upon Dr. Remak, who would be an excellent addition for Wilna. He does not yet know the Russian language, but he could teach in Latin and give his explanations in Polish (for the moment); later, Russian could be the language of the pupils. The honorable President of the Academy, Mr. de Kuczkowski, as I understand, will be in St. Peterburg in October. His influence may support the action which I have dared to submit to the Minister of Public Instruction, who is always inclined to encourage talent.

Please accept

le Baron de Humboldt.

Sansouci, 8th of September, 1839.

P.S. Mr. Remak passed the main examinations here, and the Minister has recognized him as a practicing physician and surgeon, licensed for the State of Prussia.

In spite of this remarkable letter even Humboldt, at that time probably the most outstanding and the most influential man among physicians and scientists in all scientific circles of Europe, was not able to dispel the prejudice of the Russian Government against Jewish scholars. Professor Mianowsky, mentioned in Humboldt's letter, was a friend of Remak and one of the official opponents at the occasion of his graduation. Remak was not called to Wilna as professor and had to face the fact that in Germany he, as a Jew, was officially and by law barred from every path leading to an academic career. At that time France was not only a flowering center of medical research and scientific progress; it was friendly to foreigners and especially

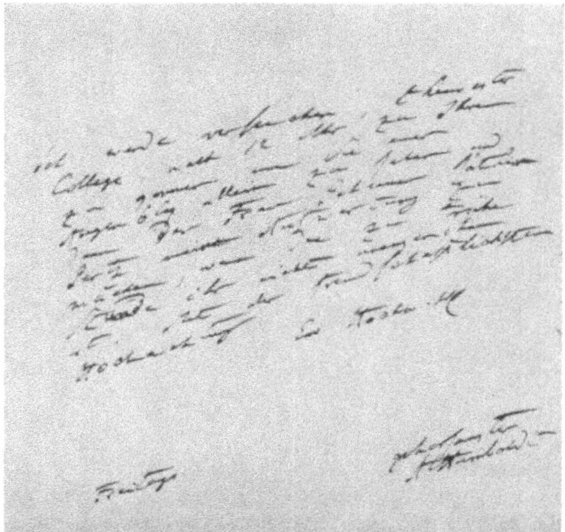

FIG. 47. A typical letter of Alexander von Humboldt. No salutation, date only: Friday. From the author's collection.

benevolent toward citizens of maltreated Poland. Remak, therefore, seriously considered leaving Germany and emigrating to France, particularly to Paris. He must have written about his plans to Humboldt and also probably apologized for having caused Humboldt the trouble of supporting his endeavors to be called to Wilna. Humboldt answered in a letter of 1839, discouraging Remak from emigrating (21).

Like all the following letters of Humboldt to Remak, this letter has, as was Humboldt's habit, no salutation and also no date. They are written in a slanting hand, often difficult to decipher; but their tone changes, very noticeably, with progressing years, showing how the relationship between the two men grew closer in the years between 1839 and 1855. The first letters use the formal terms, "Euer Wohlgeboren"; the later ones, "Dear Remak" or "Dearest Herr Doctor," and finally he closes his letter of January, 1855 with the phrase, "With old enduring attachment in friendship." This feeling of sympathy toward the young scholar already speaks out in Humboldt's answer to Remak's disclosure that he intends to go to Paris. After Remak's disappointment over the professorship at Wilna, Humboldt writes in 1839 (21: 117):

> With me, you don't need any justification. I, too, believe that the negative answer from Petersburg has as its reason only the systems, which prove to be different. In Petersburg they seem to have decided in favor of un-Christian intolerance to exclude Jewish scholars, whereas in Wilna they display a more liberal attitude. I would not advise emigrating to Paris. The practice there is extremely overcrowded and you will not gain anything from your work already published. A. von Humboldt.

Remak followed Humboldt's kindly advice and remained at Berlin, where the friendly interest of Humboldt, Ehrenberg, and Johannes Müller in his fortunes promised at least facilities for research, even though it could not obtain for him a suitable academic position. But Remak's interest in the scientific life of Poland and in the Polish medical schools never ceased.

Eleven years later, in 1850, Remak was in fact offered a chair of physiology, anatomy, general pathology, and semiology at the University of Krakow. It is indicative of his sincere devotion to his work that, in spite of the bad experiences he had already had at Berlin at that time in connection with his career, he did not accept the call, which would have given him the possibility of independent work. In his reply to Krakow University, which was written in Polish, and which in 1925 was in the possession of Wrzosek (85) he acknowledged the offer very thankfully, but he did not feel able to accept it because an extensive piece of embryological research prevented him from leaving Berlin for the next years. The work he mentioned here was his fundamental book on the development of the tissues of the embryo, with which he led to up-to-date, modern embryology. This decision may also have been influenced by the fact that in the meantime he had married the daughter of a distinguished Berlin family and was thus settled in the Prussian capital.

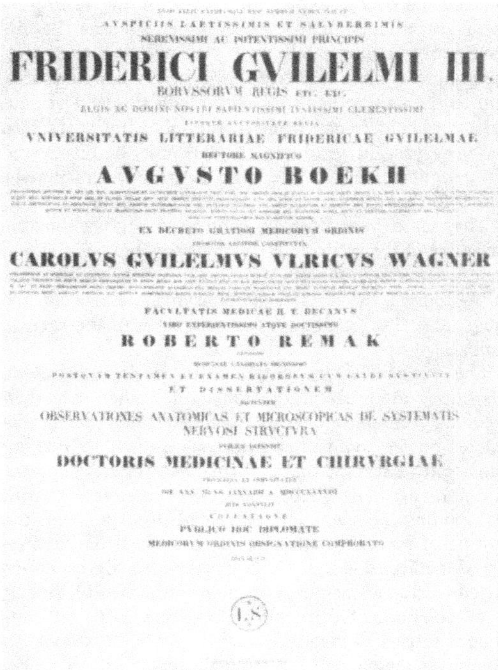

FIG. 48. Doctoral diploma of Remak (Jan. 30, 1838). Duplicate as usually handed to the young doctor in several copies with the original diploma. Courtesy of University of Berlin.

THE FIRST YEARS AS A DOCTOR

We have gone far ahead of our story and return now to the time of Remak's graduation as a doctor. He received his degree of doctor of medicine and surgery from Berlin University on January 30, 1838. Both of his parents were still alive at that time. Not many doctoral theses have ever been written that have had such an epoch-making influence on contemporary medicine. The discovery of the axis-cylinder of the medullated nerves, which is the essential part of the nerve fiber; the discovery that the nerve fiber stems from a ganglionic cell and that therefore the ganglionic cell and the pertinent nerve fiber are automatically a unit, and the description of the unmedullated nerve fibers (Remak's fibers), which are the fibers of the sympathetic nerves, all these details, which he had already published in part in 1836 and 1837, were now connected into one fundamental work.

Among the abundance of new material and observations accumulated in the thesis, these three facts are most outstanding. Each of them would have justified for the discoverer a place of honor in the history of medicine. Other minor observations, such as the discovery of ganglionic cells with two nuclei in the spinal ganglia, fade when compared with the three main points, and so do many other contributions to the field of neurology, which Remak made in the following years. In the very year he graduated as a doctor, he discovered the ganglionic cells in the heart of man and mammals, which to this day are called Remak's ganglion.

The same year Remak conducted studies on the structure of the retina. He also discovered ganglia and ganglionic cells in the intestines, and in 1840 and in 1841 in the tongue, the larynx, the pharynx, the bronchi, the lungs, and also (in 1852) in the stomach of the various animals.

The young doctor continued to work in Müller's laboratory after his graduation, and Müller, who had previously supplied him with valuable material for his studies on the sympathetic nervous system by making him a gift of several sharks,[13] followed the development of one of his most gifted pupils with interest and with his guiding advice. He entrusted Remak with the writing of several articles for the encyclopaedic dictionary of medical sciences, which appeared in Berlin under the editorship of members of the medical faculty, among them Johannes Müller himself. From 1839 he continuously tried to inspire Remak to write a textbook on general pathology (73). Remak really set to work, and the manuscript was well along, but he did not feel like finishing it, even though Müller, who had himself published an outline of general pathology, repeatedly tried to encourage him to complete the project, using the ample material of the famous Berlin clinician's Schönlein's hospital wards for this purpose. But this task was a disagreeable one for Remak. It was, as he expressed it, "to be suspended between heaven and earth." This meant only to meditate on problems and conditions when such meditations had no scientific value, and when material research and helpful endeavors were urgently needed for the patient (66).

STRUGGLE FOR RECOGNITION

The significant characteristic of Robert Remak's life as a scientist was just the opposite of Valentin's. His most brilliant discoveries met with distrust, contempt, and acid criticism on the part of the prominent representatives of the profession. From the start of his career as a scientist to the very day of his death, Remak's life, like that of his contemporary Semmelweis, was a struggle for the recognition of his discoveries. Among them his work on embryology met the least opposition.

Generally speaking, E. Michaelis' judgment of Remak, made in 1877 in Albrecht von Graefe's biography (50), is correct; he calls him a man whose merits in histology as well as in the field of pathology were never adequately acknowledged, either by his contemporaries or by posterity. That was true during all of Remak's lifetime, and it is true to this day.

When Johannes Müller finally gave Remak credit for his discovery of the unmedullated nerve fibers, he even expressed, in his *Archiv* in 1838 (pp. c and ff.), a kind of apology, stating that while the early opposition to Remak's work may have been justified, even necessary, to prove its real value, now everyone had the opportunity to convince himself, by investigating the appropriate material suggested by Remak, that he was correct in his discovery of the unmedullated nerve fibers. This remark by Müller is indubitably meant as a defense of his pupil against the critical attacks of Valentin (see p. 166).

Recognition by Müller was the highest reward for Remak, especially in view of the continuous opposition of Müller's most intimate friend, Henle. It was written in a tone of respectful acknowledgment of an outstanding pupil by his great teacher. Nevertheless, there is not the warmth with which Müller had previously, in his yearly reports, defended his close friend and pupil Henle against attacks, nor the enthusiasm with which he always speaks of his pupil Schwann's achievement. A genius like Müller, who, in 1837, glowingly praised the discovery of the fibrillatory movement in vertebrates by Purkinje and Valentin, was surely aware of the far-reaching implications of Remak's work but no enthusiasm can be felt in his announcements of the results in his annual reports.

There was some tenseness noticeable in the relationship between Remak and Müller's school. Was it Remak's peculiar attitude and character? Was it Henle's opposition? Was it Müller's inability to be pleased by his pupil's discovery of facts which the master had officially doubted before? Who can tell! Du Bois-Reymond, in his eulogy for Müller (11), does not hesitate to declare that Müller had the reputation of envying others for their scientific achievements. Only a few days before his death Müller confessed to Du Bois (11: 153): "My envy changed to admiration. But this is nobility of character which one attains only gradually." An insignificant proof of this attitude of Müller shows in a letter, in this writer's possession, congratulating his friend Henle on the occasion of the latter's accepting a call to the University of Heidelberg. This letter mirrors the close friendship of both. Müller, who never was connected with Heidelberg University writes: "I always felt to have missed a main part, because I never have lived and worked there [in H.] neither as student nor as teacher. It is evident that I would grudge many a person such a position but of course not you."

Should a discovery that necessarily would make the discoverer world renowned be less reason for envy than the call to a professorship?

Surely this young student Remak revealed unusual qualities. It was indicative of his acquaintance with

[13] Froriep's *Notizen* 3: 150, 1837.

scientific literature and of his sincere integrity that when publishing his discovery of the axis-cylinder he should cite the otherwise unknown fact that Fontana, in a publication on viper venom (16: 369) may have already had the right idea about the structure of nerve fibers. Of course, Remak here gives more credit to Fontana than the latter really deserved (80).

Here is another example of Remak's somewhat strange behavior. Remak was an eager microscopist in those years of his neurological studies, but as mentioned above, he did not limit his interest to neurohistology. He investigated the most diversified material. For instance, he was the first to study carefully the histology of condyloma, a wart-like growth or tumor. Two years later G. Simon[14] wrote concerning this work: "The only exact investigation on this topic was performed by Remak, who had his observations published by Gonzenbach." Probably every ambitious student of Remak's age of twenty-one would have been eager to publish such basic studies and discoveries himself. Remak did not care; he gave the material to a fellow student, O. De Gonzenbach, who included it in his doctoral thesis (Berlin, 1837), where it may be found on page 8. This was not the only such incident. At the same time Remak studied microscopically the diseased skin of favus patients and saw there peculiar structures like rods and buds. He did not care to publish this important discovery himself, and we find it mentioned only in the doctoral thesis of his friend and fellow student Xaver Hube, who gave him credit for it.

Such an attitude, to be expected in a distinguished chief of a laboratory, is strange in a student of twenty-one, who has not yet graduated; it was likely to create the impression of snobbishness and to produce a somewhat cool relationship between him and other young competitors for fame in Müller's laboratory.

It was also unusual not to dedicate his doctoral thesis to one's parents or, like Henle, Schwann, and Helmholtz, to their famous teacher Müller; Remak dedicated it to an unknown young Polish doctor friend of his. Among his three opponents, all of the Polish nationality, one was a professor and one a count studying law. All these rather extraordinary acts probably created a tense atmosphere between young Remak and the other members of Müller's laboratory and perhaps, also, between him and his chief.

This tension became stronger the following year. Remak was already well known in the scientific world. Carus, the famous scientist, master of comparative anatomy, court physician to the king of Saxony, painter and natural philosopher, asked him in a letter for certain information on the histological structure of the retina. The manner in which Remak answered this letter was unusual. He did not publish his findings on this subject in a paper, but Müller published Remak's reply to Carus in his *Archiv* in 1839 as a letter written by Remak to Carus. To this letter is added a short contradictory remark by Müller's right hand man Henle, who, in the meantime, had taken over from Müller the annual reports on antomy for the *Archiv,* and had been made a lecturer at the University since 1837.

In denying the facts accepted by Remak, this paper by Henle was, if not hostile, at least written in an unfriendly spirit, and Müller's own report on Remak's publications sounds still cooler this year than it did in 1838. Henle, in order to understand the situation well, as managing editor of *Müller's Archiv* had received Remak's manuscript from Müller before its publication, so that he was able to publish his opposition simultaneously. These remarks, added to Remak's five-page article, were also five pages in length. Henle not only objected to Remak's questioning of the connection between the rods in the retina and the nerve fibers, adhering to Treviranus' opinion that these were the terminal parts of fibers of the optic nerve; he also took the occasion to introduce polemical remarks about Remak's discovery of the axis-cylinder of the nerve fibers, which he, Henle, at the time regarded only as the empty sheath of the nerve fibers, thus siding with the hostile Valentin.

This kind of polemic was no doubt an open attack on Remak. Th. Bischoff, Müller's pupil and a highly esteemed professor at Heidelberg and later at Munich, wrote in the same volume of *Müller's Archiv* a report on the discoveries in physiology during 1838.[15] He too made official attack on Remak's discovery of the unmedullated fibers, concluding (p. 163) that he, the reviewer, agreed with Valentin that these alleged fibers did not exist at all. He even implied that Remak had mistaken certain epithelial formations for the supposed sympathetic nerve fibers. In the following year the same Professor Bischoff, in his annual report in *Müller's Archiv,* remarked only briefly that more and more scholars were agreed on and had proved the fact that there was no such thing as Remak's organic nerves (the unmedullated nerve fibers).

In that year the worst blow to the young scholar's reputation came from Müller himself who, in his *Archiv* of 1839, reviewing Remak's Polish publication on his findings in neurology, raised his mighty voice against one of the most outstanding discoveries of his pupil and said in so many words (p. 204): "Concerning the direct connection of ganglionic globules with the gray fibers, I never was convinced of that, in spite of the fact that Remak demonstrated to me often enough during his investigations the processes of the ganglionic globules."

Everyone in those early years seemed to agree with Valentin, who stubbornly rejected all of Remak's neurological discoveries concerning the unmedullated fibers and the connection between nerve cell and nerve fiber. It certainly needed a strong character to resist such

[14] *Müller's Archiv* 1839: 17.

[15] *Ibid.*, 123.

concentrated attacks against his own fundamental discoveries and to continue his work indefatigably as Remak did, in spite of being handicapped and depressed by an apparently serious chest condition. But only three years later came the fundamental corroboration of this discovery from Müller's own laboratory by his pupil Helmholtz (30).

How great was this period and how great these personalities! Remak, the young student, resisted abandoning an opinion, which his admired and beloved teacher, Johannes Müller, the greatest anatomist and physiologist of Germany, did not share. Müller, on the other hand, did not hesitate to publish in his own journal, out of due respect for the firm conviction of a reliable and sincere research worker, the work of his young assistant, in spite of the fact that he himself was not at all convinced that the observations reported and the conclusions drawn were really valid.

How much could we, in our time, learn from them!

All this happened when Remak had little hope concerning his future scientific career and none with regard to his health. He was certain, as he wrote Valentin at the peak of their fight (see p. 166), that he did not have much time left to do research work and wished, therefore, to utilize his days as well as possible for his studies and to live in peace with everyone.

His controversy with his own teacher, however, did not result in a break in their relationship; both Müller and Remak wanted only to find the truth. Their disagreement therefore impresses us, who live in a time of very different standards.

Remak was not defeated by all these controversial opinions and polemics nor by his political and physical handicaps. He must have worked day and night at that time. In those critical years in addition to his original research work, he wrote many articles for the German *Encyclopedia of Medical Knowledge,* edited by some members of the Berlin Medical Faculty. One of these articles was ordered by mistake and was never printed by the encyclopedia, because another author had already been assigned to the subject. It was an article on menstruation, which led Remak to various investigations of his own. These were published in 1839 and during the years following. But the histology and the physiology of the nervous system and the fight for recognition of his discoveries continued to be the main focus of his interest during those years. When he published his important findings in 1838 in the Polish language, he did it in order to acquaint the physicians among his compatriots with his new outlook. Here he stated, in defense of his own priority, that Fontana, whose description of nerves in the second volume of his book on snake venom [16] he had previously declared to be a forerunner of his own discoveries, really had an entirely erroneous view concerning the axis-cylinder. This was confirmed sixty years later in a critical study by Stieda (80), and must be evident to everyone who cares to read Fontana's fundamental publication.

Recognition of the existence of Remak's fibers (his "organic fibers") was not general up to the middle of the last century. J. Budge still wrote in 1847 in Wagner's *Handwörterbuch:* [17] "The so-called organic, gelatinous or Remak's fibers seem not to belong to the real nerve fibers." Rudolf Wagner himself wrote in 1847 in his *Handbook* (p. 390): "The fibers described by Remak and designated with his name I never accepted as nerve fibers." Even the critical and cautious Carl Ludwig, in his textbook on physiology, still doubted in 1858 whether Remak's fibers were really nerve fibers.

In all these cases the opposing authors could claim that their attitude was one of bonafide criticism. It was different with Henle; at first he denied categorically the existence of Remak's primitive band (axis-cylinder) in the nerves. However, when this fact was increasingly acknowledged, and Purkinje gave the band the name axis-cylinder, to which name Remak unhesitatingly agreed, Henle tried to assert that Purkinje's axis-cylinder was entirely different from Remak's primitive band. This was not a *bona fide* statement, and Remak contradicted this trick repeatedly. He did it first in *Müller's Archiv* in 1843 (p. 199), and when Henle continued, against his own better knowledge, to attribute priority for this discovery to Purkinje, Remak published all the details [18] of how in Henle's presence, he gave Purkinje the first demonstration of the axis-cylinder (discovered by Remak in "May or June, 1837") when Purkinje visited Johannes Müller's laboratory and his famous pupil Remak in Berlin in December 1837. He quoted verbatim what Henle said on this occasion.

Similar to the alleged difference between Purkinje's and Remak's axis-cylinder was Bidder and Volkmann's position in their book on the sympathetic nervous system published in 1842 (6). There they agreed with Valentin and Henle that Remak's organic fibers are no nerve fibers at all, but that, on the other hand, the organic fibers described by Purkinje, Rosenthal, and Pappenheim (p. 15) are something entirely different from Remak's organic fibers. Henle used this same objection against Remak's discovery later. When Remak, in 1842, reported in Canstatt's *Jahresberichte* on the recent physiological literature, he protested against this conclusion (p. 23) and also against Bidder and Volkmann's statement that he had investigated only mammals. He emphasized that the structure of the sympathetic nerves is basically the same in all vertebrates and described in a footnote his demonstration for Purkinje, adding that, when he himself visited Purkinje in 1840 in Breslau, there was no disagreement between them as to the identity of Remak's and Purkinje's organic fibers. But all this did not help, as mentioned above. Years later the greater number of Remak's

[16] **16**: 205, 1787.

[17] **3**: 408, 1847.

[18] *Müller's Archiv,* 469, 1844.

enemies still did not recognize his fibers. It must have been a great satisfaction, therefore, for him to read the following statement by Henle on page 42 of Canstatt's *Jahresberichte* of 1849. He said (in translation): "By and by all opinions agree that Remak's fibers of the branches of the sympathetic nerves have to be regarded as real nerve fibers. Koelliker is still of the opposite view."

The hostility toward Remak and his discoveries passed from generation to generation. Bidder was a close friend and collaborator of Volkmann. Remak's opponent in these years. Stieda's historical article of 1899, on the development of our knowledge of nerve cell and nerve fiber (80) still shows a vestige of this attitude, but he had to admit Remak's importance even for the modern theory of central ganglionic cell and neurite. Yet he repeatedly states, in this otherwise good article, how wrong Remak was to believe at first that the axis-cylinder was a flat band. That Remak was really the discoverer of the axis-cylinder and with that discovery revealed the true structure of the nerve fiber seems, in Stieda's presentation, unimportant as compared with the terrible mistake made by Remak in first supposing this structure to be flat instead of cylindrical.

In spite of all controversies, however, Remak's great discoveries soon made his name well known all over scientific Europe. Alexander von Humboldt and his and Goethe's friend, the famous C. G. Carus in Dresden, and other outstanding scholars were cognizant of the great development in all science and medicine, which began at that time with the use of the microscope for scientific purposes. The devotion of men like Valentin and Purkinje in Breslau and of Ehrenberg, Müller, Remak, Henle, Schwann, and others in Berlin to the use of this instrument for the advancement of medicine initiated an epoch of precise, objective observations. Such a movement necessarily spelled the doom of the spirit of "Naturphilosophie."

Berlin, in the first half of the nineteenth century, became, through Johannes Müller and the clinician Schönlein and their pupils, a leader in the revolutionary struggle of objective science versus the philosophical school of interpreting forms and events in nature in a symbolic, philosophical way. The greatest minds of the previous period were such natural philosophers (Naturphilosophen), and they boasted of names like Hegel, Schelling, Oken, and even Goethe, and young Johannes Müller was regarded as inclined in their direction. In this struggle of views, the microscopists played a major part. In the early nineteenth century Schelling and Hegel were still highly admired, and the last outstanding scientist representing the old school and denying the new way was Carl Gustav Carus, Professor and later Director of the Medico-Surgical Academy in Dresden, court physician to the King of Saxony, and author of important works on anatomy, comparative zoology, craniology, and psychology. His report on his meeting with Purkinje and Remak, both of whom visited him in the fall of 1841 in Dresden, is extremely interesting (10). In his autobiography he writes how impressed he was by the reports of these two outstanding physiologists on their microscopical discoveries. Full of interest as this great man was, he wrote:[19]

> Two fine physiologists, Purkinje (still in Breslau) and Remak (from Berlin), came to see me late in the fall, both of different points of view, mainly microscopists. Day after day various controversies arose, as can be well imagined, but both were serious, gracious personalities. I willingly followed their objections and tried to do them justice. In this way I became more and more acquainted with the material.

At that time Carus was writing his textbook on *Physiology,* still entirely from the point of view of natural philosophy, and he thought it important to maintain the balance of ideas by warning against overestimation of rising microscopical research.

How highly young Remak was regarded by a man like Carus becomes clear from his remarks (10: **3**: *227*) recognizing that he himself should not have yielded to his publisher's demand in 1847 for a second edition of his *Physiology*. Carus, now aware of the importance of the new discoveries, writes (p. *227*): "It was not my business nor my profession to delve into all microscopical, microchemical, and physical material accumulated at that time in huge amounts by people like Valentin, Müller, Remak, and others."

There is no question that Remak was, at that time and in this respect, considered the equal of Valentin and Müller and an outstanding representative of the new school of Berlin.

THE HISTORY OF THE DISCOVERY OF THE GANGLION-NERVE CONNECTION

By the middle of the nineteenth century the struggle against Remak's great neurchistological discoveries was over. One by one of those who had ridiculed them and accused Remak of fundamental mistakes and ignorance yielded to the increasing pressure of facts: first, Johannes Müller, then Purkinje, finally Valentin, and most reluctantly Henle. The facts became standard knowledge and teaching material, and their discoverer was no longer mentioned. This holds true largely for the fundamental fact of the origin of nerve fibers in ganglionic cells. One after another of Remak's followers and former opponents soon claimed for himself the great discovery. Modern textbooks, as a rule, do not place great stress on careful historical research, merely copying statements one from the other or omitting the historical part entirely. A detailed report of the facts is therefore justified.

In 1849 Koelliker, in the first volume of his *Zeit-*

[19] Carus, C. G., *Lebenserinnerung* **3**: 132, Leipzig, Brockhaus, 1866.

schrift für wissenschaftliche Zoologie (p. 135) was the first to claim for himself, in an article entitled "Neurologische Bemerkungen" the credit for this discovery. He writes:

> Concerning the origin of the nerve fibers, it is well-known that in 1845 I was the first to discover in vertebrates the connection of real nerve fibers with the pale processes (Fortsätze) of ganglionic cells (42). Previous investigators found that these processes of ganglionic cells are very long in invertebrates and that probably there is a transition into the nerve fibers.

In support of his claim Koelliker quotes Bidder, who says (5: 10) that Koelliker's statement met "with great and definite confidence and had extraordinary success." Koelliker asserts that he was the first to see the connection and transition of ganglionic cells into fibers, unmistakably dark-margined nerve fibers, which we call today myelinated nerve fibers. Koelliker mentions that neither Hannover nor Will nor Helmholtz were able to prove the connection of nerve fibers with ganglionic cells, although Hannover claimed that discovery for himself even in vertebrates (27). In this article of Koelliker, Remak is mentioned only on page 142 as the last among those (Hannover, Will, Helmholtz, and Remak) who described for invertebrates ganglionic cells from which originate single fibers ("einfachen Faserursprung").

Another claimant for the great discovery was Rudolf Wagner, leading anatomist and physiologist of his time. In his *Handwörterbuch der Physiologie,*[20] where he still denies (1846) that Remak's organic fibers are nerve fibers (pp. 390 and 408), he emphasizes that on November 15, 1846 he observed the origin of primitive fibers of nerves from ganglionic cells in the torpedo fish and that he reported this fact before the scientific society in Göttingen on December 31, 1846.[21]

According to this article by Wagner, Remak deserves no credit at all in neurohistology. What he saw were fringes around ganglionic cells of which he could not make head or tail, and his other supposed discoveries were only misinterpretations of microscopical pictures. Modern textbooks usually name Waldeyer as the father of the so-called neuron doctrine. Most of them, however, in dealing with the neuron and the nervous tissue, do not even refer to the history of our knowledge in this field. Only J. F. Fulton, very much interested in the historical aspect, mentions in his *Physiology of the Nervous System*[22] that Remak in 1838 postulated that the unmyelinated nerve fibers arose from the cells in sympathetic ganglions.

The entire disregard of Remak's contributions as the real basis of the modern neuron doctrine is understandable. Koelliker, who claims this credit for himself, was the head of a great and influential school from which many leading anatomists and zoologists and writers of textbooks of succeeding generations came. The same was the case with Bidder and Volkmann and with J. Henle, Remak's famous enemy of long standing. Henle, in his *Handbuch der Nervenlehre*[23] still says six years after Remak's death: "In 1847 R. Wagner discovered simultaneously with Bidder and Robin the processes of cells in spinal ganglia of fish which turn ('übergehen') into dark-margined nerve fibers." On page 26 he summarizes the opinions about the connection of nerve cells and nerve fibers in the spinal cord and brain as follows: "On this problem, too, Koelliker was skeptical for the longest time, whereas R. Wagner and his pupils repeatedly reported the transition of pale cell processes into dark-margined myelinated fibers." After again mentioning Wagner's discovery of 1847, he finally adds (p. 27) that in 1854 (!!) Remak made similar findings in the spinal cord of oxen.

That is all that Henle had to say, the man who witnessed Remak's discoveries in Johannes Müller's laboratory in 1837 and 1838, being Müller's assistant at that time, who knew Hannover and his work very well, and who saw Remak's struggle for recognition against Henle himself, against Bischoff, Valentin, Purkinje, and many others. Forgotten was the fact that Henle himself, in 1840, in his *Pathologische Untersuchungen,* had extensively reported (p. 87) on Remak's concept of the origin of organic nerve fibers from ganglionic cells and his own doubts as to the correctness of this idea. In 1841 the same Henle, in his *General Anatomy,* mentioned repeatedly (pp. 633, 635, 789) Remak's allegedly erroneous idea of the origin of his "organic nerve fibers" from ganglionic cells and Valentin's and his own opposition to such a concept. That Remak had the same conviction concerning the nerves of the central nervous system is also attested to by Henle himself in his *General Anatomy* (p. 674) where he wrote: "Of course, it should not be overlooked that Remak expected to find in the brain the same origin of the nerve fibers from ganglionic cells as he imagined he established in ganglions."

Now that more than a hundred years have passed since Remak's doctoral thesis was published, an unbiased evaluation of the facts seems indicated.

First, we have to bear in mind that photography was invented only in 1839, and that it took years before photomicrography was well enough developed to permit appropriate publication of objective findings. Every statement concerning microscopical findings made before this modern time is the subjective opinion of the observer. Every published picture before 1839 is not an objective document, but subjective testimony of what the research worker was certain he saw. This holds for the pictures published by Remak as well as for those

[20] 3 (1), 1846.
[21] 3 (1): 361, 1846.
[22] Fulton, J. F., *Physiology of the nervous system,* 190, New York, Oxford Univ. Press. 1943.
[23] 3 (2): 16, 1871.

published by Koelliker, Henle, Valentin, and the contemporaries.

When Remak started his work in 1836, the prevailing opinion was Valentin's concept of the juxtaposition of nerve cell and nerve fiber, without any organic connection with each other. Purkinje, in his report at the meeting of German Scientists and Physicians in Prague, 1837 (59: 179), made the statement: "Nothing definite could be ascertained about the connection between ganglionic cells and nervous or cerebral fibers."

Remak, as early as 1836, 1837, and 1838, had the revolutionary vision of the ganglionic origin of nerve fibers. He tried fairly and honestly to show in his drawings (see p. 239) what he saw and to explain clearly his evaluation of what he saw. How shameful it was to create the impression, as Koelliker, R. Wagner, and others did, that Remak did not have the vision and understanding for such a discovery, for Remak's results are excellently attested to by the man with whom Remak daily discussed his conclusions, though at first he did not succeed in persuading him of their correctness. This man was his teacher Johannes Müller.

Müller, in reviewing the literature of 1837 and 1838, wrote a report of Remak's views in his *Archiv*[24] summarizing Remak's paper written in Polish. Müller states that since he was unfamiliar with this language, he received from Remak, for this review, a translated abstract of the paper. What Müller reports here, not as a statement of his agreement, but as an unbiased reviewer, must therefore be regarded as authoritative. Literally translated, it reads as follows:

> The organic fibers [Remak's fibers], however, originate from the ganglionic cells ['Ganglienkugeln'] themselves. Therefore the ganglia have to be regarded as the real origin of the gray or organic nerves, so that this system has its centers in the ganglions of the sympathetic nerves and in the ganglions of the posterior roots of the spinal nerves. The amount of nerves which appear in the peripheral part of the sympathetic nerve seems too large to reduce them like other nerves to the elements of spinal and cerebral roots. But because the white fibers pass only through the ganglia, it was difficult to imagine any reason for such an increase of mass. The investigations of the author [Remak] explain these facts.[25]

This review of a critical and interested teacher is in fairly literal agreement with the text of Remak's publication in 1837 in Froriep's journal.

Other witnesses to the fact that Remak was the first to dare to present findings on nerve-cell-fiber unity can be found in the publications of his opponents of the period before his theory was accepted. When Valentin, for instance, sharply criticized all Remak's discoveries in 1839[26] he stated: "Remak asserts in the text of his paper as well as in the explanation of the figures that his organic fibers . . . originate from the ganglionic cells themselves. . . ."

The first to confirm Remak's discovery was A. Hannover, a personal friend of Remak, and later a famous anatomist in Copenhagen. Hannover wrote a letter to Professor Jacobson and this letter was published in part by Johannes Müller in the last issue of his *Archiv* in 1840 (p. 552). The main statement in this publication (27) is: "The origin of the brain fibers from brain cells and their lifelong connection with those central parts ('Centralgebilde') is for me more than probable." Hannover, who investigated the cerebrum and cerebellum of vertebrates with the chromium method, states that as a rule two fibers originate in one ganglionic cell; he also confirms definitely the existence of Remak's primitive band (axis-cylinder) which at that time was still regarded by some scholars as another daydream of Remak. He does not quote Remak, but that is not necessary in a short private letter, and there is no doubt that at that time he was well acquainted with Remak's theories. Remak himself resolved all doubt on this question when, in 1841[27] he published a paper which he had read on December 15, 1840 to a meeting of the Friends of Science in Berlin. In this paper he announced the presence of a white layer of nerve fibers on the surface of the brain; he discovered it in the summer of 1839, when he was studying the nerve fibers in the brain, and Hannover, too, was doing research in Müller's laboratory.

Remak writes (p. 506):

> I noticed it ("die weisse Rindenschicht") in the summer 1839, when I followed the course of the primitive tubes in the cortical substance by means of the microscope, and communicated that observation to my friend, Dr. Hannover, who was then present in Berlin and was engaged in similar investigations. This scholar, whose exactness I estimate very highly, immediately confirmed my observations."

Concerning the cerebral nerve fibers, Remak, careful as always, states on page 510:

> I cannot assume with certainty whether they, the primitive fibers of the cerebrum, show a transition into the elements of the gray substance ganglionic cells and their processes. Hannover also favors the probability of such a transition *Müller's Archiv*, p. 555, 1840. But on the basis of my experience I am suspicious ("misstrauisch")

[24] *Müller's Archiv*, 1838: cii.

[25] Because of the importance of this witness, we quote here this passage from Müller in the original also:

"Die organischen Fäden aber entspringen von den Ganglien Kugeln selbst. Daher sind die Ganglien als die wahren Ursprünge der grauen oder organischen Nerven zu halten, so dass dieses System in den Ganglien des n. Sympathicus und in den Ganglien der hinteren Wurzeln der Spinalartigen Nerven seine Centra hat. Die Menge der Nervenmasse, die sich im peripherischen Teil des N. Sympathicus entwickelt, scheint zu gross um sie, wie bei den anderen Nerven auf die Stammelemente von den Spinal- und Cerebralwurzeln zu reducieren. Da nun aber die weissen Fäden durch die Ganglien bloss durchgehen, so war es schwierig sich einen [*sic!*] Vorstellung von der Ursache einer solchen Vermehrung der Masse zu machen. Die Untersuchungen des Verfassers klären dieses Verhältnis auf."

[26] *Müller's Archiv*, 1839: 151.

[27] *Ibid.*, 1841: 506.

concerning the *immediate* [italics by Remak] transition of the dark-margined, i.e., myelinated primitive fibers into the cells of the brain ganglionic cells; for me it is much more probable that the dark primitive fibers show a transition into the longer or shorter pale processes of the brain cells.

From this remark in Remak's paper (December 1840) it is clear that Hannover's conviction concerning the nerve-cell fiber connection (late in 1840) is based on knowledge of Remak's work and conclusions. The end of the above quotation from Remak's paper presents another excellent observation by this critical scholar; today we know very well that the myelin sheath does not start *immediately* at the nerve cell.

Of course, Hannover was very well acquainted with Remak's previous work and ideas, being in daily contact with him over many months.

In 1838 the Royal Society of Sciences of Denmark arranged a competition, offering a prize for the best paper on "Which conclusions could physiology draw from the recent microscopical researches concerning the nervous system?" No question that by "recent researches" were meant those of Ehrenberg, Valentin, and Remak as the most spectacular.

Adolph Hannover, a twenty-five-year-old student from Denmark who had just graduated in March, 1839 as Licentiate in Medicine, came to Berlin with the intention of participating in this competition. There in the same year, 1839, he continued his studies in anatomy and physiology in Johannes Müller's laboratory (27). Müller gladly admitted the talented young foreigner to his institute. Hannover was not just a beginner; in 1837 he had won a Gold Medal from the University of Copenhagen. The subject of this competition had been "Exponatur structura gangliorum systematis nervosi."

With this award Hannover was well introduced to Müller, who extended to him every courtesy, placed his fine microscope at his disposal, and encouraged him to enter the new Danish competition. Hannover remained in Berlin for nearly nine months up to the spring of 1840,[28] and thus had plenty of time for close contact with his young co-religionist Remak and, as Remak himself put it, to become a friend of his. Remak, from whom we know that he was always on especially good terms with the foreigners (94) on Berlin's Medical Faculty, perhaps on better terms than with the native members of Müller's laboratory, was almost the same age as Hannover, and that too drew the two young scholars together. As we learn from his compatriot, Solomonsen, Hannover found the general atmosphere in the Berlin laboratory not very much to his liking (77). Remembering the days he spent later studying in Breslau, he writes to Solomonsen: "The Breslau people were congenial folk, a complete contrast to the dry people of Berlin."

[28] *Müller's Archiv,* 1840: 320.

In 1840 Hannover left Berlin for a trip through Germany, Italy, and Switzerland where he visited Valentin, the other outstanding scholar in the field of neurohistology. He submitted a paper on the history of the microscopy of the nervous system during the past ten years to the Society of Science in Bern, which awarded him a prize, and he returned to his homeland in 1841, where he submitted to the Danish Society of Science a paper on his investigations. This paper, written in Danish, has a preface dated "1840 and 1842." It was published in 1843 in the *Proceedings* of the Danish Royal Society of Sciences (28). The following year it was published as a book in a French translation. Unfortunately, in this book the previous literature is not reported or criticized. Hannover shares very decidedly Remak's point of view concerning the origin of the nerve fiber, but without mentioning Remak's name. The second paragraph of the book makes a very definite statement beginning with the words: "Les fibres cérébrales ont leur origine des cellules cérébrales" (29).

No bitter rivalry ever existed between Hannover and Remak. They were on very friendly terms, as we can see, not only from the way in which Remak writes about Hannover in 1841 as a "highly esteemed friend of his," but also from Hannover's attitude towards Remak, which was equally cordial. This is indicated by Hannover's signature in a copy of his book on the *Microscopy of the Nervous System* (1844), which he dedicated to Remak. This copy is preserved in the Seguin Collection of the Department of Pathology of the College of Physicians and Surgeons in New York. Reproduced as our figure 49, it shows that the friendship between these two famous pupils of Müller continued for many years after their personal contact in Müller's laboratory. A further consideration is the fact that in the German language the word "friend" is used much less casually and less non-committally than in any other language. Therefore, Hannover's affectionate dedication of his book on the nervous system, years after Remak's statements on the history of the great discovery, demonstrates the lack of any resentment or claim for priority on the part of Hannover. That Hannover, indeed, only confirmed and elaborated on Remak's findings is again attested to by their teacher, Müller, who was most familiar with the work of both of them. He writes in the fourth edition of his *Handbook on Physiology:* [29] "Hannover confirmed the observations of Remak concerning the connection of the processes of the ganglionic cells with the gray fibers. . . ."

In Bern, Hannover found Valentin, whom he visited after leaving Berlin, very congenial and friendly, and they remained lifelong friends. What Hannover reported concerning his sojourn in Berlin must unquestionably have influenced Valentin's later opinion on Remak's discoveries.

[29] 1: 528, 1844.

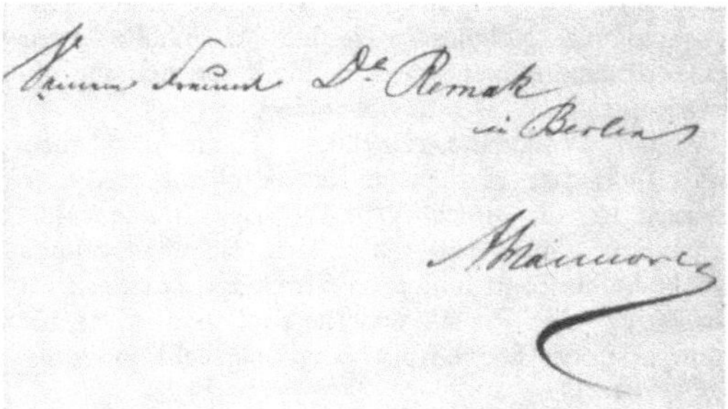

FIG. 49. Personal dedication of the Danish anatomist, Hannover, in a copy of his book on the nervous system. Courtesy of Columbia University, New York.

How little J. Henle, as late as 1845, appreciated Remak's and Hannover's work in neurohistology is apparent from his critical remarks in Canstatt's *Jahresberichte*,[80] where he reviewed the histologic literature of the year 1844. Of Remak's organic (unmedullated) nerve fibers he writes there that "except for Hannover and Remak himself nobody believes any longer" in their existence and he adds that Hannover "again puts forth the view, long ago disproved by Valentin, that the organic nerve fibers originate in the ganglionic cells."

Müller, though in the early forties he had not yet been converted to the new gospel, was not only eager to publish the important statements of Hannover and of Remak but he was also anxious for a final solution in his *Archiv*. Therefore he also persuaded one of his most brilliant younger students, Hermann Helmholtz, to investigate the problem in invertebrates. Helmholtz, as mentioned above, confirmed Remak's findings convincingly, publishing his own investigations in 1842 in his doctoral thesis dedicated to Johannes Müller.

The next year brought another confirmation of Remak's findings. Friedrich Will, lecturer on the medical faculty of the University in Erlangen, published in *Müller's Archiv*[81] a paper on the structure of ganglia and the origin of the nerves in invertebrate animals, as a preliminary report. He does not quote any literature, but he probably was well acquainted with Remak's and Hannover's previous publications in the same journal. Will's final conclusion on page 92 reads as No. 6 of his summarizing statements, that "the nerve cells with simple tube-like processes are to be regarded as the origin or terminal of primitive nerve fibers."

The evidence was growing and was soon overwhelming, when Koelliker in 1844 published his observations. The best impression of how, in 1845, this new, convincing addition to Remak's discovery was received by the profession may be gained from a handbook article by A. W. Volkmann on "Nervenphysiologie," published in 1845 in Wagner's *Handwörterbuch der Physiologie*. This article was written in 1844 before, and partly amended in 1845 after, Koelliker's publication. Volkmann, who with Bidder (6) had published excellent investigations on neurohistology, writes (p. 481): "In short, we do not know the origin of nerve fibers and we probably never will know it . . . ," and he continues:

> All doubts concerning the possibility of finding the origin of nerve fibers would disappear if, as Remak, Helmholtz, Will, and Hannover assert, the fibers have their origin in the ganglionic cells. However, I could persuade myself as little as Valentin or Henle that the processes, occasionally originating from the ganglionic cells, could be regarded as nerves.

Of course, in 1842 Volkmann and Bidder (6) had seen the origins of sympathetic nerve fibers from ganglionic cells but had misinterpreted their findings entirely. Remak, in reviewing this work, pointed out his own priority with respect to the correct view (66).

On page 498 of his above quoted paper on Nervenphysiologie, cognizant of Koelliker's new publication, the same author, Volkmann, says:

> True, Remak has already stated that the organic fibers stem from ganglionic cells, but these nerve fibers . . . were apparently nothing else than the fibers named after him, a kind of cellular tissue, but no nerves. After him Helmholtz, Will, and Hannover tried to prove the same thing, but I at least, was not impressed by their argumentation.

Here is another opponent of Remak, who frankly admits his priority of the great discovery. In 1844 he still doubts the validity of Remak's conclusions, but in 1845 he already admits to having seen in the heart of frogs the origin of nerve fibers from ganglionic cells (Nervenphysiologie, 613, footnote). That Koelliker was no more than the most impressive in the line of Remak's followers is very clear from the following passage in Volkmann:

> On repeating the observations on the frog, I too found similar pictures, but I would not have dared to regard them as nerve origins. It seems that it was Herrn Koelliker's privilege to decide the matter by asserting [!] that he found that those thick, fairly formless processes of ganglionic cells, if followed further away from the place of their origin, form unquestionable fibers.

Volkmann is critical and fair enough to summarize the state of affairs in 1845 as follows (p. 565): "The discoveries of Koelliker *and of his predecessors* [italics are mine] make it probable [!] that the nerve fibers originate from ganglionic cells." How little Koelliker was justified in claiming for himself the credit for this discovery can be proven from his own publication of 1844 (42). After having emphasized that each nerve fiber stems from a nerve cell, he says on page 19, as a kind of excuse for this daring new concept: "What in former days was already suspected, mainly that the nerve fibers stem from the ganglionic globules, seems recently,

[80] 1845: 25.
[81] 1844: 76.

to be more and more recognized as a general law. I am not the only one nor the first who reports observations thereon." He then quotes Helmholtz, Will, and especially Hannover. Remak's statements on the same problem are disregarded because Koelliker in his paper of 1844, like Volkmann, was still of Valentin's opinion that "Remak's fibers" are no nerve fibers at all.

Of course, even Koelliker did not convince everyone. In spite of his publication of 1844, R. B. Todds, in 1847, still came to the conclusion in his *Cyclopedia of Anatomy and Physiology* [82] that the connection between nerve fibers and nerve cells is an entirely unexplained problem.

Finally came Rudolf Wagner, who confirmed the now, well established fact in the selachian fish Torpedo in 1846 and 1847.[83] In his *Handbook* [84] he manages an incredible degree of distortion, saying:

> In spite of the fact that Remak saw in the brain and in ganglions of invertebrates thread-like processes of ganglionic cells, without suspecting that they are the origins of primitive fibers, one is convinced from his drawings that he did not know the real origins of primitive fibers from ganglionic cells.

How confused Wagner was himself, in contrast to Remak, concerning the entire problem can be seen in his short paper, "New Investigations on the Elements of the Nervous Substance," in Canstatt's *Jahresberichte*.[85] After a good description of his own findings, he adds a postscript (p. 83) criticizing Bidder and Volkmann. Meantime Volkmann had already been convinced of the nerve ganglionic cell connection and had published his corrected conclusions in Wagner's *Dictionary of Physiology*. Therefore the latter probably refers in his polemic remarks to Volkmann's and Bidder's original view (1842) that the ganglionic cells were only imbedded in nerve substance but were not the origin of nerve fibers. At the same time Wagner says on page 83 that the origin of the fibers in the cells cannot be conceived in the way that Volkmann and Bidder have done. That makes confusion complete because Volkmann and Bidder originally did not speak at all of the origin of the fibers in the nerve cells, and later (1845) Volkmann agreed with Remak's opinion even though he did not mention Remak.

It was only in 1847 that Johannes Müller himself investigated the problem, and he writes about it in a letter to his friend, the anatomist Anders Retzius in Stockholm, dated December 16, 1847 (74: 58). He reported on an excursion to Helsingor in the fall of 1847 to do research on rays. "I also investigated the connection between nerve fibers and ganglionic globules and found the discovery of R. Wagner and Robin correct. The axis-cylinder of the nerve fiber is connected with the inner part, the nervous tube with the outer part of ganglionic globules." Neither Helmholtz's nor Remak's name is mentioned in this letter, and the observation, as it is stated, is not correct.

Wagner, Volkmann, Koelliker, Henle, and their pupils took care to deprive Remak of the credit he deserved for the discovery of the basic fundamentals of modern neurology. Only Max Schultze admits frankly in his contribution to Stricker's *Textbook on Histology* [86] that Remak was the first to discover the origin of nerve fibers from ganglionic cells in vertebrates.

To eliminate forever any doubt as to whether Remak had clearly in mind the origin of the nerve fibers from the ganglionic cells, his opponents would only have had to read carefully Remak's doctoral thesis of 1838 (64). There on page 9, paragraph 13, he says (in translation):

> But one thing that is unquestionably most important to recognize with respect to the nature of the ganglionic cells, the investigator mentioned [Valentin] did not recognize and could not recognize. *The organic fibers originate from the substance of the nucleated globules itself.* In spite of the fact that this observation is very difficult and requires great dexterity in preparation as well as observation, it is so well founded that it already would not be possible to doubt it. [Italics are Remak's.] [87]

This quotation needs no further explanation. We only add what Remak also put in italics in paragraph 15 on page 10 of his doctoral thesis: *"The sympathetic ganglion has to be regarded as the real center of the organic nervous system."* [88]

Sir W. Osler, discussing to whom credit for introduction of surgical anesthesia should go,[89] quotes Francis Darwin as saying: "In science the credit goes to the man who convinces the world, not to the man to whom the idea first occurs." This is a statement of how things are; it should not be regarded as the standard for what is just or for the way things should be.

FUNCTION OF THE ORGANIC NERVOUS SYSTEM

A comprehensive and, so to say, final statement of Remak concerning the entire problem of the unmedullated nerve fibers appeared in the German language in 1840 in Ammon's *Monthly for Medicine, Ophthalmology and Surgery* as an article of over forty pages. At the time when Bischoff, Henle, Volkmann, Wagner, Valentin, and other outstanding anatomists still consistently

[82] 3: 646, 707, London, 1847.

[83] *Handwörterbuch* 3: 361, 1847.

[84] 3: 390, 1847.

[85] 1847: 81.

[86] S. Stricker *Handbuch der Lehre von den Geweben,* 126, Leipzig, W. Engelmann, 1871.

[87] The Latin text reads: "Sed rem haud dubie gravissimam ad gangliorum naturam cognoscendam investigator ille non cognovit neque cognoscere potuit. *Fibrae enim organicae ab ipsa globulorum nucleatorum substancia oriuntur.* Quae observatio quamquam dificillima sit magnamque et praeparandi et observandi dexteritatem requirat tamen ita constat, ut jam de illa dubitare non liceat."

[88] *"Ganglia sympathica pro veris centris systematis nervosi organici habenda sunt."*

[89] *Ann Hist. Med.* 1: 329, 1917.

denied the existence of the "organic nerve fibers," Remak was already concerned, in his article of 1840, not so much with new proof of their existence, but with the investigation of their physiological function. He firmly rejected the opposing views of Henle and Valentin and built up a theory of the physiological function of the entire organic nervous system.

This classical paper of Remak's was far ahead of his time, and consequently was never properly evaluated and appreciated. When, in the twentieth century, the organic nervous system, or as it is now called, "the autonomic nervous system," was studied and its importance and function rediscovered, Remak's work was already long forgotten, although many of the new basic discoveries were important corroborations of his original statements.

The new and fundamental point in Remak's work was his theory that the differences in the structure of his organic nerve fibers (Remak's fibers) correspond to their different function, different from that of the other nerves in the body. This explained his distinction between the "animalic nervous system" and the "organic nervous system." The latter, in his opinion, originated, not like the first in the brain, but in ganglionic cells of the peripheric ganglia. Another fundamental conclusion of his was that the physiological function of the organic nerves was to influence: (*a*) involuntary muscle movement all over the body, and (*b*) secretion all over the body.

When Remak published this paper in 1840, he had just added the discovery of ganglia in the bladder to the many other places where he had previously found ganglia of organic nerves. On page 257 and the following pages he summarized his opinion based on his own anatomical findings and on experimental results. He stated that the organic nerve fibers influence the function of heart, vessels, lungs, spleen, stomach, intestines, liver, pancreas, kidneys, mucous membranes, serous membranes, and probably also the skin. In all these organs these nerves control involuntary movements. Because the liver is generously supplied with such nerves, but not with any considerable amount of involuntary muscles, Remak drew the excellent conclusion that this alone is proof that the secretion of the liver and the other glands is controlled by the nerves too, for the liver is an organ of excretion and not of movement.

On page 259 is one of the most astonishing and excellent statements of this genius, in which he emphasizes that the organic nerves only influence and moderate the autonomic function of these, mentioned organs, and further that the function does not stop entirely in the absence of the nervous control. On page 264 he postulates organic reflexes and reflex influence on the secretion. It was a long way from there to Pawlow's systematic proof of this postulate, but Beaumont's experiments may have already exercised an effect on Remak's opinions and ideas. We know definitely that they did influence Purkinje in his experimental investigation of digestion. Purkinje reported on these researches, referring to Beaumont, at the Convention of German Physicians and Scientists in Prague in 1837, and his address was published in 1838.

Remak based his opinion, not only on anatomical findings, but also on the clinical observation that affections of the nerves, as well as such remedies which influence the nerves, change the secretion. He connected the so-called "sympathies of the tissues," or what the old physicians called the "consensus partium," with organic reflexes, mentioning his own observations on the effect of localized stimuli on the intestines and arteries, even coming extremely close to the idea of axon reflexes. He also emphasized that the organic nerves influence, not only the quantity, but also the quality of secretion. It does not detract from our admiration of such a vision that Remak considered the effect of the organic nerves on the secretion as largely an indirect effect, arising from their influence on the vessels.

This paper of 1840, really the classic fundamental work on the function of the autonomous nervous system, appeared at a time when outstanding colleagues of Remak—Henle, Bischoff, Valentin, and others—still regarded his organic nerves as artifacts or a kind of connective or epithelial tissue. Among the leaders in anatomy, Johannes Müller and Purkinje gave Remak credit for his great discovery, though without any conception of its overwhelming significance, which Remak alone saw and emphasized in his paper of 1840. Of course, some previous experimental observations had been made on the effect of certain nerves on the contractibility of involuntary organs, like the heart (A. v. Humboldt), the intestines (Johannes Müller), and the vessels (G. Valentin), but all these experiments had been performed with regard to certain specific nerves. Remak was the first to recognize the general law embracing all his "organic nerves" in a system with the general function of controlling involuntary muscle action and secretion.

All his experiments and his observation that most nerves are mixed, containing medullated as well as organic fibers also led Remak to the conclusion that there is a double innervation of the voluntary muscles, one spinal, the other sympathetic, the latter being mainly responsible for the tone of muscles. This interesting concept of muscle physiology, too, was taken up again decades later in modern times.

Finally, Remak set forth, in the *Deutsch Klinik* [40] a hypothesis of central regulation of sympathetic effects. He observed that after sympathectomy the narrowing of the homolateral pupil is accompanied by a widening of the contralateral pupil. The homolateral widening of the vessels and increase of the temperature of the ear

[40] 7: 295, 1855.

in such cases is coupled with opposite effects on the other ear. But he also emphasized as a central result the antagonistic effect of muscle contractions in cases of paralysis of certain muscles and groups of muscles in the face, neck, body, and extremities. In this field he was a forerunner of Sherrington. These experiments and observations by Remak led him to the kind of clinical activity that kept him busy in the last period of his life, the period devoted to galvanotherapy.

Volkmann in Wagner's *Handwörterbuch d. Physiol.* followed in Remak's footsteps four years later (1844), when he also arrived at the conviction that the sympathetic nerves have motor functions with relation to involuntary muscles. He denies however (p. 605) their effect on voluntary muscles. He concedes the importance of Remak's discovery of ganglia in the heart and the intestines, which he calls "one of the most interesting anatomical discoveries of modern time" (p. 614), because since Bichat, the ganglion was regarded as a kind of central organ. This opinion was also supported by Ehrenberg in 1833 (13).

JAMES JOHNSTONE'S IDEAS ON THE USE OF GANGLIA

Indeed, Remak had only one important predecessor in the concept of the function of the sympathetic nerves and ganglia. But this man's ideas were not sufficiently appreciated by his contemporaries and apparently were long forgotten in Remak's time.

James Johnstone, a physician born in Annan in 1730, studied chiefly under Whytt in Edinburgh, where he graduated in 1750. After a visit to Paris, he settled in 1751 as a physician in Kidderminster, later moving to Worcester (1783), where he died in 1802. According to Davenport's *Dictionary of Biography* (London, 1831), Johnstone was the first to use mineral acid vapors to counteract contagion. Johnstone twice reported in the *Philosophical Transactions* of the Royal Society of London on his concept concerning "the use of the ganglions of the nerves." Not being a Fellow of the Royal Society, he wrote a letter on November 24, 1763, to Charles Lord Bishop of Carlisle, F.R.S. (36), which the latter presented at the meeting of May 31, 1764.

Johnstone mentions that Lancisi and Winslow already regarded the ganglia as a kind of subsidiary brain. He points out that the organs which work involuntarily, like the heart, intestines, pupil, blood vessels, Fallopian tubes, uterus, liver, spleen, kidneys, are supplied with nerves rich in ganglia, whereas motor and sensory nerves, viz., olfactory, optic, auditory nerves, and the nerves of voluntary motion, have no ganglia. He concludes (36: 181):

> May we not then reasonably conclude that ganglions are the instruments by which the motions of the heart and intestines are from the earliest to the last periods of animal life rendered uniformly involuntary, and that to answer this purpose is their use, which they subserve by a structure unknown to us, no less than that of the brain, though it seems not improbable the first may be analogous to the last?

Johnstone, unjustly forgotten in the history of medicine, was as much ahead of his time as Remak. His theory was not accepted and he comes back to it in a second paper (37) which three years later, on March 5, 1767, was read at the meeting of the Royal Society. There he (this time his name is written J. Johnston, M.D.) defended his theory against all objections of his adversaries. In a sound and very logical manner he refutes the arguments of his opponents and adds to his theory only the new aspect, that the ganglia and their nerves "may be supposed to have some use in glandular secretion" too. His final conclusion (37: 131) is: "The ganglia according to their structure may justly be considered as little brains, or germs of those nerves detached from them."

The idea of the special function of the ganglia of the nerves captivated Johnstone's imagination from 1763 to the end of his life. He summarized his new opinions in a book of ninety-six pages, sold for two shillings in 1771 (38), which he republished with additions in 1795 as the first chapter of his book, *Medical Essays and Observations* (39).

This remarkable physician's life, his original ideas, and his excellent observations in clinic and experiment are valuable enough to warrant an extensive biography and ergography to secure for him a deserved place in the history of medicine at least 150 years after his death. He was among the first, after Withering's publication of 1785, to use digitalis extensively. In 1795 he gave a classical, short, and clear description of the symptoms of digitalis poisoning (39). He was probably the first to administer digitalis by enema (39: 161), and even suggested to his patients that they smoke digitalis leaves instead of tobacco. He corresponded with Haller concerning his own opinion about ganglia and kept himself informed on the German medical literature.

Johnstone's contribution to the problem of the "use of ganglions" was his recognition of the importance of the ganglia of the nerves for involuntary organs generally. In 1795 he summarized in detail his views (39: 108) as follows:

> The ganglions are organized for the purpose of separating from the power of volition all the organs moved by stimuli acting on irritable parts in the vital and other involuntary organs: the heart, the intestines, the abdominal viscera and glands in general, the Fallopian tubes and uterus, the iris.

This was an important start on the solution of a great problem. Of course, it was only a start, but the insight into the fact that all organs with involuntary functions are supplied with ganglionated nerves is a cornerstone in the structure of our modern knowledge of the autonomous nervous system.

Johnstone also conducted experiments and summarized his novel methods of research in the second chapter of his book that appeared in 1795. Its title shows the original mind of the author, for it reads: *Cui bono? or Physiological and Pathological Observations on the Function of the Visceral Nerves.*

What this protagonist of modern experimental medicine and pharmacology has to say at the age of sixty-five about the reception of his ideas and experiments by the profession (39: 100) sounds sad but at the same time very up-to-date and familiar: "My opinion has been silently attacked and as silently adopted without any explicit acknowledgment of the author or any direct quotation of his work."

Not only in England and Switzerland (Haller) was Johnstone's work known, but he mentions that his system was also adopted by one Frederic Casimir and published in Mannheim (Germany) in 1774. He also refers to a German translation of his 1771 book by one Dr. Kolpin entitled *Versuch über den Nutzen der Nerven Knoten, von James Johnstone* (Stettin, 1787). He probably knew Kolpin personally or through correspondence because this booklet of 104 pages, published by Johann Sigismund Kaffke in Stettin, does not bear Kolpin's name; only the preface is signed A. K. However, all this ephemeral literature was soon forgotten.

Unquestionably Johnstone's excellent observation was unknown to Remak as it was to other scholars of his time. Remak would not have hesitated to quote this opinion, just as he did not hesitate to cite the observations of Fontana when he published his own discovery of the axis-cylinder.

Johnstone did not have any histological or microscopical facts to offer to support his theory and, aware of this shortcoming, he confesses (36) that in connection with strict proof of his opinion, difficulties arise "from our imperfect knowledge of the nerves, in general a terra incognita, which remains to immortalize the name of some future discoverer in anatomy."

Seventy years after Johnstone's second publication this prophecy came true.

REMAK STUDIES "HORNER'S SYNDROME" FOURTEEN YEARS BEFORE HORNER

A final contribution to the physiology of the sympathetic nervous system was made when Remak in 1855 [41] demonstrated through experiments on cats, dogs, rabbits, guinea pigs, and sheep, that cutting the cervical sympathetic nerve produces a prolapse of the nictitating membrane, constriction of the pupil, and narrowing of the palpebral fissure, owing to a ptosis of the upper and slight elevation of the lower eyelid. This happens, of course, on the homolateral eye only. Electrical stimulation of the peripheral section of the severed cervical sympathetic nerve made all these symptoms disappear. The latter experiment can be repeated on the same animal time and again.

[41] *Deutsche Klinik* 7: 294, 295, 1855.

This experimental observation with excellent details was not an original discovery of Remak, but neither was it that of the Swiss ophthalmologist Johann Friedrich Horner, with whose name this syndrome, as a clinical entity, is connected to this day. In two papers (17, 18) J. F. Fulton dealt with some foreshadowings of Horner's discovery.

My own checking on the subject (41) produced the following picture: After the well-known first experimental observations of Parfour du Petit (1727), the question of the influence of the sympathetic nerve on the eye was repeatedly mentioned in literature. The doctoral thesis (Pavia, 1846) of S. Biffi from Milano should be mentioned. Ruete, Professor at the University of Göttingen, wrote in the same year (1846) an article on "Physiology Applied to Ophthalmology" for Wagner's *Handwörterbuch.*[42] There he states, from clinical and experimental observations, that the pupil becomes wider if the sympathetic nerve is stimulated but smaller if the sympathetic nerve is paralyzed. He compares these effects with the effect of the nerves on the heart. Budge and Waller reported in 1851 and 1852 in the Paris Academy of Sciences on animal experiments, showing not only constriction of the pupil after severance of the homolateral sympathetic nerve, but also on the opposite effect when the nerve was stimulated. They also conducted the latter experiment on the head of a newly decapitated criminal.

A very thorough description of what happens when the cervical sympathetic nerve is cut as well as stimulated was given by Claude Bernard in 1852 in repeated presentations at the Paris Academy of Sciences. These experiments were unquestionably known to Remak. He met Claude Bernard personally at that time (1852) in Paris. At the meeting of August 6, 1855, at the Paris Academy, Bernard presented Remak's paper on the motor effects of the "grand sympathetique," and in the same year Remak dedicated to Claude Bernard his book on the methodical electrical stimulation of paralyzed muscles. In his paper Remak quoted both Petit's and Bernard's findings (the years given are 1712 and 1849).

A new fact in Remak's observations was the influence of the sympathetic nerve on the nictitant membrane and the emphasis on the tonic effect of the sympathetic nerve on striated muscles, which according to Remak, have a double innervation. Of interest also is his remark that he used to show this experiment to his students in his lectures on experimental pathology. More and more clinicians now became aware of the importance of the facts observed, yet they were still only isolated cases (15). Heineke in Greiswald (1860) made a pertinent observation in a patient with a tumor on the left side of the neck. Verneuil in Paris in 1864 observed myosis, heat, congested vessels, and sweating on the side of the face where a parotis tumor gave reason

[42] 3 (2): 234, 1846.

to ligate the carotid artery. Demme in 1862 found mydriasis and exophthalmos in a patient with goiter.

In 1863, finally, Weir Mitchell, Morehouse, and Keen (57) observed in this country with masterly preciseness and published in 1864 an extremely interesting case, in which gunshot that penetrated the right side of the neck of a soldier led to the development of a syndrome exactly like that described by Horner six years later. Because this contribution of the American authors seems to be entirely forgotten, we quote literally from Weir Mitchell, Morehouse, and Keen's Book.

On page 40 the authors describe as follows their findings in the patient, a soldier twenty-four years old, when the wound had already healed for some weeks:

> The pupil of the right eye is very small, that of the left unusually large. There is a slight, but very distinct ptosis of the right eye and its outer angle appears as though it were dropped a little lower than the inner angle. The ball of the right eye looks smaller than that of the left. This appearance existed, whether the eye was open or closed and gave to the organ the look of being tilted out of the usual position. The conjunctiva of the right eye is somewhat redder than that of the left and the pupil of the right eye is somewhat deformed oval rather than round . . . the right eye having become myopic.

It was observed that when this patient walked around in warm weather,

> his face became distinctly flushed on the right side only and pale on the left. He felt pain and red flashes in the right eye. In repose no difference was found in the temperature of the two sides in mouth or ear. After five months, the patient was dismissed from medical care to return to his military duties. At that time nearly all of his peculiar symptoms having disappeared, the clinical study came then to an end.

In discussing this case the authors (1864), to stress their point that all the observed signs were due to a lesion of the cervical sympathetic nerve, emphasize all the similar symptoms known from the literature to have resulted from cutting the sympathetic nerve in animal experiments. They also discuss all the other possibilities that might contribute to provoke such symptoms, for instance, spinal concussion, but their final conclusion reads: "We ourselves are of the opinion that this was a case of injury of the sympathetic nerve and if so it is probably the only one on record." The title of the chapter of their book in which this case appears is "Wound of the Sympathetic Nerve," and the authors say in the introduction to the case report: "During our long connection with this hospital we have encountered a single case of lesion of the sympathetic nerve."

In connection with this publication, there is surely no need for further comment, from the point of view of medical history, concerning any claim for priority (41).[42a]

It was only in 1864, when von Graefe published his syndrome as a sign of Graves' disease, that general clinical attention was called to the fact that a part of the eyesigns in this disease are due to increased sympathetic tone. This was first made public by von Graefe in a paper read before the Berlin Medical Society on March 6, 1864. In the discussion on Graefe's paper, Remak, who was present at this meeting, immediately reminded the gathering of his own experimental work, giving valid proof of von Graefe's view that the sympathetic nerve is involved in what today is known as Graefe's sign (24).

Five years later the Swiss ophthalmologist F. Horner (34) published his observations of symptoms caused by unilateral sympathicus lesion, today known by the name of Horner's sign, which is nothing else but a finding from clinical observation which various physiologists had obtained experimentally between 1727 and 1855, and a confirmation of the clinical observations made by Weir Mitchell and his colleagues in 1863. Horner also verified all the symptoms that Budge, Claude Bernard, and Remak had observed in the homolateral eye after severing the cervical sympathetic nerve, including the dilation of vessels on that side and increase of the skin temperature. Horner was well acquainted with the clinical statement of von Graefe, whose pupil he was, and with the remarks that Remak made during the discussion in 1864, for in his paper of 1869 he cites both sources in the literature where this discussion of Remak was published. Apparently, however, Horner did not care to look up Remak's publication of 1855, to which the latter referred expressly in his discussion. In describing the syndrome, Horner only states inaccurately on page 198:

> Here we have, therefore, the counterpart to the elevation, or better to say, the retraction of the upper eyelid into the orbita in Basedow's disease which was described by von Graefe and Remak as an effect of the stimulation of the organic fibers in the upper lid.

There is no question that Horner, had he thought to consult a physiologist, or at least to check Remak's original paper of 1855, would have realized and acknowledged the priority of Remak and the other pertinent literature with respect to this syndrome as he did for Graefe's sign. Subsequent authors, of course, took no great pains to check the original literature, and so it happens that today a group of signs are known under the name of Horner's syndrome which should rightly be called Petit's or Biffi's or Budge-Waller's or Weir Mitchell-Morehouse-Keen's or Remak's syndrome.

[42a] W. W. Keen left an account of this discovery in his *Surgical reminiscences of the Civil War* (W. B. Saunders & Co., Philadelphia 1905), where on page 436 he reports how he made the diagnosis and how he later called Claude Bernard's attention to this observation. Keen mentions how the reminiscence of a picture of a cat with cut right cervical sympathetic nerve in Dalton's old textbook of physiology led him immediately to the right diagnosis. This author appreciates that his attention was called to Keen's report by Dr. Walter J. Freeman from Yale University.

RESEARCH VERSATILITY

In the meantime Remak had settled in Berlin as a practicing physician.

All his struggle, all the public criticism of his work, without even the full-hearted support of his own chief, made the prospect of an academic career extremely slim for Remak, even if he had not been a Jew. His older competitors in Müller's laboratory had already arrived at the academic goal. Schwann was called in 1839 as Professor to the University of Loewen in Belgium; Henle became Professor at the University of Zürich in Switzerland in 1840. Remak received no offer. Because he was a Jew, he was not even named successor to Henle as prosector or to Schwann as a *Gehülfe* at a salary of ten Thaler a month. A new generation of Müller's gifted pupils followed, filling the vacancies in his laboratory. Remak went into general practice in Berlin, remaining in Müller's laboratory only as a voluntary worker. However, the results of his research during the early years of his practice were so important that they secured for him the lifelong support and collaboration of his esteemed teacher, Johannes Müller.

The enormous amount of work Remak published in the years between 1839 and 1847 is really amazing, not only because of its quantity, but also because of the excellent observations and discoveries he made in very different fields. He was the first to suggest the use of the expression, "Protoplasma" for the content of animal cells, and Max Schultze, in his classic paper on "What Should Be Called a Cell" (1861), says more than twenty years later: "Remak's attempt to introduce the expression 'Protoplasma' (of Hugo von Mohl's invention) for animalic cells did not find the followers it deserved." In 1840 Remak discovered the outermost layer (of white substance) of the brain, corroborated in the same year by Baillar. In April, 1840 he had discussed his fundamental neurological discoveries in Breslau with Purkinje, whom he visited there, and his friend, the Danish anatomist Hannover, confirmed his findings. At that time he was studying the layers of the gray substance of the brain and the ganglion geniculatum. At the 1841 meeting of German physicians and scientists in Braunschweig, he reported important studies on the development of red blood cells. It was during that period that he began research to prove his theory that each cell originates from another one by cell division. A long and heated discussion followed this presentation in Braunschweig on September 20. The chairman of the meeting was E. H. Weber from Leipzig, and Remak had to continue his paper on the next day, a very unusual success.

At the same time Remak carried out microscopical investigations on certain nerves (*rami communicantes*) together with his teacher, Müller,[48] and made his fundamental statements on the influence of sympathetic nerve fibers on the secretion of glands and movements of smooth muscles. Many articles on anatomical and pathological topics, like the one entitled "Nervensystem" (1841), were written by him in these years for the German *Encyclopedic Dictionary of Medical Sciences.* For this same publication Remak wrote on the nervous system, the retina, ossification, osteosarcoma, and so on. Some of these articles are reviews of up to seventy printed pages. He discovered at the same time an unknown muscle on the operculs of the gills of fishes and in the first volume of Canstatt's *Annual Reports* (66) wrote his own programmatic review of progress in physiology in 1841, emphasizing in it that he had no time for continuing with this type of work in the future. At the same time he defended his discoveries in neurohistology against Henle, Valentin, and Reichert. He was writing in German on gynecological problems, and in German and Polish on benign and malignant tumors. In 1843 he published his first fundamental paper on embryology, and he studied the contractibility of muscle fibers.

REMAK STARTS TEACHING ACTIVITIES

Besides all the research work he did, it remained Remak's great ambition to teach and to instruct pupils in the new methods and new points of view in medicine.

It was in 1841 that he began his teaching activities. The value of microscopical investigations for clinical problems, even though not yet generally acknowledged, began to influence theoretical and practical medicine more and more. However, opportunities for a student to learn to use the microscope well were very slim. The high cost of a good microscope prevented even very interested physicians from purchasing such an instrument. Then, too, the majority of physicians were not yet convinced of its value for clinical medicine. We know, for instance, that when in 1840 Henle accepted a call to the young and unquestionably progressive University of Zürich, there was only one microscope in the anatomical laboratory, and this was of the already long outdated solar type (49: 165). Microscope building started in America with Charles A. Spencer in 1838 (97) and in New York there existed in 1847 only four or five achromatic microscopes.

In 1837 when Henle became lecturer at the University of Berlin, he gave courses in microscopic anatomy (histology), at that time an entirely new subject in the curriculum of the students. Now, in the fall of 1840, Henle left Berlin for Zürich in Switzerland. Of course, Remak would have been the most suitable person to give instruction in this field, but he was not a lecturer, and as a Jew, he was not even eligible for the position of a lecturing Privatdozent in a Prussian university. He was convinced, however, that the lack of adequate instruction in microscopy was deplorable from the standpoint of the interest of the student and a handicap to the progress of medicine. In 1841, therefore, he

[48] Nervensystem, *Encyclopedic Dictionary of Medical Sciences,* 1841.

published an article in the Berlin medical journal, *Medicinische Zeitung,* on the "Misuse of Formal Criticism and the Need for Real Criticism in Medical Science" (p. 72). In this article Remak put his finger on a growing danger in modern medicine. More and more teachers and physicians, he asserted, were afraid to be regarded as reactionary old-timers, and therefore tried to apply ideas stemming from the field of microscopy to clinical and theoretical medicine without having any personal experience in the use of a microscope or real knowledge of modern microscopy. His just demand was that not only each teacher on the medical faculty of a university, but every progressive physician, should become acquainted with the use of this instrument. To provide interested colleagues with an opportunity to learn new methods and new facts, Remak announced in a footnote to this article that, beginning on the third of May, 1841, he intended giving instruction in anatomical and microscopical observations based on modern physiological and pathological experience. Not being connected with the University in any teaching capacity, he offered these courses to interested physicians in his own apartment at Leipzigerstrasse 18 every Monday and Thursday from twelve to one.

By that time Remak was already well known to his colleagues in Berlin through his own contributions. In April, 1840, the *Berliner Medicinische Central Zeitung* announced his election as a corresponding member of the Medical Society in Warsaw. And even though he was not an official lecturer at the University, his offer to give courses was so interesting to the profession that this same medical journal also reported his plan (p. 319, 1841). It added an explanation that the anatomist Professor Berres in Vienna had offered similar instruction for a considerable time.

One of Berres's outstanding pupils in this line of study was David Gruby. We know that Gruby, who had lived in Paris since 1840, gave similar instruction there privately, though he, too, was not appointed a lecturer at the University, and that he even did this before, when he was still living in Vienna. We also know that his Paris courses were attended by the notables of the University of Paris.

Two years afterwards when Remak applied to the Minister for a lectureship at the University, he mentioned that he had already given lectures and instruction that had been attended by some of the teachers of the University. Years later, as Schönlein's assistant, Remak gave similar instruction in Schönlein's clinic; even after his appointment in 1847 as an official lecturer (Privatdozent), there was no place available in the rooms of the University for his lectures. For ten years he and his audience had to be content with his private rooms as an auditorium. Only in 1861 did the *Allgemeine Medicinische Central Zeitung* make the surprising announcement (p. 46):

It is reported that for the next term Herr Doctor Remak will give his lectures in histology and embryology in the Anatomical Museum. Up to now he was obliged to give them in his own apartment, since he did not have a laboratory. The necessary instruments will be put at the disposal of Dr. Remak for this purpose through the kindness of Professor Johannes Müller.

The journal added that it would be desirable for Remak also to use the facilities offered to him for the purpose of aiding physicians and students in independent physiological and microscopical investigations.

Probably the most famous among Remak's pupils during this time of private lecturing in his own apartment was A. Koelliker, later Professor of Anatomy and Physiology in Würzburg. Koelliker gives in his own autobiography a very vivid report of his experiences with Remak. He writes (43: 8): "A turning point in my life was Berlin. I spent three terms at this University from the fall 1839 to the spring 1841." He continues then (43: 9 and 10):

In my anatomical studies in Berlin I gained the most important inspiration not only from Johannes Müller and Henle but also from Ehrenberg, Meyen and Remak. By those scholars were revealed to me little known or unknown fields like the infusoria, the microscopic anatomy of plants and embryology. With vivid satisfaction I remember mainly a privatissimum at Remak's when this highly gifted scholar showed to a few eager listeners in his apartment his observations on the development of the embryo of the chicken, explaining his findings by demonstration of preparations and by discussions which remained for me unforgettable and which soon later were presented to the scientific world in his famous great work, which founded a new era in embryology.

ACTIVITIES IN CLINICAL MEDICINE

The humble way in which Remak began his activities as an unofficial, but inspiring private lecturer did not interfere with his interest in practical medicine, in surgery and gynecology, from which he drew his livelihood. That is evidenced by his invention of a method to stop arterial bleeding, by his designing of a special type of forceps for such purposes (1839), and by various publications on the problem of when the operative removal of a tumor is indicated and when it is contra indicated. The request of the editors of the Berlin *Encyclopedic Dictionary of Medical Sciences* led him, as mentioned above, to research on menstrual blood and to the writing of several papers and even a small booklet on the subject of the alleged toxic properties of that kind of blood. This pamphlet of about sixty pages was dedicated to the surgeon and ophthalmologist Professor J. Ch. Jüngken (1793–1875) in Berlin.

His manifold interests and activities made Remak very well fitted for the position of an academic teacher; at that time lecturing at a university was not yet restricted to a small specialty, but required a wide background of knowledge in the most diversified fields of medical sciences. Very adequate to such demands was the varied and always fruitful life of research that

Remak led from the day of his graduation up to his departure from Müller's laboratory and his entrance into Schönlein's Clinic as an assistant, that is, during the years from 1838 to 1843. It is difficult to realize that a man could accomplish what he did single-handed, in addition to earning a livelihood as a practicing physician and surgeon. Those years were years of great importance, not only for Remak personally, but also for the academic life of Berlin and for its reputation as a center of medicine in the world. It was in those years that modern medicine was born.

MEDICINE IN BERLIN AROUND 1840

The year 1839 was, in many respects, remarkable in the medical life in Berlin. Johannes Lukas Schönlein, at that time Professor of Medicine at Zürich, Switzerland, was called to succeed Professor Behrens at Berlin. He accepted this call and began his lectures at Berlin on Easter, 1840. He was welcomed with high expectations; everyone saw in him a representative of the modern trend in medicine. Immediately he instituted a reform in medical studies in Berlin in that, in contradistinction to his predecessor and to his contemporary colleague Wolff, he delivered his lectures, not in a more or less classical Latin, but in the German language. He soon also fructified all kinds of modern investigating methods and encouraged their use in his clinic, such as auscultation and percussion, thermometry, microscopy, and chemistry. For investigations of the latter type a chemist, Franz Simon, was appointed, but he died in 1843 (68).

Before long, Schönlein attracted many of the most promising young students and doctors of the University as his audience and as his assistants. Among them the two outstanding ones were Robert Remak and Ludwig Traube. Indeed, it can be said that the lustre and fame of the Berlin School of Medicine in the middle of the nineteenth century started with the activities of Johannes Müller (1833–1858) and Lucas Schönlein (1840–1859) (53). So close was the collaboration between these two eminent scientists that shortly after Johannes Müller's death in 1858, Schönlein resigned his position on the medical faculty in Berlin (1859). He did not have to retire yet, and he lived until 1864.

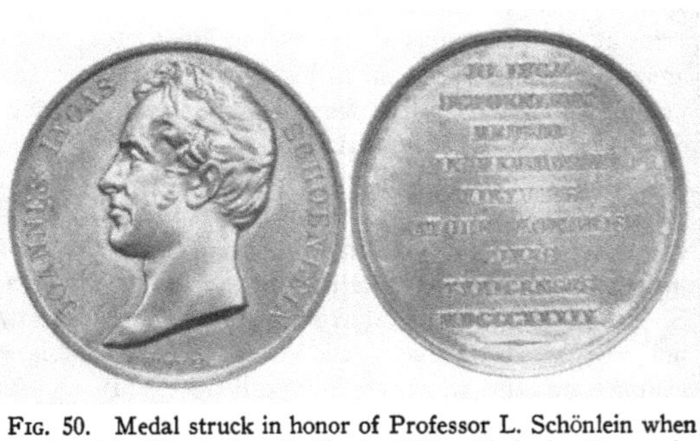

FIG. 50. Medal struck in honor of Professor L. Schönlein when he left Zürich for Berlin in 1840. Made by Bovy, the famous medalist who made a portrait medal of Goethe. This was dedicated to Schönlein by citizens of Zürich. From the author's collection.

Besides being professor of Clinical Medicine, Schönlein was adviser on medical questions to the Minister of Education of Prussia (Vortragender Rat in the Prussian Kultus-Ministerium), in which position he wielded a certain influence in the filling of vacancies on the medical faculties in Prussia. We shall remember this fact later in the story of the life of his assistant, Remak. He resigned from this position only in the summer of 1849 after the 1848 Revolution.

Another event in the fall of 1839, of great importance not only for Berlin but especially for Remak's future, was the admission of a certain young student to the medical faculty as a member of the Pepinière (the Friedrich-Wilhelm Institute), an institute and medical school for military surgeons. He was Rudolf Virchow, the son of a farmer in Schivelbein in Pomerania, a very gifted, eager, and assiduous student, no less ambitious than Remak, but with certain special attributes that gave him, even as a young man, a definite advantage over the already famous scholar Remak. Virchow's family was acquainted with many of the leading Prussian military medical men from North Prussia. A brother of his father, living in Berlin, was a well-known, high-ranking officer in the Prussian Army, Johannes Christ Virchow by name. A brother of his mother, Ludwig Ferdinand Hesse, was an outstanding architect in Berlin. Among his main architectural creations were the new Charité Hospital, the Veterinary School, and the Elizabeth Hospital (60). Though young Virchow never had a great deal of money at his disposal, he had all the necessary push and pull for a career worthy of his abilities, and, as we shall see, used his connections very well to serve his high ambitions.

Something else occured in Berlin in 1839 that soon revolutionized all medicine and biology, and again it was one of Johannes Müller's paladins who started this revolution. There lived in Berlin at that time a young man of thirty-five who had a very unusual educational background. Born in 1804 in Hamburg, the son of a physician, he studied law and settled, with the degree of doctor of law from the University of Heidelberg, as an attorney in his home town of Hamburg. A failure and dissatisfied with this type of pursuit, he resigned from his profession at the age of twenty-seven and made an unsuccessful attempt to commit suicide. After that he started out on a new life as a medical student at Göttingen and at Berlin. Here, under the influence of his uncle, the physiologist and botanist Johann Horkel, he was soon attracted by the beauties of botany, the *scientia amabilis,* and became a botanist. Fascinated chiefly by general problems in botany, he wrote a few important articles on cell production and fructification in plants. His "Beiträge zur Phytogenese," which appeared in 1838 in *Müller's Archiv,* was outstanding among them. On the basis of these first publications he was called in 1839 as an Associate Professor to the Medical Faculty of the University of Jena. Here he taught up to 1862, when he accepted a call to the University of Dorpat as Professor of Anthropology. Soon he left this position also. Later, having retired from university life, he lived in Dresden, Wiesbaden, and finally Frankfurt a.M., where he died in 1881 (53).

This man, Jacob Schleiden, was the first clearly and effectively to spread the idea that each plant consists of cells, each cell being characterized by a cell nucleus (cytoblast). In this theory he surely had predecessors in the Italian Malpighi, in Robert Hooke in England, and in the German Hugo von Mohl. But only Schleiden realized the importance of the concept of the cell theory and was able to make the necessary generalization of it. He also, realized that the biology of the individual cell was of paramount importance for botany, as well as for comparative physiology.

During his residence in Berlin, Schleiden lived next door to a young physiologist (53) who was a member of Johannes Müller's group of pupils, by name Theodore Schwann (1810–1882). Both met repeatedly and enjoyed scientific discussions. Schwann eagerly accepted Schleiden's new theory of the importance of cells and their nuclei and immediately grasped the consequences of this new gospel for animal anatomy and physiology. After a few months of intensive work, he published his famous *Microscopical Investigations on the Conformity in the Structure and Growth of Animals and Plants.*

REMAK'S THEORY OF CELL PROPAGATION

Schwann's publication, as is well known, was epochmaking in biology and medicine. As a pupil of Johannes Müller, Remak knew him well, and this young doctor, probably one of the best microscopists among the crowd around Müller, immediately became as everyone else greatly interested in Schwann's new theory.

It is to a great extent overlooked that Schwann's cell theory really consists of two different parts. The first part is the statement that all living beings are made up of cells, each cell being characterized by a nucleus. With this part of Schwann's theory Remak agreed fully. The second part of Schwann's theory concerned the origin of all these animal cells. On this point Schwann had the idea that the unorganized fluid in the body might be the matrix in which all cells are formed. This matrix was called the cytoblastem. Schleiden, on the other hand, favored the idea that cells are built within other cells, just as the embryo is formed in the uterus. Remak disagreed with this part of Schwann's theory from the beginning. In 1842 he wrote for the first volume of *Canstatt's Annual Report on Medicine in All Countries* (66) the report on progress in physiology during the year 1841. There he already emphasized strongly his objections to this part of Schwann's theory, while J. Henle in his *Textbook on General Anatomy* still[44] asserted that in animals the creation of cells by cell division had never been proved. A. Koelliker, in his *Embryology of the Cephalopodes*, published in 1844, reported observations that also pointed to the creation of cells by division, but Henle rejected any generalization of this view. In his report in Canstatt's *Jahresberichte* (1845) on the progress of histology in the year 1844, Henle takes a firm stand against abandoning the concept of free cell creation in a formless cytoblastem.

On page 8 of his 1842 report (66) Remak says: "The special kind of origin of all animal cells is not yet well known; one has to be cautious, however, in accepting statements that cells are created in a cytoblastem outside all the cells." His ideas were well grounded in observations and experiments that went back to the time immediately after the publication of Schwann's fundamental and soon generally accepted theories. Schwann did not know anything about proliferation of cells by cell division. The first to emphasize this fact was Remak, who observed it in red blood cells of embryos in 1841.

Remak never abandoned the problem of where cells might originate but returned to it time and again. His intensive studies on the embryology of vertebrates, which occupied him for the next several years, made him certain already in 1851 (71) that each embryonic cell stems from another cell by division. He had previously established the division of embryonic blood cells; he had observed the division of muscle cells; and now, being certain that this was definitely the law among animals, he presented it clearly in a classical paper that appeared in *Müller's Archiv* in 1852 under the title of "The Extra-cellular Creation of Animal Cells and Their Multiplication by Cell Division" (71). Here he emphatically rejected Schwann's idea of the creation of cells out of a formless cytoblastem, insisting on cell division as the only source of cell production. And he does not limit this statement to embryology, but goes on to make the very interesting and important comparison that this notion is just as absurd as the idea of the spontaneous generation of animals. He says, in literal translation: "For myself the extracellular creation of animal cells has been, since this cell theory was made public, as incredible as the *generatio equivoca* (spontaneous generation of organisms)."

Contrary to the well known anatomist Reichert, Remak even noticed that each nucleus, in the progredient development of the embryo, comes from the first nucleus of the fertilized cell by a continuous division. So Remak maintained and proved years before Virchow not only what was later known as "Omnis cellula e cellula," but also what was later called "Omnis nucleus e nucleo." At the conclusion of this article (71) Remak made the following fundamental statement:

[44] P. 176, 1841.

After the confirmation of my doubts, which I have had for many years, I dare to express the opinion that pathological tissues are as little created within an extracellular blastem as normal ones are, but they are derivatives or products of the normal tissues of organisms.

This was unquestionably a conclusion referring not only to embryonic, but to all normal and pathologic tissue, and the basis of everything that was later proclaimed as the cell theory of Virchow. It is incomprehensible, indeed, how anybody who read the original papers of Remak could doubt this historic fact. For those who still are uncertain whether Remak really meant his cellular theory only for embryonic cells or generally, the concluding sentence of another paper, printed in *Müller's Archiv* in 1852, may settle the matter. This was an article on the development of connective tissue and cartilage, and the last sentence reads: "After this report any part which extra-cellular substances may take in the creation of tissues must appear entirely doubtful." In the field of general biology and cytology Remak must therefore be regarded as the real creator of the modern concept of cell production and his publications show that he built up this concept carefully since 1841 and probably since the publication of Schwann's theory.

We now present a few statements which, long after Remak's fundamental publications, young Rudolf Virchow still had to make on this problem. In a paper concerning the alteration of pathological and therapeutical points of view as a result of microscopic investigations, written in 1847, (81) Virchow was still a strict adherent to Schwann's cell production theory. On page 218, in talking of carcinoma, he set up a few "laws." They read:

1. All organization happens through differentiation of formless material blastem.
2. All blastem comes out of the vessels primarily as fluid, exudate.
3. All organization begins with the creation of cells (Müller's law).

This is a literal translation of Virchow's "laws." They are a repetition of Schwann's ideas and strictly in contradiction to the correct, revolutionary opinion of Remak.

To understand how much Virchow, already deeply involved at that time in pathological investigations, was still influenced by the ideas of natural philosophy in medicine, one needs only to read page 219 of this paper, which gives Virchow's position on the cell theory at a time when Remak had already published his well-founded doubts (81). Virchow writes: "Everywhere, ruled by the same law of differentiation, there occurs a separation of heterologous different substances in the form of round, in most instances probably pustulelike bodies out of a formless homogeneous material. This may be free or contained in pre-existing cells." Such a statement represents a confession of adherence to Schwann's as well as to Schleiden's theory of free cell creation. How far Virchow's fantastic ideas went even as late as 1847, we can judge when we learn that he compared this supposed fact of free cell creation with the creation of cosmic bodies and nebulae out of a kind of "universal blastem," and with the formation of crystals out of a concentrated solution, and, believe it or not, with the development of the soul.

In his conclusion he said: "There is one unique great law of nature to be recognized in the entire world of matter as a general principle of movement and formation."

Like Johannes Müller and Virchow, Henle, too, in 1846 still rejected Remak's point of view that every alleged free production of cells had to be criticized sharply. He too regarded as erroneous Remak's idea that cells were created by cell division only.

G. Gluge, well known Professor of Physiology and Pathology at the University of Brussels in Belgium, published in 1850 a two volume atlas of pathological anatomy. In this atlas (22) and in the English edition that was published in Philadelphia in 1853 (23) the creation of cells out of cytoblastem was strongly emphasized. Leidy's translation reads (23: 31): "The coagulable liquid which exudes from the blood vessels is called cytoblastema . . . in it are formed the . . . elements of the tissues." And on page 32 it says: "Cells appear rarely to increase by division in the animal . . . and an undoubted instance I have not observed. . . ." That was the prevailing opinion among anatomists still in the middle of the last century.

In 1852 we find this fantastic idea strongly emphasized by Professor Wunderlich in the second edition of his widely used *Handbuch der Pathologie und Therapie* (Stuttgart, Ebener & Seubert, 1852). There, in the first volume, on pages 391 to 405, he describes in detail how the cells of the body are created out of a liquid *blastem.* Like Johannes Müller, he is of the opinion that this kind of creation is valid not only for normal tissue but also for malignant tumors. Like all of his contemporaries, he does not believe in any cell division. He does not in this chapter mention Remak but, time and again, quotes the romantic opinions of Virchow and others and, on page 402, he makes the remark: "Propagation of cells or nuclei (Körperchen) by cleavage (Zerklüftung) or splitting has not up to now any practical interest." In the middle of the last century Professor Wunderlich not only taught this opinion to scores of German students at the University of Leipzig but also, by means of his book, many interested physicians.

In 1854 Remak published a final statement, so to say, on the entire problem in the journal, *Deutsche Klinik.*[45] This was a paper he had read on March 27, at a meeting of the Berlin Society for Scientific Medicine. The title was "A Contribution to the History of the De-

[45] 6: 170, 1854.

velopment of Carcinomatous Tumors." In this paper, written with classical clearness and decisiveness, he attacks Schwann's as well as Virchow's theory on the basis of his own observations.

"The extracellular cell creation," he says (p. 173), "as postulated by Schwann can not be proved. The cells, of which the animal germ consists, multiply, by continuous division which starts at the nucleus as I have observed it. Never could the creation of cells in a free cytoblastem be observed. The same holds for tumors." He denies every free creation of nuclei, too, and emphasizes the fact that malignant tissue originates from normal tissue. Tumor tissue is not a new creation but only the transformation of normal into pathological tissue.

This statement was opposed to the dominant opinion of Johannes Müller, Henle, Virchow, Bischoff, Koelliker, and every outstanding figure in medicine. There cannot be any doubt that this paper by Remak was well known to Virchow, too. Since his name is mentioned in it and his theories are contradicted, we may even suppose that Remak, in accordance with the custom among scientists, sent a reprint to Virchow in Würzburg, where the latter, whom Remak knew personally, had meantime established himself as a professor, being highly interested in the problem in question. Virchow reviewed this paper by Remak in the *Jahresberichte der Medicin pro 1854,* on page 38. The last sentence of this review reads: "He [Remak] finally insists, as before, that no free nuclei exist, nor any extracellular creation of cells." To this statement Virchow does not add any personal comment or his own opinion.

Remak's conception and proof of the only way of cell propagation was generally rejected. Bischoff, professor at Münich, strongly opposed it and expressed his disapproval in 1852 in his *Embryology of the Guinea Pig* (pp. 19–21), and again in 1854 in his *Embryology of the Deer* (pp. 11, 12, 30); even Koelliker, broadminded and open to accept new ideas and points of view, disagreed with Remak's statement about cell propagation in his *Gewebelehre* (p. 36) even in 1852.

HOW VIRCHOW ADOPTED REMAK'S THEORY

Remak's repeated objections to Schwann's theory of cell production, his conclusive observation, and his emphatic statement that each cell stems by division from another cell, finally evoked the interest and the attention of other scholars. In the first volume of Virchow's *Handbook on Special Pathology* (82), we see how deeply Remak had already impressed him. Here Virchow gives full credit to Remak (p. 329), quoting him as a proponent of the opinion that free cell formation out of a formless cytoblastem must be doubted altogether.

In 1854 Virchow made the following statement, thus tacitly admitting Schwann's, Müller's, Henle's, and his own earlier misconception: "First of all we agree with Remak in that nowhere in the body do there exist primarily free or naked nuclei." This sentence shows that Virchow understood well the significance of Remak's statement, which was no less important for modern biology than the first part of Schwann's theory, namely, that all animals consist of nucleated cells. But in 1854 Virchow was still not yet entirely convinced of the complete correctness of Remak's opinion, and he still discussed four possible methods of cell formation, among them, as No. 3, the creation of cells within existing cells, a theory already discussed by Schleiden and Schwann. Virchow took pride in this idea, which he incorrectly stated was "first described by Virchow." He did not discard this type of free cell production within a cell, but now, finally, he doubted with Remak, whose paper of 1852 (71) he quoted (p. 326), the existence of free cell production in intercellular cytoblastem.

Virchow's view and attitude towards Remak with respect to giving him credit for this idea only changed a year after Remak's conclusive paper of 1854, and in the year 1855 when the last installment of Remak's work on the embryology of vertebrates was published, containing an extensive and classic chapter on the cell theory and its history.

It took Virchow eight years really to understand and accept Remak's theory in its full importance; in the meantime, he had reached his goal of full professorship at the University of Würzburg, while Remak was still Privatdozent (lecturer) at Berlin. Finally, in 1855, Virchow, definitely and strongly supported Remak's theory in the eighth volume of his *Archiv,*[46] but now he preferred not to mention the name or the priority of Remak. In an article on "Cellular Pathology," Virchow used the famous phrase, "Omnis cellula e cellula." This article and Virchow's lectures on cellular pathology, published in book form, are the principal reasons why, to this day, Virchow as a rule is undeservedly credited with having established and expounded the fact that each cell comes from another cell (2).

There can be no doubt that Virchow was well acquainted with Remak's work. He knew Remak, and nobody will hesitate to believe that he carefully read each article in Johannes Müller's *Archiv.* In 1854 he quoted Remak and his 1852 paper, and finally, he reviewed Remak's paper of 1854. Virchow not only knew Remak, but as a young beginner he had come out ahead of Remak in the matter of replacing Froriep as prosector in the Charité Hospital in Berlin, despite all Remak's merits, because he, Virchow, had better personal connections. Just when he published his famous "Omnis cellula e cellula" article, Virchow again was afraid of Remak's competition in his drive for a professorship at Berlin. This we know from Virchow's own letters to his father, of which we shall speak later

[46] 1855: 1.

in connection with Remak's fate. So it was that in this year of 1855, Virchow, determined to outstrip Remak in a great career, found it better not to mention that the idea he was expounding here in a stentorian voice as his own was really the work and theory of Remak.

Everyone, meantime, knew of Remak's crusade against free cell production. Reichert, even though he disagreed on this point with Remak, discussed it in his annual report published in *Müller's Archiv* in 1853 (p. 18). He quoted with disapproval Remak's comparison with the *generatio equivoca* and his emphasis on cell division as the only sources of normal and pathological cell production. Summarizing and disapproving he made this statement: "For him [Remak] there exists only one kind of cell production, the one by cell division."

There cannot be any doubt that in the year 1853 Virchow read this annual report, written by a well known author, on the progress of anatomy.

One small psychological matter is proof that Virchow's omission of Remak's name was not an innocent oversight, but that Virchow, while writing his article on cellular pathology, really had in mind Remak's articles of 1852 and 1854.

We have previously called attention to the fact that Remak, when he rejected Schwann's theory of free cell generation in *Müller's Archiv* in 1852, made the point which apparently impressed Reichert, too, that free cell production had to be discarded as definitely as the old idea of the spontaneous generation of organisms. It is surely not a coincidence that Virchow, in his article of 1855, declares in exactly the same way as Remak that the spontaneous generation of organisms is as little to be believed as the free generation of cells, but this time without any reference to Remak. Immediately following this statement, he used the short, good Latin expression, "Omnis cellula e cellula."

Only Virchow's famous colleague on the Würzburg faculty, Albert Koelliker, in a decent and honest way, gave due credit in his textbook to Remak. Shortly after Virchow's article, "Cellular Pathology," appeared and after Virchow had succeeded in becoming full professor at Berlin, Koelliker wrote in the third edition of his *Handbook on Histology* in 1859 (p. 720): "The credit for having pressed cell division in its widest meaning as the only form of cell multiplication has to go to Remak." Remak's priority is similarly mentioned in S. Stricker's *Handbuch der Lehre von den Geweben* (Leipzig, 1871). It was only human for Koelliker, in writing his autobiography (43) at the age of eighty-two, to forget his statement of 1859 and to overestimate his own part in the development of the cell theory. But even here he was fair enough to point out (p. 199) that Virchow, in his important publications, omitted to mention the name of Remak (and others) who, when Virchow was still clinging to the free cell creation theory, knew the true facts, and that in this way Virchow unjustly acquired the reputation of founder of modern knowledge of cell production.[47]

REMAK TRIES TO JOIN THE FACULTY AS A JEW

Now we must again return to the years between 1840 and 1843, when Remak began his practice and continued as a research scientist. On various occasions the value of the work he was doing began to be officially recognized. He became a member of the Imperial Academy Carolo-Leopoldina of Scientists, of the Senckenberg Society of Natural Science in Frankfurt, and of the Medical Society in Warsaw (68).

The first stage of Remak's activity as a research worker for the sake of research was over after he realized that, as a Jew, he never would succeed in securing the necessary facilities for independent research in any university.

It was in November, 1843, after the death of the chemist Franz Simon, who conducted chemical and microscopical investigations in Schönlein's laboratory, that Schönlein (68) approached Remak to take over the microscopic work needed in the clinic, while the chemical work would be performed by one Dr. Heintz.

There is hardly any question that Schönlein turned to Remak either as agreed with or at the suggestion of his friend Johannes Müller. There is also no question that no official title was connected with this work, but a salary was allotted by the Minister for this position as research assistant (40). When Remak in 1845 published his investigations, which had been conducted at Schönlein's clinic (68), he called himself on the title page of this book "Practicing Physician and Surgeon in Berlin." He mentioned there all his affiliations with learned societies, but he did not give any title connecting him with Schönlein's clinic.

Unquestionably, Remak's decision to leave pure science for science's sake and to enter Schönlein's clinic as a research assistant was influenced by his bitter defeat in his first attempt to embark on an academic career in Germany.

Now Remak's name was well known; his discoveries in neurohistology and microscopy were in part accepted, in part a matter of serious controversy among the outstanding authorities. He certainly felt just as entitled, five years after his famous doctoral thesis, to an academic position as any of his former colleagues in Müller's laboratory, such as Schwann, now Professor at Löwen, and the baptized Jew, Henle, now Professor at Zürich. There is not the slightest doubt that, if Remak had been baptized, he too would have already been called to a chair at a German university or would have been

[47] In a recent paper on The Speculative Basis of Modern Pathology, Walter Pagel (58) tries to remind his readers of Remak's role in the history of the cell theory, and so does E. H. Ackerknecht in his Virchow biography (Madison, Univ. of Wisconsin Press, 1953).

the most likely candidate for a future opening. But Remak, then and later, firmly refused to take such a step. As he himself made clear, he detested changing religion for the purpose of advancing one's career, and even if he had not felt that way, he had strictly orthodox Jews for parents, and because of his love and devotion to them he would never have received baptism.

The relationship of Jews to Prussian universities, in the first decades of the nineteenth century, was still determined by bigotry, by the hatred of the German people, and by the fear of competition. The dawn of humanity, the outbreak of the French Revolution, the triumph of Napoleon I and his legislation, were not able to obliterate centuries-old prejudices and antipathies. Our own generation witnessed their violent blaze one hundred years later.

When the kingdom of Prussia was deeply humiliated by Napoleon, when Friedrich Wilhelm III, in despair and fear, needed the help and sympathy of each one of his subjects, when his country was reduced to less than half its previous size, to 158,000 square kilometers, and its population to less than five millions, in this time of danger, humiliation, and misery for Prussia, the king proclaimed in an edict on March 11, 1812, that the Jews in his country, after sharing all the duties and hardships of their fellow citizens and fighting and dying for their fatherland as the non-Jewish population had done, should receive the privileges of full-fledged citizens of Prussia. Paragraphs 8 and 9 of this edict made Jews officially eligible for teaching positions in Prussian universities. A few years later when Prussians and all other German citizens, Christians and Jews alike, helped to end the Napoleonic hegemony in Europe and the emergency was over for Prussia, the same King Friedrich Wilhelm III revoked his humane "generosity" with a decree of December 4, 1822 and again excluded unbaptized Jews from any academic career.

This does not mean that up to 1822 the decree of 1812 was seriously executed so that between 1812 and 1822 Jews would have been admitted as professors or even lecturers to the universities. One isolated case did occur in the Medical Faculty of the University of Breslau (40: 187) where a Jew, Dr. Guttentag, was admitted as a lecturer (Privatdozent). In 1822 in Königsberg a Jewish physician, Jacobson, had already passed his trial lecture for acceptance as Privatdozent and had printed and distributed his dissertation for this purpose. But the King's infamous decree was promulgated on December 20, the day before Jacobson's announced public disputation as lecturer. At the last moment he was prevented from giving his disputation, in spite of all the protests of that outstanding scholar and noble personality, Karl Burdach (8: 325).

The medical faculty of the young Berlin University had even made an unbaptized Jew full professor in 1816. But this happened only by mistake, and the new professor had to make up for the oversight in ridiculous haste by express baptism. He was David Ferdinand Koreff, the son of a Jewish physician in Breslau. Koreff studied at Halle, Berlin, and Paris, and became personal physician to Prince Hardenberg, at that time, next to the King, probably the most influential man in the Prussian kingdom where, as Chancellor, he was the leading politician. Koreff had a genial personality, he was one of the inner circle of the poet E. T. A. Hoffmann, and was immortalized in the *Tales of Hoffmann* by Jacques Offenbach. He was a stanch adherent of Mesmer's gospel of animal magnetism. His patient and friend, Prince Hardenberg, secured a full professorship for him on the Berlin medical faculty (55). The Faculty, angered that this had been done without its consent, but not daring to contradict the appointment officially, instead let the bigoted King know that the newly created professor *still* adhered to the Jewish faith. Koreff could not deny this fact, and though the edict of 1812 was still in effect, his protector, Hardenberg, ordered a quick and secret baptism for him on a trip to Dobberan in the remote, little town of Meissen. This order was carried out over night in a not very dignified way; Koreff's first name, David, was changed to Johann; and the Berlin Faculty was saved from the shocking eventuality of embracing a Jewish member.

A further incident occurred when a young doctor of philosophy, who graduated in 1823, tried to establish himself at his alma mater in Berlin as Privatdozent of mathematics and physics (40). In spite of the fact that no salary was connected with such a lecturership, nor did it have the status of a governmental position, the faculty as well as Minister Eichhorn refused to admit a Jew to it, and the Minister ordered that this decision be made known to all the other Prussian universities.

That was the position of the Jewish scientist up to the year 1842, when the government undertook consideration of new regulation of the status of Jews in Prussia.

On April 7, of that year the Berlin Academy of Sciences, by a vote of 26 to 3, admitted to membership a Jew by the name of Dr. Peter Theophil Riess, a physicist of fame, especially distinguished for his studies in the field of electricity (40).[48]

To be voted a member of this academy was one of the greatest honors to be conferred on a scientist. Proof of this is in the names of two of the three others besides Riess that were at the same time submitted to the King for confirmation. They were an architect Hagen, also to be named a regular member, the famous Gay-Lussac in Paris, and Faraday in London to become corresponding members. Minister Eichhorn, objected immediately to Riess because he *still* adhered to the Jewish faith. Riess, however, was no Dr. Koreff to undergo a high-speed baptism, and the membership of

[48] *Sulamith* 8 (2), 203, 1842.

the Berlin Academy, which had elected Riess by all but three votes (40), stood by its decision and answered Eichhorn's letter with indignation. Eichhorn reported directly to the King. The case had special significance under the decree of 1822, because the regular members of the Berlin Academy were automatically entitled to give lectures at the Universities of Berlin and Bonn. In this case, if Riess decided to do so, this would contravene the King's orders of 1822, which excluded Jews from all teaching positions in Prussian universities. In the meantime, however, a new king came to the throne in Prussia. The president of the Academy, Alexander von Humboldt, had already secured his oral approval, and on June 28, 1842 Friedrich Wilhelm IV confirmed the election of Riess despite the danger that this outstanding man might dare to use his right to lecture at the Universities of Berlin and Bonn. On July 7, 1842 the first Jewish member of the Berlin Academy of Sciences was installed.

This event undoubtedly was a sensation among the Jewish population of Prussia and encouraging to a person like Remak. King Friedrich Wilhelm IV had made his decision in spite of the fact, known to everyone, that fifty years before, King Friedrich II had twice refused to confirm the election of the Jewish philosopher Moses Mendelssohn to the same Royal Academy. Friedrich II was legendary as the most enlightened and tolerant among the German princes. Here, now, a kind of precedent was created, and a breach in the wall of the spiritual Ghetto was made. Here, too, was this wonderful personality and defender of freedom and justice for all, Alexander von Humboldt, who had been instrumental in securing royal confirmation of the election of Riess (40); he knew Remak's doctoral thesis thoroughly and was in personal contact with Remak who became his acknowledged protégé (21, 69).

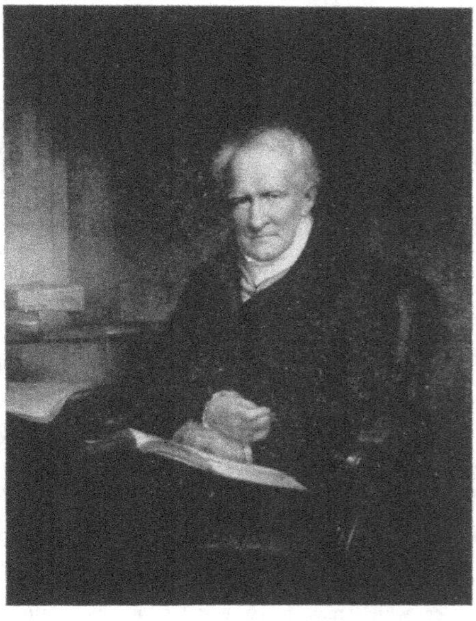

FIG. 51. Alexander von Humboldt. Portrait by J. R. Lambdin in the Hall of the American Philosophical Society.

In the year 1840, when King Friedrich Wilhelm III of Prussia died, everyone expected his successor, Friedrich Wilhelm IV, known to have expressed as Crown Prince more liberal views, to create a more liberal and just government. Remak, too, in his ambitious desire to become one of the teaching staff of the medical faculty of Berlin University thought that after the coronation it would be propitious to turn directly to the new king for permission to be admitted as a lecturer at Berlin University. He therefore communicated with Humboldt, requesting his help in this endeavor, for Humboldt, as was well known, belonged to the inner circle of the king's court. He tried to obtain an appointment to discuss the matter with Humboldt in person, but this man, whose day was too short for all his duties, wrote him a letter on August 13, 1840, disagreeing with his intentions, because he did not yet see any possibility for success, as much as he would have wished it for his protégé.

The letter (21 : 118) reads in translation:

> Of course, my busy state and my approaching departure prevent me from seeing you, Sir, at my home. In your Russian affair you had the experience that I did not spare any pains to be of assistance wherever I saw a slight possibility. I cannot agree with your present decision to turn to the King. I am afraid that this procedure will be without success. My personal position is exactly the same as it was under the last government. Propositions are not made by me; everything is in accordance with the forms that still prevail: i.e. via the cabinet and the Kultusministerium without any notification to me. You may understand how painful it is for me to give you this frank answer in spite of the esteem I have for your scientific endeavor.
>
> With the deepest respect, I am your most obedient
>
> A. von Humboldt. Berlin, 13. August 1840.

Remak could not go against this very decisive view of the most important and influential of his protectors and had to curb his ambitions for the next few years, but the new king indeed had an eye on the relationship between universities and Jews. We learn of the liberal intentions of the king from a letter, dated March 4, 1842 (20), from Moritz Veit, one of the outstanding personalities in the Jewish community of Berlin at that time, to Johannes Jacoby. In December 1841, in a personal order directed to the Minister of State, the King expressed in definite terms his opinion that Jews should be admitted to teaching positions in the medical and philosophical faculties of Prussia. A short time later in June 1842, the above mentioned nomination of a Jew to membership in the Royal Academy occurred, and now even the diplomatic and formal courtier, Humboldt, and Johannes Müller thought that Remak's chances would no longer be as bad as they had been in 1840.

On January 24, 1843, half a year after the election of Riess, Remak submitted a petition to the Minister asking to be informed whether, as a Jew, he was still excluded by the Royal Order of 1822 from becoming a lecturer at the Medical Faculty of Berlin. A few days later, on February 7, he received the Minister's decision that a Jew was not eligible to be a Privatdozent. Discouraging as such a decision by the Minister was, Remak did not give up and again turned to Humboldt, whose inexhaustible patience was again attested to by the following letter of March, 1843 (21: 121):

> It is only the volume of business which accumulated after a long absence, which prevented me from seeing you, Sir, at my home. However, I am as much disposed to be of assistance to you as before. Of course, I always discourage measures, whose success seems to me very improbable. When the question arose of a law concerning the status of the adherents to the Mosaic religion, and many important provisions appeared to me very burdensome, His Majesty indeed declared that admission to faculties should be made easier. At the moment no exception will be made because of talent; they will continue to follow the general rules. My personal recommendation, which was not wanting in your favor, was in vain because I am not present when the reports are given to the King, and could be of avail only if there were preceding cases in Prussian universities and the faculty itself did not object for reasons of intolerance. I am not able to judge to what reasons Herr Geheimrat von Ladenberg refers. If my sincerest, esteemed friend, Herr Geheimrat Müller, deems success probable, please show him this letter and let me have your petition by him in a sealed envelope with a copy. You are welcome to refer in your petition to the interest which your various works have aroused in me. But how little help will the habilitation as Privatdozent be to you!
>
> A. von Humboldt.

From this letter it can be seen that Humboldt had already previously supported Remak's application. He was alluding here either to the professorship of Wilna or the application to the Minister in January and now was again willing to help, although he did not expect much from such a procedure. The Herr Geheimrat von Ladenberg (1798–1855) referred to had been since 1839 departmental director in the Kultusministerium, repeatedly refusing to become Minister, but finally accepting the post in November, 1848. Strongly conservative and church-minded, he was the most important man to decide the personal affairs of the university. Humboldt apparently did not regard the time well chosen for Remak's application, but magnanimous as he was, he left it to the decision of Johannes Müller. The fact that Remak did submit his immediate plea to the King indicates that Müller was in favor of doing everything possible to support Remak's request. So it came about that in March, 1843 Remak, supported by Humboldt and with the necessary agreement of his teacher Müller, turned to the King personally with an application to admit him as lecturer.

All the pertinent original documents are no longer available today. They were probably destroyed by bombs or buried under the debris of the University buildings, but fortunately quotations from the original documents are preserved in a publication on the status of the Jews in Prussia, written by one Dr. M. Kalisch in Berlin in 1860 (40). They reveal Remak's ambition and also his attitude toward the Jewish religion, to which he then and all his life adhered, being a follower of the reform movement in Judaism and in later years a generous sponsor of the *Reformgenossenschaft* in Berlin (93).

Remak's application to Friedrich Wilhelm IV of March, 1843, written in the style of his time, reads as follows in literal translation:

> Great and mightiest King! Most gracious King and Lord!
>
> For eight years I have been preparing myself for the profession of an academic teacher through various physiological studies and private lectures, which have been attended even by academic teachers. However, owing to my profession of the Mosaic religion, the high ministerium of spiritual and medical matters decided, on the 17th of last month, that it was unable to permit my intended habilitation as a Privatdozent at the Medical Faculty of the Royal Friedrich Wilhelm University. Your Majesty's intention to promote every scientific endeavor encourages me to bring this matter to the steps of the throne and gives me hope that the following remarks may be accepted graciously; I am aware of their boldness.
>
> All the confessors of the Mosaic religion, especially in your Majesty's enlightened states, admit openly that they, in the midst of advanced Christian education, have furthered their long, rigid religious and moral status, and they also hope to develop it still further. Therefore, I, too, may be permitted to declare respectfully and solemnly that my education and my feeling are intimately connected with those views rooted in Christianity, which penetrate the life of science and of the state. Such an ideal accordance seems to make formal conversion to Christianity difficult rather than simple. The condition of having fewer political rights takes away from a decision first its necessary, external freedom and deprives a person, not especially occupied with religious questions, of the right to think of disposing of the dogmatic difficulties. The well known involuntary origin of such a conversion in most instances makes the social status of the converts dubious, which lessens the effect of the conversion and prevents others, who are not by external motives influenced, to follow such an example. I need not even mention the obligation of each individual to endeavor to help to advance the community given to him by nature, instead of entering another community, even though this may be for his own sincere satisfaction. Adhering to such a view, which no doubt I hold in common with many of my co-religionists, I find myself deprived of the opportunity to devote all my power to science and to the state to which I both belong and am fervently devoted.
>
> Therefore I dare to submit to your Majesty the most humble and submissive plea:
>
> > May Your Majesty decide most graciously to give an order which may make possible my habilitation as Privatdozent at the Medical Faculty of the Royal Friedrich Wilhelms University.

I hope his Excellency, the Wirkliche Geheime Rath Baron v. Humboldt, whose interest has always been won by my publications, may, through his kind intercession and representation, pave the way for me to the sphere of activity for which I ask most devotedly. If I am most graciously admitted to it, I shall prove my gratitude through the most conscientious fulfillment of my duties to the honor of God, to the advantage of the State, and to the progress of science.

Berlin, 14th of March, 1843.

This application was never seriously considered by the King. It was immediately turned over to the Minister, as had been previously a similar direct application to the King by the Jewish physician Friedrich Jacob Behrendt in 1840, and one by the Jewish historian J. M. Jost in 1841. Like both of these, it was turned down by the Minister, and Remak was notified on April 18, 1843, of his defeat. Humboldt's pessimism, expressed in his letter to Remak, unfortunately proved to be justified.

It is difficult for us who have grown up in the twentieth century to appreciate what courage and strong character it took to dare to call the attention of the King of Prussia to the fact that an extorted conversion for the purpose of a career, as daily happened in Germany, is illogical and unethical. To refuse baptism even though it meant losing a dearly desired career and to mention it to the King, whose father had revoked in 1822 promises given in 1812, was the act of a man who also dared to declare himself to be Polish when it was much more advantageous to proclaim himself German (85).

After this experience, Remak realized that in spite of Müller's and von Humboldt's support, his hopes for a scientific career as anatomist or physiologist in Germany were in vain. This fact may have been the chief factor in his turning now from pure research to clinical medicine and accepting a few months later the position of Research Assistant in Schönlein's Clinic.

ASSISTANT TO SCHÖNLEIN

Remak's activities in his new position were mainly concerned with practical clinical matters. Schönlein knew how to evaluate modern methods; he was one of those clinicians who early appreciated the importance of microscopical investigations for clinical diagnosis. The work that Remak was now expected to perform was also made available to the students of the medical faculty as part of their clinical curriculum. They were permitted to join the investigations and had to be instructed by Remak in the methods used. Thus this Jew, who was not admitted to a regular lectureship, nevertheless had to lecture unofficially. Remak's official position in Schönlein's Clinic, though it carried no official title, was that of a laboratory assistant and unofficial lecturer.

Not content to limit his work to diagnostic purposes alone, he immediately set out to widen the field of his activities, to do post-mortem examinations and to evaluate therapeutic measures. He thus created a new place for research, working in what we could call today pathological anatomy, histology, and pathological physiology. He was the right man for such a position, for since 1836 he had been busy with pathological investigations in the anatomical laboratory directed by Müller, who generously placed the facilities of the pathological museum at his disposal. The fruits of these studies by the young student were articles on melanosis, ossification and osteosarcoma, which he wrote for the *Encyclopedic Dictionary of Medical Sciences.* To be invited to contribute such articles was an honor by which Müller conferred distinction on his outstanding pupils like Schwann, Henle, Brücke, and Helmholtz.

It seems that Remak derived much satisfaction from his clinical activities. He was on very good terms with his chief, Schönlein, who gave him the opportunity for pathological observations in his own private practice, too. Remak also enjoyed attending Schönlein's clinical lectures. It was a new and inspiring experience to receive support, advice, and suggestions concerning clinical work from the man who was not only the much admired personal physician of the King of Prussia, but also the leader in clinical medicine in Germany.

There is no question that Schönlein, like Johannes Müller, coming from the underprivileged working class of Germany, wanted to be helpful in Remak's career, in spite of his faith and nationality. After the first term of his clinical activities at Schönlein's suggestion, Remak submitted a report on his clinical investigations to Eichhorn, at that time Prussian Minister of Educational and Medical Affairs. Eichhorn, an arch reactionary who a year before had turned down Remak's application for a lectureship, answered in May, 1844 in a kind way (68). He emphasized his special interest in the importance of Remak's investigations and in his endeavor to combine pathology and physiology for clinical purposes and to modernize medical instruction. Encouraged by such approval, Remak continued with his work and with his reports to the Minister in succeeding terms.

Finally, in August, 1845 he revised all the reports and put them in book form. This book, published in Berlin in 1845, was dedicated to Schönlein "with highest respect and thankfulness" (68). The book contained not only Remak's clinical and pathological experiments of the last three terms in Schönlein's Clinic, but also some of his experiments of the last seven years in Müller's laboratory, his experiences at Froriep's pathological investigations, and some of the material be received from von Graefe, Jüngken, and Dieffenbach, and also from Romberg's clinic (68). At that time friends and colleagues supported his work by giving him material and the opportunity to perform autopsies. Unquestionably, the publication of Remak's book, reporting on his activity as a clinician as well as a pathologist, anatomist, and microscopist, was undertaken with an eye on future opportunities for an appointment to a newly created position in the Charité, for which Virchow was named as a candidate by the military academy, and even with a view to the possibility of an appointment as prosector if Professor Froriep, at that time prosector (acting pathologist) of the Charité Hospital, should one day retire. The book was published at the end of 1845, and in 1846 the great competition began between Virchow and Remak for the succession to Froriep.

Schönlein originally favored Remak's candidacy for this post. All the work Remak had previously done in neurohistology, embryology, pathology, and clinical medicine made him beyond a doubt the most deserving candidate. His best recommendation for Froriep's position, which was soon to be available, was this recent book of his containing a great deal of new and valuable chemical and pathological material. Here he gave the fungus producing the favus disease the name "Achorion Schönleini," still in use, and reported his own self-experiments of 1842 through which he made certain that this disease can be transmitted by contact of the crusts with the skin of a healthy person. Showing that the "achorion" can be found in pure culture in pustules created in this way, he proved beyond any doubt that the fungus is the real cause of this disease. Only David Gruby, in Paris before Remak, had reported on such experiments in *Müller's Archiv*,[49] made with the fungus he found in the same disease, independently of Schönlein, but without positive results.

Among other things worth mentioning in Remak's book are the following. He gave the first correct description of the histology of intestinal villi, disputing the one given by J. Henle. Here he again emphasized his objections to Schwann's theory of free cell production in the cytoblastem. However, in the matter of cell production, he himself was not yet so certain and clear as he was later in his papers of 1852 and 1854. We learn (68) that since 1838, when he was graduated, he was performing experiments on horses at the Veterinary Academy of Berlin, eagerly grasping every opportunity offered to extend his research work. He was interested in and occupied with experiments on thrombosis. One is astonished at the diversity of his investigations, which were partly of a strictly clinical and therapeutic nature and partly devoted to theoretical problems. In investigating fibrin microscopically (68: 63), he comes to the very modern conclusion that the start of fibrin production may be analogous to crystal formation. He reports here his previous experiments, when he took forty to fifty pounds of blood from a horse to study successively the effect of a large phlebotomy on the regeneration of blood.

In each one of these studies, even those which might not yet have yielded definite results, we must admire Remak's keen observation and critical mind. For instance, he correctly described the histology of the pulmonic alveoli (68: 87), and reluctantly and politely corrected the erroneous concept of Henle and Valentin, who were of the opinion that a palisade layer of ciliated cells can be found in the pulmonic alveoli. Here (68: 87) we can see the way of Remak's investigations, which were not confined to microscopical observations in man, but always included comparative research and even already some embryological research. He makes the remark that no such epithelium existed, as Henle and Valentin supposed, in the lung alveoli of man, cattle, pig, or sheep, and included in a footnote his own observations, which enabled him to show from which part of the embryonic *anlage* the lungs develop.

Only a research worker with a tremendous wealth of his own experience, discoveries, and knowledge could mention in a footnote such an important discovery and allow his friends to publish in their doctoral theses discoveries of his own which even outstanding scholars would have kept for their own publications. Remak was only twenty-nine years of age when he wrote this book, which was public evidence that he was qualified to compete with anyone on equal terms for the appointment, soon to be made, of a chief pathologist (prosector) of the Charité. He even dared to object very strongly to the opinion on Discrasia of the already famous Rokitansky, pathologist in Vienna, and it is very typical that again, in disagreement with Rokitansky's "Discrasia" theory, he declared in only a few lines that the primarily diseased part in pneumonia was the epithelium of the lungs. In the same year, 1845, Remak published in Froriep's *Notizen* another fundamental, microscopical discovery. He was the first to find that each primitive bundle of the muscle is one single cell, and that part of the protoplasm of this cell is transformed into contractile muscle substance. This type of study already belongs to the period of embryological research, which filled every second of Remak's scientific life in the following ten years. However, merit alone proved not to be decisive in the matter of obtaining an appointment.

Remak's book from Schönlein's Clinic was accepted very favorably by the profession and especially by his protector, Humboldt, who, in spite of his seventy-six years, followed the studies of his young friend with eager interest and wrote two letters to Remak in connection with this publication. One (21: 122) reads as follows:

> I deeply rejoice that your interesting long-awaited "Pathogenetischen" were published, and I should like to express my deepest appreciation. At the present time, I am just returned from a short stay on the Rhine. I am disturbed anew by the arrival of the Russian court and must again occupy myself seriously with such important and new objects. Your work has for me a special attraction in the report of the puzzling creation of independent

[49] 1842: 22.

organisms by pathological factors.[50] Accept, dearest Herr Doktor, the renewed expression of esteem and attachment, which I have cherished for you already for a long time.
A. von Humboldt

P.S. My sincerest regards to Herrn Geheimrat Schönlein, whose great name surely will contribute much to attract steady attention to this work so close to medicine.

This letter, written September 13, 1845, expresses the great appreciation for and true attachment of Humboldt to the young scholar. Owing to the many obligations which the visit of the Russian court to Berlin imposed upon him, Humboldt probably forgot that he had written the above letter. Among those published by Geiger there is another written a month later (21: 123), in answer to Remak's question whether he should dedicate a copy of his work to the King.

With his thoughtful advice Humboldt thought to make sure that the book would really reach the King personally, and that it would not be held back at the office of any of the secretaries or other officials. It reads in translation:

In a very regrettable way, dearest Herr Doktor, I have hesitated from day to day to offer you the expression of my appreciation for your small but extremely sound work, which is equally important for physiology and anatomy. I hoped every week that my letter of praise would again turn up, which, in childish haste, I probably put in a different envelope. You know how much I enjoy taking an interest in your work; you also know that I blame the barbaric laws, which check beautifully aspiring greatness.[51] It will be a great pleasure for me to hand your book to the King. You only have to send it to me here with a sealed letter "to the King."

With kindest attachment, I am your most obedient
Potsdam, 16th October, 1845 A. von Humboldt.

REMAK DESCRIBES AND EXPLAINS THE PARADOXICAL PULSE

Remak soon proved to be not only the theoretician and outstanding microscopist in Schönlein's laboratory, but also an excellent observer of clinical symptoms. That is shown in his book of 1845 and also in a short, eleven page article published in 1844 under the title, "Sphygmologia," in the *Encyclopedic Dictionary of Medical Sciences* (67). This article concerns itself with pulse rate, heart sounds, pulse, and blood pressure, in so far as they were known in his time. He mentions the original statements of Haller, Magendie, and Poiseuille, that in expiration the pulse pressure may increase in animal experiments. But he adds his own observation that during deep inspiration in human beings the pulse volume (palpated at the radial artery) may decrease to the point of disappearance. This observation, the first of its kind, was made by Remak long before Williams (1850) and before Kussmaul described this fact in pathological cases and gave it the very unfortunate name of *pulsus paradoxus*. The knowledge of Remak's description of this phenomenon would probably have convinced Kussmaul that there really is nothing paradoxical in such a symptom, except for the fact that the diminishing of the pulse volume in Kussmaul's cases appeared without forced respiration in normal breathing. Remak was the first in modern times to describe what Ortner calls (1909) the *pulsus inspiratione intermittens.* He also gave the very good explanation of this phenomenon, that in deep inspiration the enlargement of the vascular bed of the lungs leads to a pooling there of the blood and consequently an insufficient amount streams into the left ventricle. This accounts for the phenomenon in the radial and in small peripheral arteries.

Probably the first to describe the symptom of a *pulsus inspiratione intermittens* was Lower in his *Tractatus de Corde.*[52] He reported it in a thirty-year old patient with adhesive pericarditis. With excellent preciseness he described the pathological findings as ascertained after the patient's death. He gave an incorrect explanation of the intermittent pulse assuming that inspiration stops the heart beat in such a case. However, the clinical symptoms of the *pulsus inspiratione intermittens* and the clinical picture of adhesive pericarditis were well observed and described by him.

REMAK AND VIRCHOW COMPETE

Since Remak was such an outstanding candidate, and Virchow was six years his junior, Schönlein opposed Virchow's candidacy for succession to Froriep's position as chief pathologist of the Charité Hospital in Berlin, and so did the Prussian Minister. But the military group supported him and so did some of the chief physicians of the Charité. In 1844 Jüngken accepted him in the surgical clinic, where he had sufficient work to do in chemical and microscopic fields. Another of his protectors was the prosector of the Charité, Froriep himself, son of an outstanding doctor in Weimar. A friend of Henle (49), he became Professor of Surgical Anatomy at Berlin in 1833 and prosector (chief pathologist) and conservator of the Pathological Museum in the Charité. Since 1836 he was a member of the Medicinal Collegium of the Province of Brandenburg. From all these positions at the University of Berlin he resigned in 1846, retiring to Weimar to take over the industrial enterprises of his father and his grandfather Bertuch, famous for his connections with Goethe.

Before Froriep's time pathological anatomy was in a very bad state at Berlin. Pagel (56) mentions that Pirogov, in a travel report of the year 1830, states that at that time a midwife named Vogelsang performed the autopsies at the Charité. It was only at the time of the cholera epidemic in Berlin (1831–1832) that the appointment of a physician as prosector was decided upon, because such a position demanded some knowledge of normal and pathological anatomy. After a short time

[50] This sentence probably refers to the Achorion Schönleinii mold and its transplantation to normal skin.

[51] This refers to the laws barring Jews from an academic career in Prussia.

[52] Chap. II, p. 106, Amstelodami, 1669.

(1831–1833), during which Philipp Phoebus, later Professor at Giessen, took charge of this post, Robert Froriep was appointed in 1833. Besides doing some work himself in pathological anatomy, he had a laudable inclination to inspire young doctors, if he liked them, to do scientific research. This he did with Virchow.

Like Remak, Virchow soon began to publish his investigations in the journal, which Froriep together with his father edited in Weimar. In 1845 Froriep informed Virchow of his plans to retire as Chief of Pathological Anatomy and to return to Weimar the following year (60: 104). He told this to Virchow in order to give the latter time to pull all the strings. Froriep admitted that Virchow, at that time twenty-four years of age, was extremely young for such a position, but he promised all his support. In a letter to his father Virchow pointed out (60) that in the event that he should succeed in obtaining this appointment, his future would be absolutely secure. This was when he had not even passed his State Board Examinations and had just begun to publish his first observations in medicine, with which he had difficulties, even in his protector Froriep's Journal.

Early in 1846 Virchow's expectations rose, it was mainly Schönlein who again placed the candidacy of Remak against Virchow. But he did not give his pupil full-hearted support in spite of the fact that the latter had just published his important book from Schönlein's Clinic, and that in the meantime such famous authorities as Hannover in Copenhagen (28: 33) and Koelliker in Zürich (42: 4) had corroborated Remak's fundamental discovery of the origin of nerve fibers in ganglionic cells. As much as Schönlein personally would have preferred Remak, he evidently was not disposed to intervene energetically for him, as we learn from Virchow's cynical remarks in another letter to his father. In May, 1846, with all Virchow's friends bringing strong pressure to bear on the Minister and his consultant, Schönlein called for Virchow to inform him that he would give Virchow's candidacy his full support. With that the entire question was decided, and a tremendous opportunity for work was lost once and forever to Remak.

There is no need to emphasize how well fitted for such a position Virchow was, how he soon gained fame within and outside the faculty as a research worker and, after he became a lecturer at the University in 1847, as a teacher in this field. But then, too, it would be superfluous to point out that Remak had already demonstrated by the results of his research that he was at least of the same quality as Virchow as a research scientist, and with more important achievements to his credit.

REMAK'S DISCOVERY OF THE "ACHORION SCHÖNLEINII"

The book just mentioned, in which Remak reported his studies in the Schönlein Clinic, is an extremely interesting document on his personality. Here, as mentioned above, he described as Schönlein's discovery a mold producing the skin disease favus, and suggested for it the name "Achorion Schönleinii," used to this day, thus making the name of his teacher immortal in medicine and mycology. This discovery and the name given to it by Remak has a special piquant aspect through a note in Remak's book relative to the Achorion mold. A physician by name Xaver Hube, who in 1837 wrote his Berlin doctoral thesis, "De Morbo Scrophuloso," was a friend of Remak from his home town of Posen, another of his close friends from Poland. In this thesis he made the statement that already in 1837, while working in the Children's Clinic under Barez in the Charité, Remak discovered in the substance of crust-covered places in favus disease spherical bodies and ramified fibers to be found as a typical constituent of these favus products. On page 19 of his doctoral thesis Hube wrote that Remak did not care to publish these special findings but permitted them to be included in his, Hube's, thesis.

Unquestionably, therefore, Remak was the first to observe this interesting phenomenon and the cause of the disease in favus. However, in 1842, when he proved the infectiousness of the favus condition, and again in this publication from Schönlein's Clinic in 1845, he expressly and sincerely denied (p. 193) having originally recognized the nature of these structures as being ramified molds. I am not inclined to agree with Rille (75) in doubting that a keen observer like Remak, who at that time had already discovered and correctly interpreted the most difficult details in microneurology would indeed have been unaware that those spherical bodies, rods and ramified branches, which he discovered in favus were of a special nature. I cannot agree with Rille when he says that Remak, four years after the publication of the fundamental discoveries of Gruby, with all the evidence for the parasitic etiology of favus, denied his own priority just to praise and to flatter his teacher and protector. It is true that immediately after Virchow's first success in obtaining an appointment at the Charité in 1844, Remak at the time when he was considered by Schönlein as Froriep's successor, gave all credit for this discovery to Schönlein, eliminating himself from all claims to priority. What he writes in his 1845 book is not different from what he wrote in 1842, when he was able to prove that favus is a communicable disease. He does not make a secret of the fact that he was the first to see the fungus, but with admirable sincerity he emphasizes that he did not realize that he had seen a fungus. It was before Agostino Bassi discovered that the so-called Muskardine disease of silk worms was a fungus disease of these animals, and it was Bassi's discovery which put Schönlein on the right track. Remak disclaimed all credit for this in 1842, prior to his connection with Schönlein and his clinic.

REMAK BECOMES PRIVATDOZENT AND IS DEPRIVED OF A PROFESSORSHIP

All this did not really influence Schönlein in 1846 to support his assistant in his efforts to secure the appointment as pathologist (prosector) of the Charité Hospital; twenty-five-year-old Virchow became prosector of the Charité and in the following year, 1847, a lecturer (Privatdozent) in the Medical Faculty of Berlin University. Schönlein was not able to prevent this, and as Virchow wrote in a letter to his father in 1846, Schönlein decided like a clever general actively to support the winning side (60).

Remak had instructed students in Schönlein's Clinic for three years and here at least, in spite of the defeat of 1843, was a possibility to do his activities justice. As a Jew he was not permitted, as we already know, to apply in the regular manner for an appointment as a lecturer, but Schönlein, who without question favored Remak and even allowed him to take part in his private practice (68), now became really helpful on behalf of his assistant. As personal physician to the King of Prussia and official adviser to the Minister on Medical Affairs, he was probably instrumental in Remak's new effort to obtain a royal decree from Friedrich Wilhelm IV through which, for the first time in the history of Berlin's University, an unbaptized Jew was made a Privatdozent in its Medical Faculty. That actually occurred finally in the year 1847, when Remak's career competitor, Virchow, was appointed lecturer, too. Undoubtedly Remak's appointment was connected with this event, the intention being to reward Remak and to compensate him at least in part for his disappointment in the Virchow affair. Instrumental in this unprecedented success of Remak's was another personality who was extremely influential at the court of the King. This was, of course, Alexander von Humboldt, for forty years an intimate friend of the poet Goethe, and throughout his lifetime a helpful friend to every gifted scientist.

Remak was the same ardent worker and fanatic research scholar after the defeat of 1843 as he was before. Not only did he publish the results of his research in the German language and his doctoral thesis in Latin, but he also took care to publish the results of his research in Polish and in French. He was serious in his statement, made in his application to the King of Prussia in 1843, that it was everyone's duty to be faithful to his own nation. He also felt under an obligation to inform his Polish colleagues of the progress of medicine in Germany and even to help develop the technical terminology of the Polish language in accordance with modern requirements (85).

Remak also supervised the translation into Polish of a 514 page textbook for midwives, which was published in Berlin in 1841. All these activities repeatedly called the attention of scientific circles in Polish universities to their successful young compatriot in Berlin.

In 1839, as already mentioned above, the Faculty of the Medical Academy at Wilna in Russia recommended Remak as Professor of Physiology to the Russian Minister of Education, von Ouwaroff. This is not a mere legend as Wrzosek (85) says, but we have the reliable testimony of Humboldt for it (21; 40: 23), who recommended the young scholar for this position on the excellent reports of his teachers, Ehrenberg and Müller.

This was certainly a great honor for a young man only twenty-four years of age, but, of course, the Russian government was the last in the world to consider the appointment of an unbaptized Jew to a prominent position or, indeed, to any governmental post at all. So, this was another disappointment Remak had to face at the start of his career.

Indefatigable, he continued with his work of research and in 1847 published a large volume with two plates on the nervous system of the intestines. Grateful for all that Humboldt had done for him, he wanted to dedicate this book to his fatherly friend and protector, and he asked his permission to do so. But again Humboldt advised Remak most unselfishly to include in the dedication either of his teachers, Schönlein or Johannes Müller, and he did it in the most tactful manner, careful not to hurt Remak's sensitive feelings. On January 23, 1847, he wrote to Remak (21: 124):

> I scarcely have enough spare time to thank you for your kind offer, but would it not be possible to dedicate the book at the same time to me and to Schönlein or Johannes Müller; such an *Accomplement* with learned friends would be very agreeable to me.
> With sincerest esteem,
> Your most devoted
> A. von Humboldt.
> Friday, Berlin, 23rd January, 1847

Just two years before, Remak had dedicated a book to his teacher, Schönlein, but he had never so honored Johannes Müller, not even in his doctoral thesis. He therefore followed Humboldt's advice and dedicated the book on the nervous system of the intestines, "in deepest esteem and sincerest thankfulness," to Humboldt and Johannes Müller.

On receiving the first copy of the book in the middle of February, Humboldt writes to Remak on the fifteenth of that month (21: 124):

> The dedication of such an important and wonderfully artistically printed work as your "Darmnervensystem" was a great honor and pleasure for me. Please, dearest Herr Doktor, accept with my sincerest thanks the renewed expression of the respect I have felt towards you already for a long time. I was stimulated especially by what you say on page 6 and 12 concerning the nucleated, winding fibers with dark contours, and I was reminded of your previous work. May I ask you humbly to give me, if it is possible for you, the pleasure of your instructive visit on Thursday. I wish not only to see you, but to have various things explained first-hand about the figures.
> With excellent and high esteem,
> A. von Humboldt
> Monday (15 February) 1847.

It is really astonishing not only with what eagerness Humboldt, at the age of nearly eighty years, immediately began to study this scientific book, but also how he perceived at once the relationship to previous work of Remak over the past eight years; now he was anxious to see the author at his home in order to receive from him detailed explanations. It was not only for that reason that Humboldt wanted to see Remak personally; Humboldt was to see the King a few days later and wished to discuss with Remak possibilities that were now presenting themselves so that Remak's desire to become a member of the teaching staff of the Berlin University might finally be realized. After he had made certain that this time the King was really willing to make an exception in the case of Remak, he did not hesitate to take things into his own hands. We know from notes in Remak's own hand (21: 128) that they both, Humboldt and Remak, met on the 23rd of February at the home of Johannes Müller who that year happened to be the dean of the medical faculty. They discussed the necessary steps to be taken, and Humboldt, careful as he was, dictated to Remak while he was there how he was to write his immediate application to His Majesty. Even prior to this meeting between the three men, Humboldt, after having discussed everything with the King, hastened at once to inform Remak in a special letter, which reads in translation as follows (21: 127):

I am glad to inform you, my dearest Herr Doktor, that I already prepared the King yesterday evening concerning your application to be granted the habilitation as a Privatdozent at the University. He answered me in the most friendly way in the affirmative. Nothing was spoken about any new legal regulations but about condescending in individual cases. This I achieved even without showing your beautiful etched drawings, on whose support I had unnecessarily counted. You will not be surprised that I also mentioned the approval of a great name, that of my friend Schönlein, in this matter. Since you are supposed to take official steps with the King and Minister, please come to see me Tuesday at half past one so that we can discuss the form. You see, I always find time when meritorious scientific activity, such as yours, is involved and a principle of political progress.

With excellent and high esteem
A. von Humboldt

21 February 1847

It is, indeed, touching the way in which Humboldt does not spare time, conferences, or interventions, and sees ministers and the King himself, to fight for Remak's good cause. This explains the lifelong devotion and esteem of the latter for this great personality.

In 1847 when Remak and his protectors deemed it propitious to repeat a direct appeal to the King and Humboldt succeeded in his preliminary efforts, times and conditions had changed a good deal since Remak's defeat in 1843. Through political events, especially those in France since the days of Napoleon, it became evident to everyone at that time that no government in Europe could feel secure in the future if it tried to bring back political conditions to the status of the prerevolutionary eighteenth century. The population in all parts of Germany, especially the intelligentsia, felt disappointed and politically cheated after Napoleon's downfall, and resolved to do something about it. The many German princes and kings began to feel uneasy between their dissatisfied subjects and their greedy ruling classes.

The Jews in Prussia, too, had changed considerably in the thirty-five years since the edict of 1812. The younger generation was eager to acquire secular knowledge and to adapt themselves to their non-Jewish environment. Imbued with the historic Jewish sensitivity for right and justice, they were ready to strive, to agitate, and if need be, to fight for their own rights and for the rights of other underprivileged groups. Karl Marx, the baptized Jew, began his radical activities in Cologne in 1841. A group of Jewish and non-Jewish poets, including Heine, Börne, Herwegh, Freiligrath, was politically active. Each one of these had the same ideal of humanism and freedom, but there were controversies and struggles among themselves. The early glow of the twilight of the gods of 1848 appeared on the political horizon.

Under such circumstances the unbearable injustice of the status of Jews as third-class citizens and the need for revision of their legal rights and special privileges became more and more urgent and remedial measures were in the preparatory stage in 1847. A pertinent law was submitted for consideration to a meeting of the Erste Vereinigte Landtag, a kind of House of Representatives assembled in Berlin, and was discussed from June 1847 on. These discussions aroused the most lively interest and violent party feeling among the population, Jews and non-Jews alike.

It was on February 24, 1847, in this atmosphere of political tension and excitement, that Remak submitted to the King his second direct application to be held eligible for a lecturership. This application, though written with all due devotion to the King, had a different tone and less of the servility that was customary before then. It reads, in literal translation:

Most serene King!

For the last eleven years I have been occupied with physiological and pathological investigations which would already have opened an academic career for me more than six years ago if I, as a Jew, had not been prevented through the highest Cabinet Order of August 18, 1822 from setting out on it. Conversion to Christianity was impossible for me because of the orthodoxy of my parents, to whom I owe reverence and love. Also, I have always had the greatest disgust for the idea of securing external advantages by a change of religion.

Because, therefore, the prescription of the law up to now has prevented me from joining the ranks of academic teachers, I dare to make this most humble plea that your Majesty most graciously permit me to enter a teaching position at one of our own universities.

His Excellency, Herr Baron von Humboldt will be gracious enough to hand your Majesty a copy of my work ... as a sign of my deepest respect, in which I remain,

Berlin, 24th February, 1847.

This application (40) is very different from the first one four years previous. It is much more concise, and its tone is that of manly pride and self-consciousness. In view of the times and the manner of addressing a king, it is a most courageous demand for a merited right. In an unmistakable way it indicts the infamous 1822 order of the King's father, and it brands the conversion to Christianity, imposed by the government as prerequisite to an appointment, as unethical from every point of view and revolting to a real man. It also refers to the intervention of the sympathetic Alexander von Humboldt, who always had the ear of the King.

How seriously Humbolt, at that time seventy-eight years of age, meant his support of Remak's just cause can be judged by the fact that he not only talked over the problem with the King effectively and persuaded him, but he himself served as courier to deliver the new application and Remak's book. Kalisch does not mention its title (40: 23), but according to Humboldt's accompanying letter, it must have been Remak's book of 1845. The new publication mentioned by Humboldt was the still unpublished book on the nervous system of the intestines, which was dedicated to Alexander von Humboldt and to Remak's teacher Johannes Müller.

Humboldt did more than act as intermediary; he accompanied Remak's short application with a long letter, which reads as follows (40):

Your Royal Majesty!

You were gracious enough to express your views to me in such a definite and gracious way, when I ventured to speak in my own name and in the name of my distinguished friends, Geheimrath Schönlein and the anatomist Johannes Müller, of Dr. Remak of Jewish faith, noted for his important anatomical discoveries, that I do not hesitate to accompany the most humble application of this young scholar with these lines.

Dr. Remak was born of very orthodox and poor Jewish parents. A prize essay of his found public recognition already in 1835 at the University in this city. When, in 1839, he was submitted to the Russian Ministry by the Medical Academy of Wilna as Professor of Physiology, I recommended him strongly to Minister von Uwaroff because of the reports which I received from Müller and Ehrenberg. This was unsuccessful because of un-Christian religious intolerance, in which the Minister himself, as he wrote me expressly, by no means joined.

Remak's fine microscopical investigations, his entirely independent and very talented work, led Geheimrath Schönlein to appoint Dr. Remak as a research assistant paid by the Ministry at his clinic. Since 1843 the students of Geheimrath Schönlein have participated in his demonstrations at the Charité. Devotion to his very aged, still living parents and his aversion to a change of religion for the purpose of receiving material advantages barred a man who is not only very promising but for the past ten years has been very productive, from an academic career, in accordance with prevailing legal orders. Your Royal Majesty was gracious enough to tell me that you would now like to favor a very distinguished Jewish scholar with a dispensation and I therefore renew my most humble plea that your Royal Majesty may graciously permit Dr. Remak to enter an academic teaching position at one of the universities in this country.

The enclosed publication is important also from the point of view of clinical pathology, and adorned with extremely fine plates. It will soon be followed by a larger one for which many anatomical plates are already engraved. They demonstrate a progredient and continuous activity.

Berlin. February 27th, 1847.

Remak's application to the King had been handed to Humboldt only two days before, on the twenty-fifth of February. He acknowledged receipt of it in the following letter (21: 128):

I have your treasures and you will surely not doubt that I shall deliver everything with the greatest sympathy. I had to open your letter to the King in order to put it in an envelope with my handwriting and my seal, adding a letter of my own in which I spoke of Schönlein, Johannes Müller, and my own judgment, especially of the beautiful work you have done. I shall prepare the Minister by a personal visit, but that probably will not be before Sunday, and I shall write you after it has taken place.

In friendship yours,
A. von Humboldt

Thursday, 25 February 47.

P.S. I also wrote in your behalf to Schönlein. His word is important with the King, and I sincerely would not like to overlook anything.

How painstakingly careful Humboldt was can be seen not only from his own letter, but also from his personal visits to the Minister, the fact that he wrote to Schönlein, and his remark added to this letter, explaining why he thought he had to open Remak's letter and put it in another envelope. He wrote:

I was obliged to do that because, incidentally, you wrote on the letter that I was supposed to submit, "through His Excellency," but in matters directed to the King, no servant of the state (Minister or Field Marshall) is given the title excellency.

Finally, Humboldt handed Remak's application together with his own supporting letter to Councilor Illaire. He reported immediately by letter to Remak what he had done and that he had also made a special call on one extremely important man in the entire affair, the Minister of Education, Eichhorn, an outspoken reactionary who actually, as we shall see later, tried to do his utmost to keep Remak from any success in his career. Humboldt writes (21: 129):

On Friday I brought your application and my very extensive letter to the King to Herrn Geheimen Kabinettsrath Illaire so that he, which is most advantageous, may submit both on Saturday in his report. This actually took place, and yesterday evening the King told me in a very friendly manner and without my asking him: "I immediately approved the case of your Dr. Remak." I can't say whether it now goes first to Minister Eichhorn, but the first thing today, Sunday morning at half past eleven, I went to see Minister Eichhorn to show him your "Nerves of the Intestines." He promised me most definitely not to put up any obstacles in this matter. On the contrary, he appeared very interested. You may now write directly to him. You see, my dear Remak, that I am one of the few who like to be active where they see scientific activities and where principles can be defended.

Yours
A. v. Humboldt

28 February 1847

With this letter of Humboldt's Remak was informed that he had reached his goal, that the King had decided his case favorably, and that he himself should now communicate with the Minister by suitable letter. The letter that Remak wrote, which he thought proper, almost spoiled everything at the last moment and may explain, at least partly, all the ensuing difficulties that Remak encountered in spite of the King's decision. Unfortunately, we have no copy of Remak's letter to Eichhorn, but from the following letter from Humboldt, dated March 10, we can infer that Remak may have been hesitant to trouble Humboldt again and to impose on his time by first submitting to him an outline of his letter to Eichhorn. That was a pity, though a very understandable consideration for the fact that Humboldt was always very busy. Surely the wise and experienced courtier would never have permitted such a letter to be dispatched. Remak made the very unhappy decision to write now to the Minister a programmatic statement on the rights of the Jews and on religious tolerance; he may have tried to discuss with the Minister all the rights and privileges of a future Jewish member of a faculty, and he may even have had it in mind to obtain a full professorship at one of the Prussian universities, for instance at Bonn, where once his master, Johannes Müller, had been professor. This undiplomatic procedure, without first consulting Humboldt, even though surely done in ignorance and without realizing the possible bad effects, made Humboldt completely desperate. After this occurrence, he wrote Remak the only reproachful letter, among all those extant, which reads as follows in translation (21: 129):

What an unhappy idea, dear Remak, that you start a religious discussion with the Christian Kultusminister, and make difficulties for me after I have expended my sincerest good will and my most precious time. It would have been so easy just to give him your new book and just to ask him for support of your application to the King, as I did. You are not yet Professor Extraordinarius and yet you now already discuss whether you will be able to become Rector or Dean. I deeply regret this incident. . . . [These dots are Humboldt's.] You know yourself that the King will not give orders to make you Professor, for instance at Bonn, and now you stir up untimely, general questions.

In friendship your most devoted
A. v. Humboldt

Berlin, Thursday, 10th of March, 47.

In spite of this unfortunate outbreak of Remak's temper in the letter to the Minister, this time, finally, the concentrated efforts of Humboldt, an old friend of the King, Schönlein, his personal physician, and the world renowned Johannes Müller, succeeded in persuading Friedrich Wilhelm IV. On March 8 a Royal Order in favor of Remak was directed to the Ministers Eichhorn and Von Bodelschwingh.

This decision of the King in Remak's case was greatly influenced by the political situation and by the pending intention of arranging a new deal for the Jewish population of Prussia. This is apparent from the following text of the King's Order directed to Eichhorn, which reads (in translation):

Because the question concerning the admission of Jews to public teaching positions is connected with the regulation of the conditions of the Jews as citizens and therefore may not be decided in the very near future, it seems to be suitable for me to open a way for it to go ahead. Having already expressed my intention not to exclude the Jews from this part of public activity, I shall do it by admitting individuals through special dispensation.

In accordance with this point of view, in answer to the pertinent application of Doctor Remak, which I am sending to you enclosed with the recommendation of the acting privy counsellor von Humboldt, I wish to empower you, State Minister Eichhorn, to admit the petitioner to an academic teaching position at one of the universities of this country for which he is qualified, except for the confessional requirements, unless you have some special objections of which notification should be given.

Berlin, 8th of March, 1847

Thus, finally, the royal decision was made concerning the admission of Remak as lecturer at a university and concerning other to-be-selected Jewish petitioners, but the dissenting and, owing to Remak's letter, indignant Minister by no means followed this order immediately. The King's Order was put *ad acta* by him without further action. Soon the Minister of the Interior, probably influenced by Humboldt or Schönlein or another of Remak's protectors, brought up the matter again, asking Eichhorn on April 30, 1847 either to follow the King's Order or to report to His Majesty on this matter, in which case he as Minister of the Interior would decide upon his own procedure (40: 25).

Eichhorn's answer was a new delay of the entire matter, with the obvious intention not to carry out the order. He replied that as he understood, Dr. Remak's appointment should be effective as soon as there was an opportunity, but there being no opening at any of the universities, he, Eichhorn, did not see any possibility of reporting to the King or notifying Dr. Remak, but he deemed it advisable to await the development of the new projected regulation of the status of the Jews in Prussia.

It was clear that this attitude was intended to defeat the purpose of the King to make a decision in the case of Remak before the new status of the Jews was legally decided, and in this way, through the public expression of his own view, to influence the decision of the Landtag concerning the new Jewry law. This law, which was discussed in the country's Assembly in June, 1847, aroused controversies and varying opinions and attitudes not only in the entire population, but also in the Landtag itself. Progressive and reactionary views clashed strongly, and it was by no means the unanimous feeling of the Prussian conservative Junkers that the Jews should be granted, in addition to all the duties of citizens and taxpayers, also the legal rights of citizens. Among the representatives of the country at these famous meetings was a young man, exactly the same age as Remak, a Prussian Junker and country nobleman. He had studied at the University of Göttingen in the years during which Remak began his fundamental research work, and while there he was a specimen of the strong, conceited, dueling, drinking, and pipe-smoking type among the German students. From his father he inherited the Schönhausen estate, from where he came as a deputy to the joint Landtag. His name was Otto von Bismarck, and he was the man who later molded the mighty position and the will to power of the German Reich and the mental attitude of most of its citizens. This young man who, with many of his type and age, was to decide the future of the Jews in Germany, after having discussed the problem in question, made the following concluding statement, which was included in the minutes of the meeting of June, 25, 1847: "It was exclusively my intention to deny that it would mean progress to emancipate the Jews."

Surely von Bismark was not the only Prussian legislator who felt this way. Consequently, Eichhorn's opposition to notifying Remak and the faculty of the King's more magnanimous attitude could expect to have the support of many politically important circles. But the matter was not left to itself, and we would not be wrong in assuming that again the wonderful Humboldt was the driving power behind events, when finally Eichhorn received another very brief letter from the King's Cabinet saying:

> His Majesty the King at the conference yesterday, made mention of a previous order given to your Excellency concerning the granting of an academic chair to a Jewish scholar, Dr. Remak, and he asked for information whether this Order has already been carried out. His Majesty regards this appointment as a very suitable transition to the principles adopted in the project of a Jewry law and therefore wishes it urgently.
>
> Because this matter was entirely unknown to me up to now I can only confine myself to asking Your Excellency kindly for information at your earliest convenience.
>
> Berlin, May 15th, 1847.
> Tiele.

Now Eichhorn was really compelled to act quickly; therefore on May 23 a letter signed by Eichhorn was sent to Remak in which he did not discharge the instruction of the King to bestow on Remak a chair on a Prussian Faculty, but merely informed Remak of the decision of the King to admit him to an academic teaching position at a Prussian University for which he would be fitted. He also requested a reply from Remak as to "whether he still wishes to become a Privatdozent," in which event he, Eichhorn, would arrange everything with the Rector and Senate of the University and with the Dean of the Medical Faculty. This procedure was definitely a fraudulent act on the part of the Minister, because the unmistakable intention of the King, especially emphasized in the Cabinet's Order of May 15, was to give Remak a chair on a Medical Faculty, which meant a full Professorship, and not to make him a lecturer. That Eichhorn really knew that he was cheating Remak can be seen from a letter to the King, written on the same day, May 23, 1847. In this letter he reported that he had informed the practicing physician and surgeon, Dr. Remak, that his appointment as Privatdozent at the Medical Faculty of Berlin was now possible, and he added:

> Since a certain teaching position, which could be given to Remak, is not available, I had to restrict myself to this announcement, because I may suppose that it fulfills the highest intention of Your Royal Majesty that Dr. Remak may acquire the claim to an extraordinary or ordinary Professorship in the same way as it is open to other competitors for academic teaching positions.

This was a cheap pretext on the part of the Minister to pretend not to know Remak's qualifications for a chair at the university, testified to not only by Humboldt, but by the three most outstanding members of the Medical Faculty at Berlin, Ehrenberg, Müller, and Schönlein, and attested to also by the fact that a foreign university had recommended Remak, when he was only twenty-four years of age, for a full professorship. Malevolence, bias, and hypocrisy were again able to triumph over merit and justice, and this, among other similar experiences, makes it understandable that Remak later became more and more the bitter personality that he appears to be in some of the polemics of his later years.

It must have been Remak's letter replying to the notification of Minister Eichhorn, which he wrote in accepting, *faute de mieux,* the position of Privatdozent, and probably also an apology to Humboldt for not having followed his advice on this or on the previous occasion in March, which made Humboldt write the following letter to Remak in June, 1847. The latter was now officially admitted as Privatdozent, at a time when the political question of officially changing the status of the Jews to full citizenship had everyone in Germany in a state of excitement. It seems that Remak, informed concerning the King's much more generous original decision, requested in his new letter to Eichhorn a higher position than that of a Privatdozent. Johannes Müller supported this plea, whereas Schönlein apparently was not informed, because Remak already planned, if he were successful, to give up his position at Schönlein's Clinic. Humboldt writes (21: 130):

> I thank you, my dear Remak, for your frank information. How could you ever be suspicious that my wish to be helpful to you and to secure for you a position which

satisfies your desire could become cooler because of an unjust demand, because you do not prefer to do something which initially seemed to me to be more advantageous. I know much better how to respect the deep feelings and differing opinions of those for whom I have the high esteem I feel for you, and I never permit myself to limit anyone's individual liberty. I am glad to hear that my noble friend, Geheimrath Müller, now also agreed to your last step. Your beautiful work can receive no higher consecration than the benevolent approval of a man who, with his mental and scientific greatness, combines the most noble human feelings. Your last answer to the Minister Eichhorn, of the 20th of June, falls at a time when the activities of the parliament involving the edict concerning the Jews and the periodicity [?] here in Berlin have produced much irritation and oscillation. Such hot days are just not favorable for considerations that are supposed to decide something of individual importance. However, now my dear Remak, after your latest answer has been dispatched, I promise you solemnly that I shall definitely manage to see Minister Eichhorn personally one of the next days, and I shall negotiate entirely in accordance with your desires. I shall not mention to Geheimrat Schönlein the information you gave me yesterday, nor anything about the procedure I have in mind if an urgent reason for doing so does not arise. It cannot be my desire to produce a new and entirely superfluous complication. A separation from him before your situation becomes independent could only be of damage for you. I shall not write to Minister Eichhorn. Being dogmatic concerning acquired rights only deflects one from one's purpose. I was sorry that yesterday, when you so kindly intended to visit me, was the day of the military festival in the new palace. Of course, I shall forward your plea concerning the dedication, but the days before the adjournment of the parliament should not be chosen.

Most kindly,
A. von Humboldt.

Potsdam, 21st of June 1847

From about the same time is a letter from Humboldt without a definite date, though Geiger reasons it was June 22, 1847 (21). It again refers to Remak's projected letter asking for a higher position than that of a Privatdozent. It reads:

My visit to Minister Eichhorn would not touch on your new application. You may submit it now or later on. First, I have only to find out of what mind he is and what can be expected from him. The Minister will not enter into any discussion, my dear Remak, concerning your rights, which to me are by no means doubtful. Would you be kind enough to visit me Sunday at half past twelve in *Berlin?* According to the explicit declarations of Herr Brüggemann in the Parliament (Kammer), you are not entitled to ask for a professorship at Bonn. At the moment they will not make exceptions *for your sake* or change a decision once made.

Yours,
A. von Humboldt.

Potsdam, Tuesday.

This letter again shows that Remak's demand and endeavor was for an appointment as full professor, if possible at Bonn, and not simply to allow himself to be put off with the position of a Privatdozent in Berlin, and that Müller and Humboldt supported this demand which they, too, considered justified. Theodor Brüggemann (1796–1866), referred to in Humboldt's letter, had just delivered a speech in the parliament concerning the admission of Jews to full professorship in the field of mathematics, science, medicine, and philology. Since 1843, he had held a leading position in the Prussian Kultusministerium (Vortragender Rath). In his speech he discussed the by-laws of the various Prussian universities, mentioning especially Bonn, where the constitution of the University speaks only of appointing Protestant or Catholic professors. He himself was in favor of admitting Jews to full professorships in medicine, science, and geography, but not in philosophy, history, and philology. He interpreted this part of the constitution of Bonn University to mean that Jews were not eligible for professorships at that university.

Considering the political status of the Jews in the middle of the last century, even the poor miserly reward for Remak's scientific achievements and for a life successfully devoted to science and medicine—his appointment as a Privatdozent in the medical faculty of Berlin—was remarkable. On October 14, 1847 Remak, in the traditional, solemn way gave his first introductory lecture in the large auditorium (*aula*) of Berlin University (86). He had the satisfaction that both of his parents joyfully shared his success. All Jewish journals in Germany reported this unprecedented event.

Though dissatisfied with this poor academic reward, Remak did not change his scholarly attitude towards medicine. In the same year that he began his academic lectures, his important book on the nervous system of the intestines came out; on Humboldt's advice, he continued his work as research assistant in Schönlein's Clinic; and at the same time he carried forward his fundamental research on embryological problems. All these activities, in addition to his practice, soon became too much for one person. In 1849 he finally resigned his position in Schönlein's laboratory with the purpose of devoting all his research in the following years to the problems of embryology in which he now was entirely absorbed.

In spite of all the disappointments Remak had experienced up to this time, his appointment as lecturer at the Medical Faculty of Berlin was a tremendous success, perhaps the greatest in his entire academic career. The German people, more than any other, have always been impressed and influenced by an official title. By becoming the first Jewish Privatdozent of the Medical Faculty at Berlin, Remak immediately acquired a reputation as a top ranking figure among the Jewish physicians of Berlin. There is no question that such a position and title also meant considerable financial success, even though no remuneration, except the meager students' fees, was connected with the privilege of teaching as lecturer. In the eyes of the general practitioner, the Privatdozent ranked as a consultant, and his fees were automatically increased with such a title. That has always been the way in Germany, even to this day.

Schönlein and Müller surely did their best for Remak on this occasion, and that Schönlein was not biased against Jews is clear from the fact that a year later another famous Jewish assistant of his became a Privatdozent on the Berlin faculty. This man was Ludwig Traube. In the meantime, however, things had become easier, for the year 1847 brought a new regulation of the status of Jews in Prussia, and 1848 saw so many changes in Germany that things unheard of before suddenly became possible. Remak's case, meanwhile, had broken a path that was not too easy to traverse even at the second attempt.

REMAK IS NOMINATED FOR A PROFESSORSHIP

In the winter term of 1847, Remak began his official lectures at Berlin University. We know from the program book of one of his outstanding pupils, Leopold Auerbach, that Remak was giving several lectures in his first teaching term: one on histology, for which the pupils had to pay the usual fee, and one free course, a so-called *publicum*, on medical microscopic investigations. The latter may have been a continuation of Remak's instructions for students given for some time already at Schönlein's Clinic. From Auerbach, too, we know that in the summer term of the same year Remak taught embryology as a fee course.

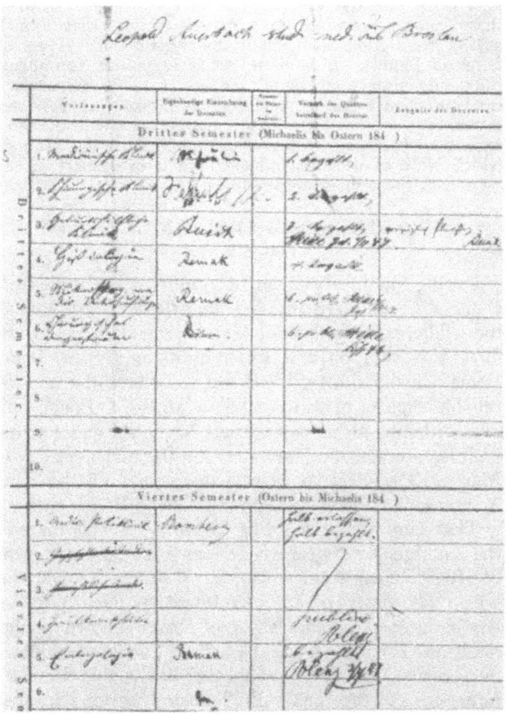

FIG. 52. Remak's signature in Leopold Auerbach's book of registered classes in the fall and spring term 1847–1848. These were the first times Remak lectured as Privatdozent in Berlin. From the author's collection.

Indeed, embryological studies were the object of Remak's main interest at all times after he had finished his comprehensive, neurological publications. Certainly, he never completely lost his interest in the field of neuro-histology. He published new studies and new discoveries from time to time in the following years, most of them in the *Archiv* of his teacher, Müller, some (since 1849) in the journal *Deutsche Klinik*. He was also interested in and devoted some work to other matters. In 1843 and later he studied the contractibility of muscle fibers; in various papers he described how, during menstruation, the epithelium of the uterus is eliminated. He emphasized in the same paper that with respect to the period of females the basic event is the periodical activity of the ovaries. In the same year, 1843, he also published a paper in *Müller's Archiv* on the development of the chicken in the egg, in which he outlined briefly the embryology of vertebrates.

In this paper a remark concerning his personal relationship with his teacher Müller, in the year in which he entered Schönlein's Clinic, is of some interest. Remak acknowledged the great advantage he had of discussing with Müller the problems of comparative anatomy. Indeed, from the beginning he included comparative points of view in his embryological work. He acknowledged that Müller generously gave him access to the objects in his museum for his investigations. It was not merely a *façon de parler* when he said in conclusion that Müller's actions towards him again secured his teacher the pupil's lasting gratitude. This attitude Remak retained all his life, in spite of divergencies in his own and Müller's opinions on some special scientific problems.

A sign of Müller's recognition of Remak's achievements and at the same time of the academic coolness between him and this pupil of his, is evident in a letter Müller wrote in the summer of 1849 to the Prussian Minister, who asked for Müller's advice on the question of calling some outstanding physiologist of the younger generation to the chair of physiology at the University of Koenigsberg in Prussia (26). The list of candidates that Müller had previously suggested is typical of his cautious and often timid character and indicative of his opinion on the members of his inner circle. Schwann and Henle were already professors at foreign universities. He therefore suggested (mainly his own pupils) in the following sequence: Brücke, DuBois, Helmholtz, and Ludwig. After a long paragraph, in which he evaluated the merits of each of them, he finally added: "On this occasion I must also mention with laudatory recognition the accomplishments of the Privatdozent Dr. Remak." Following a few more sentences on the trend of Remak's largely anatomical and embryological research, he said: "The trend of Dr. Remak in the field of physiology is exactly as much justified as the experimental one." In accordance with these suggestions, which put the candidates apparently in alphabetical order, Brücke became Professor at Koenigsberg. However, there is no question that among the five candidates named by Müller, with the exception of Helmholtz, who later succeeded Brücke at Koenigsberg, none proved as outstanding as Remak and Ludwig.

How little Remak in his career was supported by anyone from Müller's laboratory except Müller himself can be judged from the correspondence between DuBois-Reymond and Carl Ludwig published under the title *Zwei Grosse Naturforscher* by Estelle DuBois-Reymond and Paul Diepgen in 1927 (J. A. Barth, Leipzig). There, on page 49, in a letter of May 1849, DuBois-Reymond made very derogatory remarks about Remak who to his displeasure was nominated by Müller for the professorship as physiologist at the University of Königsberg. DuBois, who wanted to push the candidacy of Ludwig, was angry about Remak's nomination, mentioning that Müller "asserts that he [Remak] also is a physiologist." But he was not afraid of this competition because the faculty, adequately instructed by Brücke, would surely not nominate or tolerate Remak as professor. On page 73 of this book in a letter of October 4, 1849, Ludwig expressed a similar feeling concerning a successor of himself as professor in Marburg. He stated that it would be impossible to consider Peters, Remak, or Moleschott. These were the odds against which Remak even later in his career had to struggle: governmental bias, canonized by law, and personal antipathy of those who knew him as collaborators in Müller's laboratory, such as Henle, DuBois-Reymond, Brücke, and under their influence their personal friends like Carl Ludwig.

We have proof that Remak was not only a great scholar and research scientist but also a fascinating and inspiring teacher. Koelliker's (43) recollections of the time when Remak was his teacher were already mentioned. Concerning Remak's teaching activities in his years as Privatdozent and his influence on his outstanding pupils, we find another report in the autobiography of the famous Swiss anatomist, Wilhelm His, later anatomist at the University of Leipzig in Germany. It sounds as enthusiastic as the above mentioned recollection of Koelliker. In his *Lebenserinnerungen* which was only printed as manuscript and not sold by bookdealers we find on page 26 ff. the following:[53]

In the summer of 1851 I attended the classes of R. Remak on embryology which became important for my own later development. We were three or four students, the above mentioned Dr. Weja a physician from Greece, an Englishman, and, as far as I remember, a student from Breslau. Remak first lectured in the University but then he had us come to his apartment, Unter Den Linden, one of the main streets of Berlin, where he kept his incubators and microscopes, and sacrificed for us many eggs to give us satisfactory demonstrations. Innumerable crawfish had also to be sacrificed because Remak cleansed the embryos with the fresh blood of crawfish. By Remak too we gained insight in a developing field of science because the second issue of his great work on embryology did not yet appear. During the first lessons all seemed entirely strange and only by and by I began to understand Remak's idea of germinative layers and especially the role attributed to the middle germinative layer. Since then I was highly captivated by the new observations showing the connection between embryology and histology and the related problems.

Remak's later turning to electro-therapy and the reaction of others are also mentioned in the autobiography of Wilhelm His, in the following words (p. 26):

It is well known that Remak, after the conclusion of his great embryological investigations, turned to electro-therapy and in this field too, started new developments. His jumping into the practice after such intense theoretical activities appeared at that time startling. There were rumors that his relatives had reprimanded the financial inefficiency of his previous studies and were the reason of his transition to a more lucrative activity. I don't know how justified these rumors were. It is a matter of fact that Remak during his lifetime was greatly under-estimated. Even his fame as founder of modern embryology was recognized fully only after some time. He was a lively personality, easily carried away by his ideas in personal discussions. However, as author he is justly regarded as one of the most excellent observers. I myself owe to Remak inspirations which were of decisive influence for a great part of my own work throughout my life.

REVOLUTION AND CHOLERA IN BERLIN
1848–1849

During the time between 1847 and 1849, many events changed life in Germany and the private life of Remak too. The exciting days of March 18 and 19, 1848, the days of revolution and street fights in Berlin, found Remak involved also, if we are to believe the not too reliable reports of Motty (85). Motty, a Polish citizen, with two of his compatriots, Cybulski and Remak, both lecturers at the University, on the turbulent day of March 19 went for a private audience with the King to intervene in favor of some imprisoned Polish citizens.

That same year, according to Motty, Remak married the daughter of a wealthy German banker.[54] On May 26, 1849 Remak's eldest son, Ernst Julius Remak, was born, who later became Professor of Neurology at Berlin University and father of a well known mathematician, Robert Remak II. Tradition handed down by Remak's son to his daughters has it that Remak's father-in-law, the banker Eli Joachim Meyer, who died in 1849, gave his consent to the marriage only on the

[53] This very interesting and scarcely known autobiography was brought to my attention by my brother, Professor Guido Kisch in New York.

[54] According to personal information supplied by Remak's granddaughters, the name of his wife was Feodore Meyer (1828–1865).

condition that Remak in the future would refrain from any kind of political activity and concentrate on his research exclusively. This led to the legend, reported by Motty (1888) but rejected by the historian Wrzosek (85) and categorically denied by Remak's son, Ernst, that Remak's father-in-law made it a condition of his consent to his daughter's marriage to Remak that the latter give up all connection with his Polish compatriots and his active sympathy with the Polish cause.[54a]

That the banker Meyer's opposition to his future son-in-law's political activities was justified is proved by the fact that three brothers of Robert Remak who were involved in student political affairs in 1848 had to emigrate to America as political refugees in the same year.

The excitement of the events of 1848 and the following period of governmental reactionary measurements involved every single person in Germany, especially in the capital of Berlin, where the revolutionary events resulted in the killing of many fighters on the barricades, and in the King and Queen being compelled to pay their respects to the procession in which were carried the bodies of these fighters for freedom.

This dangerous year found Johannes Müller elected, much to his disconcertion, to the responsible and difficult position of Rector of the University.

Many of the younger physicians and young members of the faculty were subversive elements more or less deeply involved in revolutionary activities. Virchow exposed himself to a great extent and even started a special journal called *Medical Reform* to propagate in a very definite way his ideas for organizing many activities in practical medicine and for reorganizing medical education. A General Assembly of the Physicians of Berlin came into being, and Virchow and his prospective father-in-law, Mayer, were the leading personalities among those physicians, who were eager to do away with all bureaucratic shortcomings in medicine. Of the staff of the Medical Faculty, Remak was, next to Virchow, the most active member of this revolutionary group. Johannes Müller was more reluctant and cautious, and therefore in the second issue of his journal, Virchow published the following announcement under the heading "Bureaucratisches," which can best be translated by the expression "red tape." There he wrote on page 8 that the General Assembly, in which the most outstanding physicians of Berlin were united to consider medical reform, asked for an auditorium for its meetings; but its request was refused by Johannes Müller, the Rector of the University. From this remark and its tone it could be seen that Virchow was not on the best of terms with Müller at that time. From this journal, which appeared only from July 10, 1848 to June 29, 1849, we get information concerning events that occurred in the medical circles of Berlin in this year of revolution. With Virchow's departure from Berlin for Würzburg in 1849, the journal ceased to appear.

Several committees were set up within the General Assembly of Physicians to discuss various problems. Remak was a member of the committee on medical instruction and teaching. In July, 1848, Remak together with Waldeck, suggested to the Assembly that existing special schools for military physicians be terminated. This was an open attack against the Pepinière, the military alma mater of Virchow, Helmholtz, and other outstanding scholars. When, August 4, a committee of fifteen was selected by ballot to draft an outline of a law on medical institutions and all matters pertaining to medicine in Prussia, Virchow as well as Remak was among those chosen.

At the height of the political fight, and at Johannes Müller's suggestion, a proclamation of loyalty was drafted and sent to the King, signed by eighty professors but only one Privatdozent of Berlin University. As a sort of counter move a letter of approval was sent to the Constitutional Assembly, which was a progressive body in those days and extremely unpopular with the ruling circles around the King. There were only eighteen instructors at the University who wanted and dared to sign this proclamation, and of those on the Medical Faculty it was signed only by Remak, Virchow, and Leubuscher. Another document of 1848, the minutes of a meeting of professors and lecturers of the Berlin Faculty calling for freedom of assembly was signed by Remak. This document was preserved by the family and given by Remak's son, Professor Ernst Remak, to Professor Waldeyer, anatomist of Berlin University, for his autograph collection.[55]

The outline for medical reform in Prussia was finally completed on March 15, 1849. Remak's point of view with respect to a planned physicians' organization, discussed in the 1848 assembly, is interesting as the expression of his political ideal. He, like other physicians, was very much in favor of such an organization, but he was very strongly opposed to the idea of making such an organization compulsory. Again we have to admire Remak's brilliant mind, in remembering, as we do, how detrimental similar compulsory organizations were three generations later in Nazi Germany. Remak regarded any compulsory organization of physicians as the worst despotism imaginable. In Virchow's journal, *Medicinische Reform,* his statement on this question is reported in the minutes of the General Assembly of Physicians of Berlin (pp. 236–239), but it seemed important enough for Remak himself to write a short statement on this political question and to publish it as his only contribution to Virchow's journal. As he stated (p. 239), he was willing to subordinate himself

[54a] Elias Joachim Meyer (1784–1849) was the founder of the banking establishment of E. J. Meyer in Berlin. His portrait was on exhibit in 1936 in the Jewish Museum in Berlin. It was at that time in the possession of the widow of his grandson, Geheimrath Ernst Meyer (*Jüd. Familienforschung* **12**: Sonderheft 43, 1936).

[55] Information received from Ernst Remak's granddaughter.

to the representatives of the people, but not to a majority of physicians. This is really an expression of the strong democratic idea behind the sincere fighters of 1848. Remak's activities in the years 1848 and 1849, probably recorded in the files of the Berlin secret police, coupled with the political records of his brothers, may have contributed to the fact that later the Faculty had to submit his name six times for a professorship to the Prussian Minister before he finally reached this academic goal.

Apart from all the political activities of 1848 and 1849, every physician in Berlin had enough excitement and more than enough work owing to the cholera epidemic of 1849. More than 2,400 cases of cholera occurred in Berlin up to the end of November of that year and nearly 1,600 of these patients died. Though certainly kept well occupied, Remak developed steadily during this year his lecture program at the University, In 1849 he announced lectures for the summer term in histology, embryology of vertebrates, and microscopical semiotic.

STUDIES IN EMBRYOLOGY

Remak's scientific life shows three great periods, each of which is terminated by an important event in his personal life. The first chapter of his medical career was the time he devoted to learning and research in science for science's sake, and it extended from his entry into the University, when he was eighteen years of age, to the year 1843 when he realized that he would never be able to follow successfully an academic career in Germany. The early years of this period of his life were devoted to studies under the guidance of Ehrenberg and Müller; later he carried on independently successful investigations, mainly of the nervous system. This period ended with Remak's defeat in 1843 when he tried to become a lecturer and with his entering Schönlein's Clinic as a research assistant.

With that began the second period, characterized by the influence of the great clinician, Schönlein, on Remak's method of working. One of the fruits of Remak's clinical work was his book of 1845. During this period, however, which lasted until 1856, there were still two theoretical problems to which his main endeavor was devoted. Between 1841 and 1856, his ideas on cell production, opposed to Schwann's original theory, came to a final conclusion, and strong proof in support of his point of view was offered in his embryological studies. With the papers he published in 1852 in *Müller's Archiv,* in 1854 in *Deutsche Klinik,* and in 1850–1855 in his book on embryology, he laid the cornerstone of the modern cell theory in the face of the opposition of the most outstanding anatomists and physiologists of his time. By his statement that each cell of living animals and of man is exclusively produced by division of another cell, he finished what Schwann had begun. Schwann started the basic modern concept of all biology with his assertion that all animals are built up from nucleated cells; Remak completed it with the proposition that each cell is a product of another cell and that there is no such thing as spontaneous generation of cells. These two statements, the one by Schwann and the other by Remak, together constitute the modern cell theory, and it would be only historical justice to call this theory in the future, not Schwann's, but Schwann-Remak's cell theory.

The other great problem, which continuously occupied the mind and every spare moment of the practitioner Remak in those years, was the embryology of vertebrates. These studies also began in 1841 when he published his investigations on erythropoiesis (development of red blood cells). In 1843 when his interest concentrated on the development of the digestive tract of the chicken and on the development of the glands, he investigated at the same time the origin of spinal and sympathetic nerves. In spite of his personal disappointments and the excitement of his efforts to become a lecturer at that time, and in spite of the host of new impressions he obtained in his clinical work, he did not give up his embryological research, for he became increasingly aware that even the best investigators up to this time, like von Baer and Reichert, were partly mistaken, and that none of them saw the point that soon became the leading idea for Remak in his research. Remak's main problem was to find exactly the consecutive development of each single germinal layer, beginning with the earliest stage in embryonic life.

These studies started in 1842. In 1845 we find him already busy with studies of comparative embryology. He investigated in batrachians the development of peripheral nerves. However, the intensity of these studies and the necessity for earning a living were too much of a burden for him. Though the announcement in all journals that Remak was the first Jewish lecturer on the Berlin Medical Faculty may have increased his practice considerably, he gave up, not his research, but his position in Schönlein's Clinic, and concentrated more and more on embryological studies. In 1848 he published a part of his investigations in *Müller's Archiv,* where he states that he found the solution of the problem after seven years of intense research. Finally, in 1850 the first installment of his fundamental and classical work on the development of vertebrates came out, a book in folio with twelve plates. The second installment appeared in 1851, but it took four years more before the entire book was completed. Even then this master of research was reluctant to publish it, and he did so only to be rid of all the time consuming study of this kind. Because of the lack of adequate working facilities, which a theoretician needs to carry on his studies successfully, Remak was not able to devote his life to this field as he would like to have done. He therefore closed this chapter of his life of research on December 24, 1854, on which day he signed the preface to the book. It appeared in Berlin in 1855 in a folio edition with an instructive introductory section of thirty-eight pages and a classical summary, in which the cell theory is again critically and historically presented.

In 1847 when Remak fought for his right to a lectureship with the admirable support of Alexander von Humboldt, he dedicated his book on *The Nervous System of the Intestines* to his protector, von Humboldt, and to his teacher, Johannes Müller. Now, in closing the second period of his scientific life with a book on embryology, he dedicated it solely "To Herrn Alexander von Humboldt in deepest admiration and gratitude."

This book will be a landmark in the history of medicine for all times. Here is set before the scientific world in clear summary, Remak's up-to-date, valid discovery of the three germinal layers, and his proof of which organs stem from each of these layers.

With his embryological studies Remak influenced following generations profoundly. Even the most critical of his contemporaries agree on this point. A. Koelliker writes in 1861 in his *Textbook of Embryology* (p. 18), as follows: "Remak's publication can be called almost perfect in every respect; the work of this author of 1850, 1851, 1855, appears as the most excellent and perfect in the recent period of embryology since Schwann." As late as 1884, Koelliker, who was never easily satisfied with the quality of any research work, writes in his *Grundriss der Entwicklungs-theorie,* on page 5, in a historical survey:

> Remak's germinal layer theory was received with great enthusiasm, and rightly so. This theory shed for the first time a brighter light on the structure and fate of the germinal layers and on the histological connections between them and the organs of the developed organism.

J. Victor Carus speaks in his *History of Zoology* (1872) of this "classical work of Remak's," and Oscar Hertwig, in his *Handbook on Comparative Embryology,*[56] says:

> It is one of Remak's main contributions that in his fundamental work *Untersuchungen über die Entwicklung der Wirbeltiere,* he fairly correctly determined the histological products of the germinal layers. . . . In his statement Remak, who for a time was followed by most embryologists, comes nearer to the truth than C. E. v. Baer.

I found only one author who strongly objected to Remak's embryological research; this was one Professor Emil Dürsy of Tübingen. Of course, he was a pupil of Remak's old enemy, Henle, and he dedicated his book on the *Embryology of the Head* to his teacher Henle (1869).

Remak's fundamental work was dedicated to A. von Humboldt who, in spite of his eighty-six years, clearly evaluated its importance. On June 17, 1855 he wrote (21: 131) referring to Remak's dedication (p. 239) in which he expresses gratitude for Humboldt's help against bias and prejudice:

> I cannot express to you, my dear Remak, in an appropriate way my heartfelt and intense thankfulness for the honor you have bestowed on my name by this dedication of a work that will be epoch-making in the history of anatomy and physiology. You would not have been able to touch, in a more tender and for me more agreeable way, a side of my character which I do not regard as a merit of mine, but which may indicate my free and unchangeable recognition of sacrosanct privileges of mankind. I became connected with you in friendship, when you had completed only a small part of the beautiful work that has since found such general recognition. The work that you have brought so thoroughly to completion has not only the great merit of the discoveries which it reveals and the wonderful pictures, but also that of emphatic delivery and excellent clearness of style. As much as I am overburdened at this time with others' and my own work, I was fascinated by some special interests and you will guess the object, even without my mentioning it. I read on pages 128 and 172 about the fine anatomy, the rhythm of research, and the analogy of the membrane of the egg with the cuticula and the various layers of primordial cells of plants. I feel the desire to thank you personally also. Could you give me the pleasure of your visit on Sunday?
>
> In old, enduring friendship and attachment,
> Yours,
> A. von Humboldt.
>
> Berlin 17th of January 1855.

ANOTHER COMPETITION, REMAK vs. VIRCHOW

The 1855 book was also the last word in the second chapter of Remak's scientific life. The first chapter had ended with the struggle and defeat of 1846, and Virchow's triumph in becoming prosector at the Charité, for which post Remak was suggested and would probably have been the better fitted.

The second chapter of Remak's life also closed with a struggle for a position, and again with Remak's defeat and Virchow's success. During the revolutionary days of 1848 Virchow was deeply involved in political affairs. With the psychiatrist Leubuscher, he founded and edited the revolutionary journal *Die Medicinische Reform.* He was a political revolutionary, too, as well as a revolutionary in the field of science. In 1848, when the struggle and the street fights were over, he was deprived, as politically suspect, of many privileges at the Charité, and it required the influence of all his friends and protectors to prevent his dismissal from his position as prosector. In the meantime, Virchow proved through his work that he was worthy of the important position entrusted to him. But the scene of his labors became more and more unpleasant for him who had acquired the reputation of a subversive element. Consequently, he was looking around for another arena for his scientific activities. Zürich, the young university in Switzerland, became interested in this brilliant scientist, whose fame had already reached far beyond Prussia and Germany, and considered him for a professorship (7). At the same time, however,

[56] 1: 700, 1906.

he received a call to the University of Würzburg in Bavaria, which he gladly accepted, and there he engaged in outstanding work in teaching as well as in building up modern pathology.

Virchow soon played an important part in the Medical Faculty of Würzburg, but his eyes were continually directed back to Berlin and a still wider field of activity. Finally, in 1855, when Remak's fundamental work on embryology was published, there began a new competition between the two old rivals. Berlin's medical faculty needed a pathologist, and Johannes Müller, tired and overworked, planned to give up this part of his widespread realm. It became desirable and even necessary to choose a young man who could devote all his strength to pathological anatomy and experimental pathology.

Schönlein still supported Remak's claims, and this time there was no longer any legal pretext to exclude him as a Jew from the competition. Not only that, but if there was any justice, nobody would have denied that Remak was entitled to the prospective new position. The 1847 decision of Friedrich Wilhelm IV that Remak should be given the first available chair in a Prussian university was still in effect, and we remember how Eichhorn, by this time already swept off the political scene into well deserved oblivion, in 1847 deprived Remak of his right by pretending that there was no opening for which Remak was suited. Now there was such an opening and Remak, after eight years, was still an old Privatdozent. His fundamental work on embryology was just off the press, but Virchow had, in addition to his unquestionable merits, the support and the push and pull of all his friends. These friends and connections were influential, and in the meantime one was added in the person of his father-in-law, the privy counsellor Carl Mayer, an outstanding physician in Berlin, and one of the Fathers of modern gynecology and founder, in 1844, of the Berlin Gynecological Society. He had the best connections in all the influential quarters of Berlin, and so from the very outset Virchow's chances were very promising.

How eager Virchow was to return to Berlin may be judged from the fact that repeated calls to a chair at the University of Zürich had reached him in 1855 and were declined by him (7). Now early in the year 1856 the decision in this important question was near. Virchow's attitude on questions pertaining to his own career cannot be more clearly revealed than by a letter he wrote on February 15, 1856 to his father-in-law (60). It is a long letter mainly concerned with his aspirations for the Berlin position. At that time Virchow had already been contacted by certain Berlin circles as to whether he would be disposed to accept a call if he should receive it. In his letter to his father-in-law he writes that he would regard it as frivolous not to take all necessary steps to secure such a position and to take advantage of an opportunity that might not present itself again. He does not wish to take any direct steps himself, but he solicits the assistance of his father-in-law and all available friends and gives a clear outline of who should be mobilized to influence the various Ministers. Shrewdly he would like the decision to be postponed as long as possible, perhaps for an entire term, in order not to lose any possible chances. At that time the faculty, probably under the influence of Müller, had already decided for Virchow, but there still remained the decision of the Senate of the University; the Rector of the University had to have his say; and the Ministers had to be influenced in order to find Virchow, the old revolutionary, or as Schönlein called him, the "Peoples' Tribune of 1848," palatable. His uncle Emile had to be moved to action, and through him the influential military surgeon Grimm, to whom Virchow himself had just sent, as he calls it, "a very friendly letter." Everyone else who could be of assistance was mentioned in the letter, and it even contains a paragraph concerning Remak (60: 208), which reveals as much about the tragic fate of the latter as about Virchow's real character. He writes there: "Schönlein will not be too eager for Remak. I know that from olden times. He already put Remak up against me once and dropped him finally. If you should see him, you could speak with him very frankly." Virchow here hints that in 1846 as we already know, Schönlein did not mean it too seriously when he nominated his assistant for the post of Prosector of the Charité. Johannes Müller would not be dangerous, either. He had already decided in favor of Virchow.

The only faithful man who fought for Robert Remak in 1847 was Alexander von Humboldt. He was now eighty-seven years of age, but still upright and strong, highly influential in the scientific world and in the circles around the King, who at that time was already a sick man and represented by his brother, later King Wilhelm I, as regent. The sly Virchow knew this. He knew and confirmed in this letter that Humboldt really remained true to Remak, and we know that in admiration and devotion Remak had just dedicated to Humboldt his fundamental work on embryology. Virchow writes to his father-in-law as follows: "Concerning Humboldt, I think perhaps it may be possible to change his mind. I myself do not know him, but maybe Uncle Emile could speak with him." And now comes a passage concerning Humboldt, which shows how Virchow, the barricade fighter for freedom and justice for all in 1848, had a very different mind concerning justice as soon as the matter touched his own ambition. He wrote to his father-in-law concerning Humboldt: "Perhaps you know a member of the Mendelssohn family. Because it is his way to stick to the Jews, it ought to be possible to get at him with the help of Jews." [57] With this mean suggestion Virchow employed against his

[57] Da er nun doch einmal zu den Juden hält, so müsste man ihm mit Juden beikommen!

own better judgment, the same argument that later was used so often by the Nazis. It earmarked anyone who in all justice acknowledged the meritorious activities of a certain Jew, as a philosemite, as someone "who sticks to the Jews."

There is no question that Virchow not only knew, but evaluated well the enormous achievements of Remak, whose fame he had specifically acknowledged in a letter to his father nine years before. The anatomist Waldeyer, who in the same year, 1856, began his studies at the University, wrote in his autobiography that among those members of the Berlin medical faculty who were not full professors in 1856 were some "men of world fame like Albrecht v. Graefe, Robert Remak" (83). That was Remak's reputation at the time. Virchow knew Remak very well personally. When the latter discovered the syncitial structure of the heart muscle in March, 1850, he mentioned in a footnote of his article[58] that "Virchow from Würzburg" had told him that "recently" this structure of the heart muscle had also been observed at Würzburg. This footnote, further, evidence of Remak's honesty in literary matters probably refers to Koelliker's independent discovery of the same fact, published in 1852 in Koelliker's *Handbuch der Gewebelehre.*

Virchow was aware that the scientist Humboldt liked Remak, not because he was a Jew, but because of his own evaluation of Remak's contribution to modern science and medicine. But in this special case Virchow chose to interpret the attitude of this outstanding man as the not readily comprehensible philosemitism of an old fogey. Still more despicable is the way in which he tried to influence Remak's only strong supporter. Humboldt was on very friendly terms with the Mendelssohn family, one of the most outstanding Jewish families in Germany at that time (10, 33). A close friendship existed between him and Joseph, the son of the philosopher Moses Mendelssohn, and he was obligated to the family for various favors (33: **1**: 40, 198, 353). Now Virchow suggested that some member of this family should be talked into influencing Humboldt so that he would be led to think that if influential Jewish people wanted him to vote against Remak, that could not be out of any racial or religious prejudice.

A story[59] may illuminate Humboldt's relationship with the Mendelssohn family. He once came in despair to Joseph Mendelssohn. On a notice from his landlord he had to move to another apartment and was at his wits' end to know how to move his collections and library. Joseph did not say a word, but the next morning Humboldt received a letter asking him to cease worrying; he need never leave his apartment, because Joseph was now his new landlord, having bought the house over night (33).

[58] *Müller's Archiv,* 1850: 76.

[59] This story is also related by Humboldt's personal friend C. G. Carus in the latter's autobiography (10: **4**: 153).

Virchow's plan, therefore, was a clever one. The Mendelssohns would have been the best lever to move Humboldt in his favor. Long forgotten by the string-pulling Professor Virchow was his own fervid article against favoritism and nepotism in the academic world, which he had published in 1848 in his journal *Medical Reform* (p. 86). Now things were different; he was striving for his own career.

This remarkable attitude on the part of the erstwhile "People's Tribune of 1848," later a representative of democracy in the Parliament, is consonant with the fact that Virchow, in all the years that he was director of the Institute for Pathology in Berlin, never admitted a Jew as a full assistant who did not first accept baptism. I know from information supplied by my friend, Professor Carl Neuberg, that in 1898 he himself became the first unbaptized Jewish assistant in Virchow's Institute in Berlin, and that was, perhaps, because he did not work directly under Virchow, but as a chemist was assistant to Professor Salkowski, the head of the Chemical Department in this laboratory. That was the attitude of one of the once most revered of German fighters for freedom and justice. Further light on Virchow's personality is shed by the next paragraph in the letter to his father-in-law. It reads:

> My newest editorial from the *Archiv* may perhaps be useful, and because Reimer [his publisher] had the kindness to make me some reprints, I sent you a part of them. Some of them are addressed and please distribute them among the people. Four I am giving you for your disposal. Maybe you can apply one of them to Humboldt.

Here again follows another list of names of people who, in Virchow's opinion, should be influenced in his favor. The editorial he mentions is probably the one on cellular pathology, which was published in 1855, the one containing the famous expression "omnis cellula e cellula." There he states his program to base all further investigation on Remak's principle that each cell stems from another cell. Or he may have been speaking of the editorial in the first issue of 1856, which again refers to that of 1855. We can understand why he was so careful in this impressive article to omit every mention of Remak's name, in spite of the fact that he knew full well that this fundamental program was Remak's and not his.

Once more Virchow returned to the history of the "omnis cellula e cellula" principle. It was in a short paper on the division of nuclei, which he published when he was already pathologist at Berlin University.[60] Here among several lame claims for priority on minor points, he admits in a somewhat sour tone what he admitted freely in his handbook years before, that to Remak "has to go credit for having first expressed those statements in a dogmatic way." Virchow could do no harm to himself now by such a confession.

These were the ways and means used by Rudolph

[60] *Virchow's Archiv* **11**: 89, 1857.

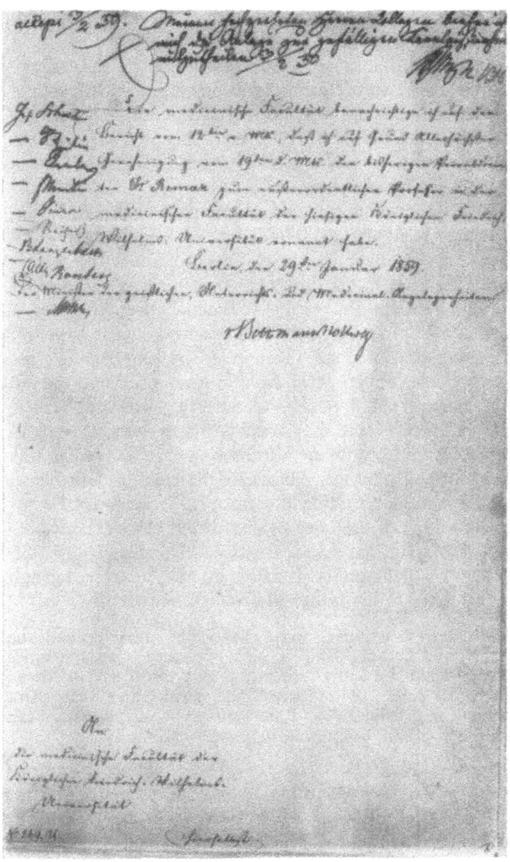

FIG. 53. Announcement of the Minister of Education, v. Bethmann-Hollweg, to the Medical Faculty of Berlin of the appointment of Privatdozent Remak as extraordinary professor. Size 10¾" × 6½". Courtesy of Berlin University.

Virchow in 1855 and 1856, and he succeeded, and he became full professor at Berlin University, and with that Remak's last opportunity to devote his life to science exclusively was gone.

From then on Remak gradually lost his best friends in the faculty. Johannes Müller, overworking and straining himself for many years, was in 1858 in a state of nervous breakdown as he had been at the start of his career. His son was summoned hurriedly from Cologne, where he was a physician, and he, his mother, and the family finally persuaded Müller to decide to give up most of his academic activities and to relax and thus regain health and strength. The next morning he was found dead in his bed (11). Nobody knows to this day the real cause of this sudden death. His assistant, Du Bois-Reymond, followed him as physiologist, and Reichert, the old opponent of Remak's ideas and discoveries, obtained the position as Müller's successor in anatomy. The face of the faculty changed quickly. One of Remak's great protectors, Schönlein, decided in the very year of Müller's death to retire (88), and the following year, 1859, resigned from his post.

Six times the faculty vainly recommended Remak for a professorship (14). Only in 1859, probably as a last favor to the departing Schönlein and to the indefatigable, marvelous eighty-nine-year-old Humboldt, was Remak made an extraordinary professor. But he never became a real full professor at Berlin University. That was the last period in the history of his competition with Virchow and his ambitions for an academic career, and the real official end of the second chapter in his life.

CREATION OF MODERN GALVANOTHERAPY

Who will be astonished now to find Remak, after all these experiences, worn out by the long illness of his son and broken by the sudden death of his wife who passed away in 1863 of pernicious anemia, taking a hostile attitude toward life and other less brilliant but more successful scientists? The third and last and very unfortunate period in Remak's life began in the middle of the nineteenth century. In his publications this last period was characterized by continuous and masterly research work again, through which he became the originator and leading figure in the clinical field of galvanotherapy. At the same time, however, his writing displayed an attitude of "I don't care." He said what he thought was right, regardless of whether his opinion hurt anyone or of whose mistakes were disclosed. He no longer spoke in the diffident manner expected in Germany by every full professor when somebody lower in academic rank addressed him or wrote about him.

More and more Remak now became a stranger among his colleagues, a friend only to a few selected persons. More and more he tried to find recognition for his clinical research abroad; at home recognition was denied to him by almost everyone. More and more frequently his publications appeared in Paris in the Proceedings of the Royal Academy. There and in the Proceedings of the Paris Biological Society we find, before the years of the Franco-Prussian War, the most outstanding German scholars represented by their articles, for instance, Valentin, Budge, Kühne, Helmholtz, Koelliker, H. Müller, R. Virchow, and A. von Humboldt. During those years Remak's papers were published in English journals and in Austrian ones, too.

Remak all his life liked to travel and to meet scientific confreres all over Europe, to learn from them, to demonstrate to them his own discoveries, and to exchange scientific opinions. As a young man, already in 1841, he participated in the Convention of German Natural Scientists and Physicians in Braunschweig, staying for some days in Dresden, where he and Purkinje were guests of C. G. Carus (10: **3**: 132). Later

Remak attended meetings in Gotha (1851), Wiesbaden (1852), Königsberg (1860), Giessen (1864), and other places. He mentioned in his early publications discussions of his findings with Purkinje in Breslau (1840) and with Weber in Leipzig and their opinions and criticisms. In 1853 and 1854 he studied the nervous system of fish in Trieste and in Hamburg. Later, when his means permitted it, he visited the famous medical centers of Europe, among them Vienna with its outstanding scientists. There he met Benedikt (4) and Carl Ludwig. Time and again he went to Paris to make contact with the scientific circles there and to bring to the attention of his French colleagues his investigations on the embryology of vertebrates and particularly the problem to which he devoted himself scientifically in the last part of his life, the method of galvanotherapy.

No less than nineteen times in the years between 1852 and 1864 we find reports on his work and claims for priority in the Proceedings of the French Academy of Sciences, beginning with Volume 35. The last of these publications was printed in Volume 61 in 1864, the year prior to his sudden death. He personally read numerous papers in the Paris Academy, or they were read by members of the Academy in his name, and repeatedly he entered such papers in competitions for Academy awards.

There is no question that in French circles Remak aroused much more interest and even more support for his endeavors in the field of galvanotherapy than he received in Berlin. The Academy of Sciences in Paris directed a Committee to study Remak's new gospel of the therapeutic efficacy of the galvanic current. French colleagues, including the famous Broca, offered him the opportunity to treat patients in their hospitals. He demonstrated his therapeutic procedures before a Commission consisting of the academicians Andral, Rayer, and Velpeau in the year 1856. He reported on these experiments personally at the Academy's meeting on September 29. Not having with him the necessary apparatus for producing a galvanic current, he was supported by Mr. Hulot, the director of the galvanoplastic work of the mint in Paris, who put at his disposal an excellent galvanic pile.

There is no evidence in the records that he ever won a prize in one of the competitions in which he participated, for instance in 1847, when he entered his studies on the nervous system of the intestines for the Academy's prize in medicine and surgery, or in 1848, when he competed for the *Prix de Physiologie Experimental* with his work on the sympathetic nervous system, or finally when, in 1862, he presented before the Academy a portable galvanic pile, competing for the award of the year 1865 given for the application of electricity to therapeutic purposes. Still, in 1864, when he personally demonstrated his portable galvanic apparatus at the Academy, Velpeau gave him permission to present demonstrations and deliver lectures during the following two weeks, that is, in December, 1864, in the Paris Hospital de la Charité. The Academy again nominated a Commission, consisting of the members Velpeau, Rayer, and Bernard, to observe these experiments and to report to the Academy. The statement made at the meeting of November 21, 1864, is the last mention of Remak's presence at a meeting of the Paris Academy of Sciences.

The story of Remak's change from anatomy and physiology to therapy was related in part in 1855 in his booklet of thirty-six pages on *Methodical Electrification of the Paralyzed Muscles* (72) and in part by Duchenne de Boulogne (2).

He apparently used the summer vacations for travel, for relaxation and for studying as well. In 1852 Remak was in Paris to present at the Convention of the Biological Society in Paris two papers on his discovery of ganglions in various organs. On this occasion in September 1852, together with the Professor of Internal Medicine, Jaksch from Prague, the neurologist Romberg from Berlin, and Hebra, the famous dermatologist from Vienna (73), he attended one of Duchenne's lectures in Paris. It must have impressed him very much, for on his return to Berlin he reported at a meeting of the Society for Scientific Medicine on Duchenne's electrotherapeutic method and recommended the use of such a method, not only in cases of paralysis, but also for orthopedic purposes as a gymnastic means.

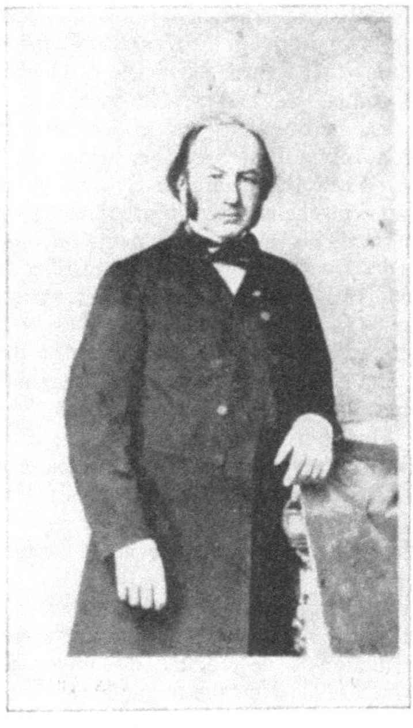

FIG. 54. Claude Bernard, one of Remak's few friends. Courtesy of the Rare Book Department, Library of the Academy of Medicine, New York.

With youthful eagerness and enthusiasm he put himself immediately to work to study the therapeutic effects of electric currents.

Like Duchenne, Remak first used faradization for treatment, and in 1855 published a small booklet of thirty-one pages on the subject of methodical electrification of paralyzed muscles (72). His method was a very systematic one. He studied each detail; he demonstrated it to his pupils in lectures on experimental pathology, which he gave during the summer term (72). It was a new field of therapeutics that Duchenne opened to the medical world in France and still very liable to discussion and criticism. Critical as Remak was, he did not hesitate in his booklet to put his finger also on some weak points in the experiments and theories of Duchenne. During the next summer's vacation he made a trip to Paris and there, at the Biological Society, presented at the meeting of August 25, a lecture and his newly published booklet. Duchenne appeared personally at this presentation, and the next day they discussed for two hours their divergent opinions in Duchenne's clinic without being able to come to a final agreement. Remak also argued his point of view with various friends in Paris, especially with Claude Bernard, to whom the booklet was dedicated.

Remak, of course, made no friends with his criticism. Duchenne was deeply insulted, and in 1856 published a very strong reply with many personal attacks against Remak in *Schmidt's Yearbook* (12). A rejoinder from Remak, which the editor of *Schmidt's Yearbook* refused to print, appeared in the *Deutsche Klinik*.[61] There is no question that Remak's criticism of Duchenne was, on some points, too hasty. He speaks of fatalities, but the case in question was in fact not a fatality, but only a cerebral hemorrhage, which occurred in a patient. Such things are surely unforgivable mistakes when someone criticizes a prominent person. On the other hand, his adverse comments on the methods described by Duchenne were partly justified, and it is at least doubtful whether Duchenne in his first publications was as clear about the differences between the therapeutic effect of direct stimulation of the muscle and that of the associated nerve, as he seems to be in his criticism of Remak, after having read the latter's booklet. However this may have been, it would be very difficult to say which of them was more right and which more wrong without a detailed study of the entire literature. In any case it is extremely regrettable that two such outstanding scientists should have become enemies.

The subject of electrotherapy however, attracted Remak's attention very intensely, and the great advance and contribution to be credited to him consist of his clear distinction between the therapeutic use of galvanization and faradization. A second edition of his little booklet was soon necessary, but he was eager to get more material for his investigations, especially when he was increasingly attacked because of his electrotherapeutic practice. His colleagues sent him cases only occasionally. Professor Romberg did, for instance, but this was only a drop in the bucket. So Remak, unfortunately, did something else that created a lot of trouble and enemies for him. He solicited patients for his investigations in one of Berlin's daily papers. In this way in six weeks time he gathered four hundred supposedly incurable patients with paralyzed muscles. We cannot judge such an act by the ethical standard of physicians of today, nor by the standard of medical ethics regarded as valid today in the United States. In Europe to this day, nobody finds it unethical, and very justly so, for a gynecologist or an ophthalmologist to state his specialty on his sign. No European physician will ever understand why it is unethical for an ophthalmologist, by his sign, to prevent gynecological patients from seeking his advice. A hundred years ago it was not regarded as unethical, and it is not so regarded in Europe today, for a physician to announce in the newspapers the opening of his practice and his specialty or his going on leave or returning. In England a century ago, ethical physicians even distributed tokens with their name and address to patients or prospective patients. So it was no crime to do what Remak did, especially in a country like Germany where in the middle of the last century, some of its universities were still notorious for selling medical doctorate diplomas to ignorant candidates from Germany and from abroad.

Of course, it did not make Remak any more popular among his colleagues that he now was not only the famous scientist without his own laboratory, but also the great practitioner, who unquestionably made more money in his practice than many of his colleagues. On August 19, 1856 he reported on the results of his treatments in the Berlin daily newspaper, the *Spenersche Zeitung,* and so little was such a step regarded as unethical that he himself quotes from this report in an article in the *Deutsche Klinik,* where he describes the effect of galvanization in contractions, paralysis, and muscle atrophy. The flood of his patients increased to such an extent that in this article of 1856 he announced that as a result of his advertisement, he was so overworked that he had to go on a vacation for some time. We may not judge such an unusual procedure too strictly today, if we consider that things like that happen in every country practically every day, though in most cases in different form. Some physician attracts the interest of a newspaper or journal, which then feeds its readers with stories about new, more or less unproved treatments of chronic or incurable diseases, with the same patient attracting results for the physicians involved. Worse than that, however, Remak, enthusiastic about his results, became somewhat careless in his scientific publications and gave his enemies wide

[61] 8: 125, 1856.

opportunities for more or less justified criticism. Among his critics was one of the rudest, Professor Ziemssen, who himself felt insulted by Remak's writing.

GALVANOTHERAPY AND ITS PREDECESSORS

Remak is justly regarded today as the founder of modern clinical galvanotherapy and really deserves all the credit for this contribution to neurotherapy. In his comprehensive book, which was published in 1858, he tried to give the details of the historical development of galvanotherapy. It should be remembered that attempts to use galvanic current for therapeutic purposes had never stopped since Luigi Galvani first published his experiments in 1791, and since Volta publicized his famous pile with all its surprising effects in 1800. These effects soon proved to be not only physical in nature, but also chemical, and excited the eagerness of physicians and laymen to try this new discovery on the human body in health and in disease. Its chemical efficacy was especially impressive, since Sir Humphry Davy was able to use the power of this pile in a magnificent way for the development of chemistry.

In his endeavor to use galvanic electricity for treatment purposes, Remak had few predecessors among physicians, and their efforts had long been forgotten by his time, but some fakes and quacks were still well remembered. The memory of them entirely spoiled the taste for this type of treatment among physicians, and Remak unquestionably suffered from these recollections of things as they were in previous times.

The history of the medical application of electricity was written in 1803 by Augustin (1) and in 1858 by Remak (73). Among serious physicians predecessors of Remak were Alexander von Humboldt (35), and especially Philipp Franz von Walther (84), who in 1803 published a booklet in Vienna on therapeutic indications and the technique of galvanic treatment. Von Walther refers to a Dr. Bremser, who previously had tried to influence a few deaf mutes by galvanic current. Grapengiesser (1801) and Max Jacobi (1802) were other pioneers in this field (73). Walther was an outstanding surgeon and ophthalmologist, professor at the University of Landshut and later at Bonn, where he faithfully and successfully attended Johannes Müller in 1827 when the latter had a nervous breakdown. In Munich, Walther became Professor and Court Physician to King Ludwig I. One of the founders of modern surgery, he also tried to treat diseases of the eye and ear with galvanic current, but in spite of the fact that he was very enthusiastic about his results, he did not find many followers, and his seriously meant efforts were soon forgotten.[61a]

Still in 1842 in an article written for Wagner's *Handwörterbuch* (1: p. 559 ff.) Valentin enumerated the conditions in which galvanization was suggested as a treatment in his times. The following may be mentioned from his essay:

1. To revive seemingly dead people (A. v. Humboldt, Bernoulli).
2. In paralytic diseases of the nerves (Valentin).
3. In aphonia (Grapengiesser, Magendie).
4. In muscle cramps, strabismus ptosis.
5. In volvulus, *intususceptio intestini,* and incarcerated hernia (Leroy).
6. In atonic constipation (La Beaume).
7. In insufficient contraction of the uterus.
8. In headaches, epilepsy, cardialgia, and hydrophobia.
9. In neuralgia of the face (Magendie, James).
10. In *tetanus traumaticus* (Matteucci).
11. In incipient amaurosis (Purkinje).
12. Against tapeworm (Busch).
13. In gout, chronic rheumatism, Asiatic cholera, amenorrhoea and dysmenorrhoea.
14. To dissolve calculi, to relieve patients with goutic tophi, to heal cataracts of the eye and turbidities of the cornea.

This abundance of supposed indications of galvanization-therapy raised the justified distrust of the profession, and soon this entire method of therapy was forgotten, especially since the more impressive faradization became known to layman and physicians.

It was different with the endeavors of quacks and business men. From early times gadgets composed of two metals were sold to gullible people, who were impressed by those inventions, having heard something about the enormous success of Galvani and Volta. They were anxious to have continuously on their body some instrument which was supposed to produce a galvanic current to treat rheumatism and other diseases. These gadgets were made in the form of necklaces or charms, or as crosses, stars, and half moons. At the end of the nineteenth and the beginning of the twentieth century, such crosses, under the name of Volta-cross,

---

[61a] In America in 1802 a book of 285 pages was printed (Troy, Moffit & Lyon), by one T. Gale, M.D., on the therapeutical use of electricity. The entire book does not make a very trustworthy impression. Its title sounds strange: *Electricity or Ethereal Fire* with a subtitle *Comprehending both the Theory and Practice of Medical Electricity.* This book on which recently Charles C. Dennie has reported (*N. Y. State Journal of Medicine* **54**: 400, 1954) is probably one of the worst in the entire literature on electrotherapy. It recommends itself on the title page as "the best family physician ever extant" and promises to be helpful, because electricity is an infallible cure of fever, inflammation and many other diseases. In checking the copy of this rare book in the library of the Academy of Medicine in New York, I found that the author indeed regards his "electric shock treatment" of highest value for rheumatism, fever, pleurisy, small pox, measles, madness, epilepsy, hysteria, palsy, dropsy, gout, dysentery, colic, asthma, diabetes, cancer, headache, deafness, cataract, hemorrhoids, and some other diseases. There is no question that such a book was not able to persuade the medical profession of the value of electric treatment as a panacea.

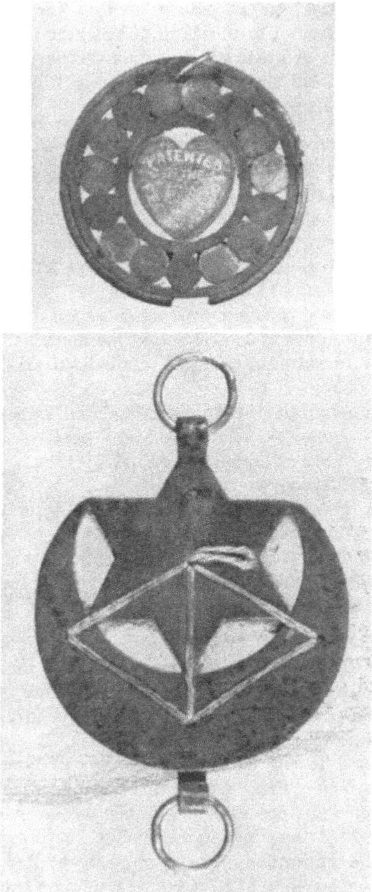

FIG. 55. Two electrogalvanic gadgets worn on the body against rheumatism. The upper American (Richardson's Magneto Galvanic Battery, patented February 3, 1880) consisting of parts of four different metals (iron, copper, tin, silver). The lower gadget, Austrian Pat. No. 50704. Copper and tin, between them felt. From the author's collection.

were sold in Austria for rheumatism, and their manufacturer was even granted a patent, No. 50704. The cross was for Christian patients, the star and half moon for Jewish patients and for those who for some reason did not wish to wear a cross on the body. In the United States a similar instrument for treating rheumatism and other diseases was patented on February 3, 1880 and sold under the name of Magneto Galvanic Battery by one Richardson; another such gadget was patented in Chicago, and was still sold in 1890.[62]

The most interesting and most lucrative business of this sort was also started in the United States, and its history was revealed in a lecture given in 1842 before the Boston Society for the Diffusion of Useful Knowledge by Oliver Wendell Holmes.

A physician by the name of Elisha Perkins, born in 1740 at Norwich, Connecticut, who had practiced his profession for many years and gained a good reputation, was inspired by Galvani's discovery to use a combination of two different metals for therapeutic purposes. He was very satisfied with the effect of his new treatment, and in 1796 he made his discovery public. His instrument consisted of two pieces of metal (iron and brass) about three inches long, which he called metallic tractors. This gadget was supposed to cure pains and inflammations, rheumatism, and tumors. The tractors were used, as Holmes reports, "by drawing them over the affected part very lightly for about 20 minutes." A patent was granted to Dr. Perkins for his discovery, and he then began to travel in order to make people acquainted with his instrument. That was the start of a kind of tractor mania, which was apparently very lucrative for Perkins and his family.

Two years later such tractors were employed in the Royal Hospital at Copenhagen in Denmark, and a son of Dr. Perkins, Benjamin Douglass Perkins, brought them to the attention of the public in London. Case reports were issued. In London in 1804 a Perkinian Institution was founded, which published its transactions in pamphlet form. Public dinners were given in London by the Perkinian Society and poems were written and published on the tractors. A satirical poem, published under the pseudonym of Christopher Caustic, had two editions in London (1803 and 1804) and various editions in the United States. In spite of its title, "Terrible Tractoration," this poem was, according to Holmes, a most zealous defense of Perkinism and a fierce attack upon its opponents, especially those of the medical profession. The greatest benefit was undoubtedly reaped by the Perkins family, for the tractors, with a real value of only a few cents were sold for five guineas ($25) apiece. A few years later the entire tractor enthusiasm collapsed. In 1811, as mentioned in the literature, the tractors were almost forgotten, and when Oliver Wendell Holmes delivered his speech on them in Boston in 1842, he had difficulty in finding even one such instrument for demonstration.

The Connecticut Medical Society expelled Perkins as early as 1797 for violating their law against the use of "Nostrums or Secret Remedies," and his book written on the tractors is today a rarity among medical bibliophilic objects. But the idea that galvanic current may have an effect on the body never died. Necklaces of various metals were sold to be worn on the body, whose moisture created the necessary wet connection between the different metals. These and the two gadgets mentioned before, patented in the United States and in Austria at the end of the last century, prove that there was a continuous market for this type of

[62] Examples of these types are in this writer's collection.

remedy among ignorant people. Remak himself mentions the wearing of small galvanic chains on the body as a therapeutic measure of his time (73), and his application, on Schönlein's suggestion in 1843, of a pair of galvanic plates behind the ears of a patient with headaches (cephalea). He also mentions in his book (73) that for many years a Berlin mechanic manufactured and sold such galvanic plates for medical purposes, and that then (1858) after his first publications on galvanotherapy, advertisements in the daily papers again offered similar gadgets. One that was used then was a combination of twenty-four pairs of galvanic plates, called "Pulvermacher's Chain"; this was sold, but was not much used by physicians in Germany and Remak doubted its value (73). However, Hiffelsheim in Paris used these chains, which were made of copper and zinc and moistened with water and vinegar before their application.

In England Pulvermacher gadgets were still used in 1870 and even later, as can be seen from a two page advertisement which I found in a book by J. Baxter Langley called *Via Medica* and published in London in a third edition in 1869. It announced: "Pulvermacher's improved patent Flexible Batteries; In the form of Chains and Bands, etc., Officially Approved By The Imperial Academy Of Medicine Of Paris, Royal College of Physicians, London, etc. etc." This Mr. J. L. Pulvermacher had a place of business at 200 Regent Street, London, W., which he called Pulvermacher's Galvanic Establishment. Here he offered to show interested persons testimonials and medical reports by eminent men of the faculty. He described his flexible chain and bands batteries in the following way:

> Disencumbered of the bulky trough of the ordinary Battery, these Voltaic Chains, of small compass and trifling weight, form a regular flexible Battery, always ready for use, capable of being set in action at any minute's notice, and carried about even in the pocket for out-door practice. By simply passing these chains through vinegar, absorbed by capillary attraction of its elements or links, a continuous electro-chemical current of high tension is instantaneously produced. These currents, methodically applied, possess curative properties, in cases enumerated beneath, surpassing those of the ordinary cumbrous and complicated medical galvanic apparatus. The Medical Practitioner, true to his mission, has (next to sufferers) a strong interest to avail himself of Pulvermacher's invention in his daily practice, especially now when a series of improvements added by the inventor to his original voltaic appliances holds out unhoped-for advantages, specified in his Prospectus and Medical Pamphlet, sent post free.

On another page of the same book Pulvermacher offers his Volta-Electric Chain-Bands in various types, for instance, narrow and broad, as chain batteries and as volta-electric bath batteries. The prices ranged from 18 shillings up to 6 pounds. The gadget was suggested for the following ailments: sciatica, rheumatism, neuralgia, gouty pains, local paralysis, and cramps in the limbs. For these the narrow Volta-Electric Chain-Bands seem to have been satisfactory, but the broad chain-bands, to be worn as a belt, were recommended for lumbago, indigestion, liver, chest and functional disorders, for nervous deafness, head, tooth, and face ache, and noises in the head; for loss of voice and other affections of the throat; for writer's cramp, trembling and nervousness; for general debility, central paralysis, epilepsy; for restoring exhausted vital energy, and for eliminating poisonous substances from the system. Of course, Pulvermacher's gadgets were not the only ones used widely in England and France as supposed galvanic batteries and as a panacea against many different diseases.

In Paris a medal-like gadget was sold under the name "Plaques galvano-electric de Mr. Castella de Paris." Its diameter was 33 mm. (95). In Austria by governmental decree No. 9692 of February 15, 1845, an electric conductor or magnetic charm was officially recognized as a remedy and preventive against rheumatism (87). It consisted of iron filings, cardboard, and oilcloth. This decree was republished in Vienna in 1855 (87).

As a rule high ranking physicians regarded such treatment only as a fake. This was the general situation when Duchenne du Boulogne in Paris started modern electrotherapy and when Remak, inspired by Duchenne's lectures, started his explorations in galvanotherapy. They were received by the entire profession with the greatest distrust and destructive criticism, in spite of Remak's reputation as a research worker. Remak, temperamental and irritable as he was, insisted on the soundness of his experiences and the observed facts with the same stubborn tenacity with which he had fought twenty years before for the recognition of his great discoveries in neurohistology. He published papers in Germany, in France, in England; he spoke in Paris at the Academy; he spoke time and again, to the annoyance of the audience, at the Berlin Medical Society and at other meetings on the effects of his galvanotherapy.

Meeting the resistance of his confreres, he carried his enthusiasm to the public, in publications in non-medical journals, and this increased the furor in the profession. Here was a doctor who, for decades, had been refused a suitable position or working facilities in the field where he undoubtedly excelled, who was not given even the title of assistant professor, and who was now a practitioner doing very well with a newly invented method attracting patients, and curing them, even though physicians of long standing were unable to do so! Now every one of the practitioners denounced Remak, asking why he did not remain in the field of his original research, but nobody came forward with an answer to the question, in which laboratory he should have continued to do research. In the worst fashion and in the strongest language, as was usual in German polemics, they accused Remak of charlatanism and ignorance. Even shortly before his death, Hugo Ziemssen dared to attack him in the *Deutsche Klinik* [63] writing: "Herr Remak is the clown in the serious circle of this Society [the Berlin Medical Society], and therefore I do not think it is necessary to take him too seriously."

Remak was cornered, driven to despair by malevolent and irritating colleagues and supported and recognized in his new discoveries by only a very few. Von Graefe, who, as president of the Berlin Medical Society in 1865, delivered a very kind and thoughtful eulogy after Remak's death, was one of these few and so was Professor Winternitz of the University of Vienna. Some outstanding men in Paris remained friendly in spite of Remak's polemic with Duchenne de Boulogne; especially Claude Bernard seems to have regarded Remak's work favorably.

Finally in 1858, in a book of 461 pages (73), Remak summarized all his experiences, opinions, and theories relative to the new method of galvanotherapy. This was his last large publication; it was followed by a summary report on galvanotherapy presented in 1864 at the thirty-ninth Conference of German Scientists and Physicians at Giessen. He published a number of reports and papers on various clinical experiences with galvanotherapy, including a summary report at the Conference of German Scientists and Physicians at Königsberg in 1860. Finally, in 1865, the year of Remak's death, his lectures on galvanotherapy, delivered at the Hôpital de la Charité in Paris, were published as a booklet of forty-one pages in French by the publisher Baillière in Paris.

THE CONCEPT OF NEURITIS

Among Remak's clinical observations and conclusions made in the last years of his life, there is still a far-reaching and outstanding one, with which he opened a new field of neurology. First in 1859, then summing it up in 1861, Remak set forth his concept of neuritis. In the *Oesterreichische Zeitschrift für Practische Heilkunde,* he summarized his experiences on this subject. Except for a few remarks by Froriep in 1837 not much was known up to that time about true neuritis. In his paper Remak now explained the differentiation between neuritis diffusa and nodosa. For the first time he discussed the concept of an inflammation of the ganglia, which he called ganglionitis. For the first time, also, he described progressive neuritis, the ascending and descending types for which he employed the name *neuritis migrans ascendens* and *descendens,* respectively. He differentiated between primary and secondary neuritis, and suggested for treatment the use of the galvanic current.

Lepelletier, Curling, Froriep, and Rokitansky were already aware of inflammatory processes in the nerves in certain cases of traumatic tetanus. Their scattered findings, however, were given no clinical application. Hermann Nothnagel rightly says in the introduction to his lectures on neuritis in 1876 (54: 823): "It was R. Remak who was the first in Germany to attach particular value to the clinical importance of neuritis."

When Remak, in the above mentioned paper, made the statement that neuritis is one of the most common and, up to this time, one of the most neglected diseases, he was correct. Later clinicians became aware of the importance of this condition, learned soon to evaluate this disease and its symptoms, even though Remak's name, as a rule, was not connected anymore with this basic discovery. Here, as with most of Remak's fundamental contributions, his findings and conclusions have stood up well under the criticism of posterity, but the man who made these contributions was forgotten.

LAST PUBLICATIONS

In the last decade of his life, Remak rarely returned to the work of his early days, except in 1861 and 1862 in short papers in *Virchow's Archiv* and in Du Bois' *Archiv.* The latter article was translated into English and appeared in 1862 in the *London Quarterly Journal of Microscopical Science.*

Refuting in a tragic way the attacks of his enemies, he later referred to the great exactness of his early discoveries as proof of his reliability in reporting experiments and observations.

Remak dedicated his 1858 book (73), faithfully as of old, to Alexander von Humboldt on the occasion of his eighty-ninth birthday. In this volume he presented an historical report on his entire electrotherapeutic work and a reprint of his previous publications on galvanotherapy, and gave a vivid description of his experiences in Paris where on September 22, 1856 he read a paper at the Paris Academy of Sciences, after spending a summer vacation at Ostende. He selected patients for his treatment in the Salpetière in Paris with the assistance of Cazalis and Moissenet, but the old grandmothers whom he found there refused very emphatically to get rid of their muscle contractions.

Despite all the cooperation of leading French physicians, Remak had the greatest difficulty obtaining patients to demonstrate his type of treatment to the commission named by the Academy to pass judgment on his statements concerning the value of galvanotherapy. At the Place Nôtre Dame, Broca and Follin were in charge of a distribution center, the Bureau Central des Hôpiteaux, where an incoming crowd of sick people was distributed to the proper hospitals, and where tickets were given to each for free baths and sulphur baths. He was warned that he would find only vagabonds and swindlers there, but instead he found a miserable crowd of really sick people, and from among them he chose a dozen "rheumatic muscle contractions" to demonstrate his method to Rayer, Brown-Séquard, and Pasquier.

[63] 1865: 159.

Not everyone in Paris was really as kind to Remak as Claude Bernard, or Broca, or Brown-Séquard, either. Dechambre made fun of his galvanotherapy in an article in the *Gazette Hebdomaire.* In November 1864 Remak demonstrated his galvanotherapy at the Charité in Paris in the presence of Velpeau and Bouillant. The government interfered, however, because Remak was a foreign physician. Some of Remak's French confreres may have been responsible for this governmental veto (91). The profession in Berlin, where Remak in 1857 reported to the Society for Scientific Medicine and later to the Hufeland Society and at innumerable discussions at various medical meetings, of course refused to accept the gospel of galvanotherapy.

In spite of all the work Remak did later, his book is his last great summary of his studies and endeavors in the field of electrotherapy. His historical survey of the subject, gives credit to everyone who deserved it. It is typical of the modern way he worked that he visualized the problem of galvanotherapy from an exact theoretical point of view and by no means confined it only to muscle and nerve physiology. In 1856 he already realized that Duchenne's important advocacy of electrotherapy, the effectiveness of which he himself had proved, needed a valid theoretical basis. With that, he began to compare the effect of the constant galvanic current with the effect of the faradic current used up to that time. He grasped the difference in their effects in the clinic as well as in physiology, and here his independent work and his foundation of galvanotherapy began. From the outset Remak emphasized that a basic understanding of the metabolic effect of the electric current would be desirable, even indispensable for further progress. In his enthusiasm he surely overestimated the rapidity and intensity of his therapeutic effects, but he proved here to be correct in his basic statements.

France at that time was far ahead of Germany in the field of neurology and electrotherapy. There, through the activities of physicians like Duchenne du Boulogne and Charcot, modern neurology was developed, and interest in Remak's work was sincere, in spite of differences of opinion. Remak and his work were treated with all the respect due an outstanding physician. But at home in Berlin he had to wage a fight against envious rivals. In London an anonymous reviewer of his book wrote (89): "This elaborate production must be considered as a curiosity rather than as a serious treatise on Medical Galvanization." This was the pattern in which Remak's work was criticized from the very beginning of his research career up to the last day of his life.

A paper by Remak published by the Viennese Academy of Sciences in 1862 is like the last flare-up of the light of a by-gone day, the final summary of his previous achievements. It is a letter to the physiologist Carl Ludwig, whom he met a few weeks before in Vienna and with whom he discussed physiological problems. Ludwig presented this communication to the meeting of the Academy on October 31, 1861, and it was published in the *Proceedings* of this scientific society (1862). Here Remak reported on some as yet unpublished odds and ends of his microscopic research, being doubtful whether he would ever find the time to finish these studies, since he was entirely absorbed in his galvanotherapeutic work. Interesting among the facts mentioned in this paper are Remak's discovery of smooth muscle fibers within the kidneys of certain animals.

DEATH

Moriz Benedikt (3) rightly compared Remak and his fate with that of Charles Bell or Marshall Hall, who, as Benedikt says, were treated in their countries as fools not to be taken seriously, up to the time that Johannes Müller gave them credit for their great merit. In the last years of his life Remak had to remind his opponents, who were seldom his equal in personality or in accomplishments in modern medicine, of his own

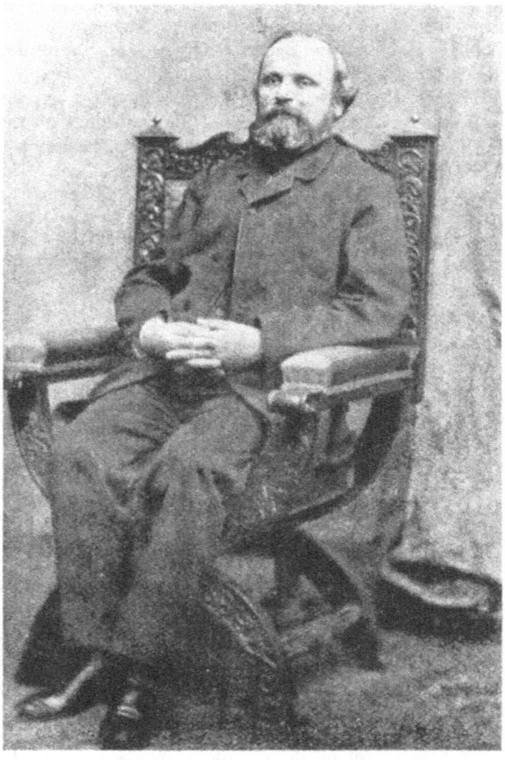

FIG. 56. Photo of Remak taken shortly before his death. Published in *Allgemeine Zeitung des Judentums* No. 30, Berlin, 1915.

scientific reliability and reputation, and of their shameful behavior.

But in spite of this struggle, he continued, undefeated, to work. In the year before his death, he demonstrated his new apparatus for galvanization at the meeting of German Scientists and Physicians in Giessen. Even in the last year of his life he was active in medical matters, reading papers and leading discussions at the Berlin Medical Society. In 1865 he actively participated in its meetings of February 8 and April 12, and 26. On March 15 and May 3, of the same year, he read papers there on clinical observations and the therapy of "cramps of the face muscles."

At that time, in spite of the fact that he still looked energetic and healthy, he had been seriously ill for the past two years. We do not know authoritatively the disease from which he suffered (4), but there is some justification in supposing that at that time he was diabetic; his nervousness, his irritability, and, finally, the cause of his sudden death, which was a furunculosis, suggests such a disease.[64] On August 29, 1865 during a summer vacation at Bad-Kissingen, he died, ending a very unhappy personal life, but an extremely successful scientific one. His last academic ambition, to become the chief of an electrotherapeutic department in the Charité Hospital in Berlin, remained an unfulfilled dream.

Though Remak had to suffer all his life from the envy and antagonism of some of his colleagues on the Berlin Faculty and from other physicians, he enjoyed the sympathy of the students. In 1861 when the University of Berlin celebrated its 50th Anniversary at a solemn ceremony on October 18, seven thousand participants were present, including students, professors, and representatives of the government. It was the greatest academic festivity Berlin had ever seen. The students themselves called for those professors whom they wished to deliver a speech. It was a spontaneous expression of sympathy by the academic people. The professors of the Medical Faculty called for on this occasion were Mitscherlich, Virchow, Remak, and DuBois-Reymond. The festivity lasted until the next morning. At one o'clock the academic teachers left their enthusiastic young students, and this may well have been the last great satisfaction Remak enjoyed as an academic teacher (90).

He was buried on September 1, 1865 at 3 o'clock in the afternoon in the Cemetery of the Jewish Community in Berlin. His mother survived her famous son.

Moriz Benedikt, founder of criminal anthropology and professor of electrotherapy at the University of Vienna, reports in several places in his autobiography on Remak and his tragic lot. Remak, he says (4: 63), who historically was the founder of galvanotherapy, was really persecuted by the matadors of science in Berlin because of this invention. Benedikt's own opinion of Remak is expressed by the answer he gave to Brücke (4). Once he was asked by his teacher Brücke, one of the younger generation of Müller's pupils, later head of the physiological department of the University in Vienna, what his opinion of Remak was.

> I told him, [says Benedikt] that in my opinion he is one of the physicians of all times, most full of genius. He sees something where nobody else does, and he has the courage to announce the most paradoxical observations and to express the most daring opinions. It has always been my experience that he saw correctly, and I am very careful not to reject even the most paradoxical of his views, in spite of the fact that some of them are really amazing. I came to this opinion in histology as well as in embryology. Sometimes it took me ten years before I was able to confirm his statements. However, I was always convinced that he had seen correctly and that this statements were correct. I was glad to assist Remak later on in Berlin to be recognized also as a galvanotherapeutist.

Benedikt met Remak personally in 1863 in Berlin. An admirer and devoted follower of Remak's work, and recognized as a Viennese professor, he tried to influence people in Berlin, like v. Graefe the ophthalmologist and Griesinger the neurologist, in favor of Remak. Indeed, we know from Remak's own remarks that in the last years of his life he was on very friendly terms with von Graefe. Friendly, too, was the spirit of Graefe's eulogy for Remak, delivered on November 15 at the meeting of the Berliner Medizinische Gesellschaft (25). What Benedikt admired especially and with reason in Remak, whom he called "the irritable and irritated man," was that Remak always saw and thought at the bedside of a patient as a physiologist, and that was what made him the great physician of his time in Berlin and likewise necessarily put him in opposition to many of his prominent medical colleagues. From their enmity, envy, and petty persecutions he had to suffer to the very end of his life. But undoubtedly Benedikt was correct in characterizing Remak in his eulogy as one of the greatest and most peculiar geniuses of modern medicine. Von Graefe, the famous ophthalmologist, spoke of Remak in his eulogy in the following manner: "If we consider the wealth of his knowledge, his mind, and his productivity, we cannot deny that with his death one of the most brilliant and gifted and most remarkable personalities disappeared from the medical world."

BIBLIOGRAPHY OF THE PUBLICATIONS OF ROBERT REMAK

The items marked with an asterisk are the only ones in this bibliography which were not checked in the original.

1836

Müller, J. Jahresbericht. *Müller's Arch.* 1836: XVIII.
Müller reports there on Remak's discovery of a ganglion at the Nervus Access. Willisii.

Vorläufige Mitteilung microscopischer Beobachtungen über den inneren Bau der Cerebrospinalnerven und über die Entwicklung ihrer Formelemente. *Müller's Arch.* 1836: 145–161.

[64] This suspicion has meanwhile been verified by Remak's granddaughter Mrs. Litthauer.

1837

*De Gonzenbach, O. De Carcinomate penis. Doctoral Thesis. Berlin 1837.
On p. 8 of this thesis Remak's microscopical investigations of condylomas are discussed.

Hube, Xaver. De morbo scrofuloso. Doctoral Thesis. Berlin 1837.
On p. 19 Remak's discovery of the microscopical findings in tinea crusts is published.

Weitere microscopische Beobachtungen über die Primitivfasern des Nervensystem der Wirbeltiere. *Froriep's Not.* 1837: **3**: 36–40.

Vermischte Anatomische Beobachtungen. *Froriep's Not.* 1837: **10**: 150–154.

Neurologische Notizen. *Froriep's Not.* 1837: **14**: 216.

1838

Über die Structur des Nervensystem. *Froriep's Not.* 1838: **6**: 342–346.

Über die Verrichtungen des organischen Nervensystems. *Froriep's Not.* 1838: **7**: 65–70.

Observationes Anatomicae et Microscopicae de Systematis Nervosi Structura. Dissertatio Inauguralis. Berlin, Reimer: 1838.
With a "Vita" and the "Theses"; otherwise same as the second edition of the same year. See next issue.

Observationes anatomicae et microscopicae de Systematis nervosi structura. Berolini, Reimer: 1838:8°VI + 41 + 1 with 2 plates. Amico suo dignissimo Alfredo de Bentkowski med. et chir. Dr.

O budowie nerwow i zwojow nerwowych. *Pamiet. Towarz. Lek. Warsaw:* **2**: 325–374, 1 plate. 1838.

1839

Mitteilung einer neuen Weise der Verschliessung durchschnittener Arterien. *Med Zeitg.* **8**: 27–28, (6. Feb.) 1839.

Nachträgliche Bemerkungen zu meiner Mitteilung über ein neues Verfahren Arterien zu verschliessen. *Med. Zeitg.* **8**: 38, Feb. 26, 1839.

Über die Ganglien der Herznerven des Menschen und deren physiologische Bedeutung. *Wschn. f. d. ges. Heilkde.* 1839: 149–154.

Über die Schädlichkeit des Menstrualblutes und über deren wahrscheinliche Ursachen. *Med. Zeitg.* **8**: 261–262: 1839 (25.XII).

Zur mikroskopischen Anatomie der Retina. (Auszug aus einem Briefe an Herrn Prof. Dr. Carus vom 27. August 1838.) *Müller's Arch.* 1839: 165–170.

1840

Über die physiologische Bedeutung des organischen Nervensystems, besonders nach Anatomischen Tatsachen. *Mschr. für Med. Augenhkde. u. Chir.* **3**: 225–265, 1840.

Neue Beiträge zur Kenntnis vom organischen Nervensystem. *Med. Zeitg.* **9**: 2–8, 1840.

Beiträge zur Kenntnis des organischen Nervensystems. *Med. Zeitg.* **9**: 73, 1840.

Zur Kenntnis von der pflanzlichen Natur der Porrigo Lupinosa W. *Med. Zeitg.* **9**: 73–74, 1840. (15.4.)

Nägel. in *Encyclop. Wörterbuch der Med. Wissensch.* **24**: 609–612, 1840, Berlin Veit et Comp.

Melanosis. in *Encyclopädisches Wörterbuch der Med. Wiss.* **22**: 693–719, 1840, Berlin Veit et Comp.

*Über Parasiten im Mesenterium der Frösche. Nov. 1840. Paper read at the meeting of Ges. Naturforsch. Freunde Berlin. Publ. in Berlin: *Vossiche und Spemersche Zeitung.* 1840.

*Über den Bau des Gehirns. *Ibidem.* Dec. 1840.

1841

Über die zweifelhaften Flimmerbewegung an den Nerven. *Müller's Arch.* 1841: 39–41. (Signed Dr. Remak pract. Arzt in Berlin.)

Über Wimperblasen und Hornfäden. (Signed R. Remak pract. Arzt in Berlin.) (Mitgeteilt in der Gesellschaft naturforschender Freunde in Berlin, den 17. November 1840.) *Müller's Arch.* 1841: 446–453.

Anatomische Beobachtungen über das Gehirn, das Rückenmark und die Nervenwurzeln. (Mitgeteilt in d. Ges. naturf. Freunde in Berlin 15. Dec. 1840.) *Müller's Arch.* 1841: 506–522.

Über die Entstehung der Blutkörperchen. *Amtl. Ber. über d. 19. Vers. Deutscher Nat. Forscher u. Aerzte.* Braunschweig Sept. 1841: 66–67. Braunschweig 1842.

Über die verschiedene Form der Körperchen im Blute und im Chylus. *Amtl. Ber. der 19. Vers. deutsch. Nat. Forscher u. Ärzte, Braunschw.* 91 (20–22. Sept.) 1841.

Discussion über Operierbarkeit der Geschwülste. *Amtl. Ber. der 19. Vers. deutsch. Nat. Forscher u. Ärzte, Braunschweig* (21. Sept. 1841): 120.

* Nauka potoznicza dla akuszerek w Pańtswie Król.-Pruskiem z 32 tablicami ryzin. Berlin, 514 pp. German text by Jos. Herm. Schmidt. Translated into Polish language under supervision of Dr. Remak.

Nervensystem (histologisch). In *Encyclopädisches Wörterbuch der med. Wissensch.* **25**: 129–152, 1841. Berlin, Veit et Comp.

Nervensystem (physiologisch). In *Encyclopädisches Wörterbuch der med. Wissensch.* **25**: 152–195, 1841. Berlin, Veit et Comp.

Netzhaut. Same *Wörterbuch.* **25**: 209–210, 1841, No. 33, 34 and 35 are signed: R.R-K.

Über den Missbrauch der formellen und über die Nothwendigkeit der realen Kritik in den Medicinischen Disciplinen. *Med. Ztg.* **10**: 72, 1841 (14.IV).

Über die Anzeigen zur Ausrottung krankhafter Geschwülste. *Med. Ztg.* **10**: 125–127, 131–133, 135–136. 1841.

Über die Entstehung der Blutkörperchen. *Med. Ztg.* **10**: 127, 1841.

Ossificatio. In *Encyclopädisches Wörterbuch der Med. Wissensch.* **26**: 114–148, 1841. Signed: R-K.

Osteosarcoma. In *Encyclopädisches Wörterbuch der Med. Wissensch.* **26**: 187–257, 1841. Signed: R-K.

1842

Über Menstruation und Brunst. *Neue Ztsch. f. Geburtskunde.* **13**: 175–233, 1842.

Die abnorme Natur des Menstrualblutflusses. Erläutert von Dr. Robert Remak. 8° viii + 58 Berlin, A. Hirschwald. 1842. Reprinted from Busch's *Neue Zeitschrift f. Geburtskunde* 13, 1842. Dedicated to Geheimrat Prof. Dr. Jüngken. Dekan der Berliner med. Fak. on occasion of his 25th anniversary as physician.

Gelungene Impfung des Favus. *Med. Ztg.* **11**: 137, 1842.

Bericht über die Leistungen im Gebiete der Physiologie im Jahre 1841. *Canstatts Jahresber. der Ges. Med.* Erlangen, 1842.

Peyersche Drüsen. In *Encyclopäedisches Wörterbuch der med. Wiss.* **27**: 26–39, 1842.

Über pathologische Verknöcherung. *Magazin f. d. ges. Heilkde.* **59**: 95–122, 1842.

1843

Über die Zusammenziehung der Muskelprimitivbündel. *Müller's Arch.* 1843: 182–190.

Bermerkungen über die äusseren Atemmuskeln der Fische. *Müller's Arch.* 1843: 190–196.

Über den Inhalt der Nervenprimitivröhren. *Müller's Arch.* 1843: 197–201.
* Uwagi nad wskazaniami do wyniszszenia wyrósli rakowých i nierakowych. *Pametnik Towarz. Lekars. Warsaw* **6**: 280–294, 1843. With date: Berlin, grudniu 1840.
Über die Entwickelung des Hühnchens im Ei. (Briefliche Mittheilung an Herrn Professor Dr. Jan van der Hoeven in Leyden.) *Müller's Arch.* 1843: 478–484.

1844

Neurologische Erläuterungen. *Müller's Arch.* 1844: 463–472.
Sphygmologia. In *Encyclop. Wörterbuch der Med. Wissensch.* **32**: 46–57, 1844.

1845

Diagnostische und pathogenetische Untersuchungen, in der Klinik des Herrn Geh. Raths Dr. Schönlein auf dessen Veranlassung angestellt und mit Benutzung anderweitiger Beobachtungen veröffentlicht. 242 p. 1 plate. Berlin, Aug. Hirschwald. 1845.
Über die Entwicklung der Muskelprimitivbündel. *Froriep's Not.* **35**: 305–308, 1845.
Über Wimperbewegung in den Canälchen des Wolffschen Körpers bei Eidechsenembryonen. *Froriep's Not.* **35**: 308–309, 1845.

1847

Über ein selbständiges Darmnervenssystem. Berlin, G. Reimer. 1847. Folio. iv + 37 + 1 with 2 plates. Dedicated to A. v. Humboldt and Joh. Müller.
M. Remak addresse dans le même but une analyse de son travail sur le développement du poulet et notamment sur le développement du système nerveux intestinal. (Pour le prix de Medécine et de Chirurgie.) *C. R. Acad. Sci. Paris.* **24**: 369, 1847.

1848

*Uber die Function und Entwickelung des oberen Keimblattes im Ei der Wirbeltiere. *Mon. Ber. Ak. Wsch. Berl.* Oct. 1848: 362–365.
M. Remak prie l'academie de vouloir bien admettre au concours, pour le prix de Physiologie expérimentale, son travail sur un système nerveux indépendant. Cet ouvrage avait étè dejà, a l'époque de sa presentation renvoyé a la commission chargée d'examiner les pièces du concours de 1847. *C. R. Acad. Sci. Paris* **26**: 264, 21. Feb. 48.

1849

Berichtigung. *Die Medizinische Reform* No. 43: 240, 1890.
Über die genetische Bedeutung und Entwicklung des oberen Keimblattes im Ei der Wirbelthiere. (Aus dem Monatsbericht der Akad. der Wissenschaften in Berlin October 1848 p. 362–365). *Müller's Arch.* 1849: 75–78.
Sur la fonction de la cauche superficielle du germe. (Extrait d'une letter de M. Remak à M. Flourens.) *C. R. Acad. Sci. Paris* **28**: 89, 1849.

1850

Über den Bau des Herzens. *Müller's Arch.* 1850: 76–78.
Histologische Bemerkungen über die Blutgefässwände. *Müller's Arch.* 1850: 79–101.
Über die Zeichen der Phtisis aus den Sputis. *Allgem. Med. Central Ztg.* **19**: 439–440, 1850.
Über blutleere Gefässe (Lymphgefässe) im Schwanze der Froschlarve. *Müller's Arch.* 1850: 102–110.
Nachträgliche Bermerkung zu dem Aufsatz: Über die blutleeren Gefässe (Lymphgefässe) in dem Schwanze der Froschlarve. *Müller's Arch.* 1850: 182–183.
Untersuchungen über die Entwicklung der Wirbeltiere. Lfg. I 1850, Berlin, G. Reimer.

1851

*Über die genetische Bedeutung des oberen Keimblattes im Eie der Wirbeltiere. Monatsber d.k. Akad. d. Wiss zu Berlin, Jan. 1851: 25–28.
Über die genetische Bedeutung des oberen Keimblattes im Eie der Wirbeltiere. (Aus dem Monatsber. der Kgl. Akad. der Wissensch. Berlin Jan. 1851, p. 25–26.) *Müller's Arch.* 1851: 208–210.
Über die sogenannten Blutkörperchen haltenden Zellen. *Müller's Arch.* 1851: 480–483.
Über den Rhythmus der Furchungen im Froscheie. *Müller's Arch.* 1851: 495–496.
Über den Bau der Blutgefässwände und ihren Anteil and der Blutbewegung. *Allg. Med. Central Ztg.* **20**: 3–5, 1851.

1852

Über extracellulare Entstehung thierischer Zellen und über Vermehrung derselben durch Theilung. *Müller's Arch.* 1852: 47–57.
Über die Ganglien der Zunge bei Sängetieren und beim Menschen. *Müller's Arch.* 1852: 58–62.
Über die Entstehung des Bindegewebes und des Knorpels. *Müller's Arch.* 1852: 63–72.
Über runde Blutgerinnsel und über pigmentkugelhaltige Zellen. *Müller's Arch.* 1852: 115–162.
An ergography of Reinhardt, given at the meeting of March 22nd of the Ges. F. wiss. Med. in Berlin. *Allg. Med. Central Ztg.* **21**: 20–203, 1852.
*Über den Entwicklungsplan der Wirbeltiere. *Ber. über d. Vers. deutscher Aerzte u. Nat. Forsch. Wiesbaden.* Sept. 1852: pp. 178–180.
Über die Contraction des Ganglienstranges beim Blutegel. *Ibid.* 181–183.
Note sur le devélopement des animaux vertébrés. (Commissaires M. M. Flourens, Serres, Coste.) Mémoires lus. *C. R. Acad. Sci. Paris* **35**: 341–344. 13. Sept. 1852. Also reprinted Berlin, Unger frères. 1852.
Note sur le ganglions nerveux des parois de l'estomac des mamifères. *C. R. Soc. Biol. Paris* (12. Sept. 1852) **4**: 138–139, 1852.
Des ganglions microscopiques sur le trajet des filets du nerf pneumogastrique dans les parois de l'estomac. Par M. le docteur Remack [*sic!*] (de Berlin) (11. Sept. 1852). *C. R. d. Soc. Biol. Paris.* **4**: 153–155, 1852.
Über die Furchung des Froscheies. *Rheinl. u. Westphal. Verh.* 1852: 64–66.

1853

**Ber. ü. d. Vers. deutsch. Aerzte u. Nat. Forsch. Gotha.*
Über gangliöse Nervenfasern beim Menschen und bei Wirbeltieren. *Mon. Ber. Kgl. Akad. d. Wissensch. Berlin,* 12. Mai 1853: 293–298.
Sur des fibres nerveuses ganglieuses chez l'homme et chez les animaux vertébrés. *C. R. Acad. Sci. Paris* **36**: 914–917, 1853, 23 May 1853.
Sur la structure de la rétine. (Note addressée par M. Remack [*sic*] a l'ocassion d'une communication récente de M. Kölliker.) *C. R. Acad. Sci. Paris.* **37**: 663, 1853, **37**: 725, 1853 (31 Oct. 53).
**Amtl. Ber. Vers. Deutsch. Nat. Forsch-u. Aerzte. Wiesbaden 1853:* p. 182.

1854

Über Multipolare Ganglienenzellen. *Monatsber. K. Akad. d. W. Berlin,* Januar 1854: 26–32.
Über vielkernige Zellen der Leber. *Müller's Arch.* 1854: 99–102.
Über Wimperblasen. *Müller's Arch.* 1854: 184–185.
Über Eihüllen und Spermatozoen. *Müller's Arch.* 1854: 252–256.

Über die Zusammenziehung des Amnions. *Müller's Arch.* 1854: 369–373.

Über den Entwicklungsplan der Wirbeltiere. *Müller's Arch.* 1854: 374–375.

Über die Theilung thierischer Zellen. *Müller's Arch.* 1854: 376.

Über den Bau der Retina des Menschen. *Allgem. Medic. Central Ztg.* **23**: 1, 1854.

Ein Beitrag zur Entwicklungsgeschichte der Krebshaften Geschwülste. *Deutsche Klinik* **6**: 170–174, 1854.

Über den Bau der Retina und der Ganglien. (Ges. f. Wiss. Med. Berlin.) *Deutsche Klinik* **6**: 177–179, 1854.

**Mon. Ber. Kgl. Ak. d. W. Berlin,* Jan. 1854.

1855

Experimenteller Nachweis motorischer Wirkungen des N. sympathicus auf willkürliche Muskeln. *Deutsche Klinik.* **7**: 294–295, 1855.

Über centrale Ausgleichung sympathischer Wirkungen. *Deutsche Klinik.* **7**: 295, 1855.

Über das Verhalten der Irismuskeln bei seitlicher Beleuchtung der Netzhaut. *Deutsche Klinik.* **7**: 295, 1855.

Über den Bau der grauen Säulen im Rückenmarke der Säugetiere. *Deutsche Klinik.* **7**: 295.

Über Methodische Electrisierung gelähmter Muskeln. Berlin, A. Hirschwald 1855, 24 pp. 8°. The same [with Anhang], Berlin, A. Hirschwald) 31 pp. 8° 1855. Dedicated to Claude Bernard. Seconde édition see 1856.

M. Rayer en présentant la troisième livraison d'un ouvrage de M. Remak de Berlin intitulé Recherches sur le dévelopement des animaux vertébrés donne dans les termes suivants une idée de ce travail (Feb. 19, 1855). *C. R. Acad. Sci. Paris* **40**: 421, 1855.

Note sur les fonctions motrices du grand sympathique. (Présentée au nom de l'auteur par M. Cl. Bernard.) *C. R. Acad. Sci. Paris.* 6 Aug. 1855. **41**: 180–181, 1855.

Note accompanying his "Memoire sur l'electrisation méthodique des muscles." (Aug. 27, 1855.) *C. R. Acad. Sci. Paris.* **41**: 355–356, 1855.

Untersuchungen über die Entwicklung der Wirbeltiere. Berlin, G. Reimer, 1855. Folio 6 + XXXVII + 1 + 194 pp. with 12 plates. Dedicated to Alexander v. Humboldt.

**Monatsber. K. Ak. d. Wissch. Berlin.* Juli 1853.

Sur des Contractions toniques des muscles pendant la galvanisation des nerfs antagonistes. *C. R. Acad. Sci. Paris* **41**: 1089–1091, 1855, 17. Dec. 1855.

Neurologische Beobachtungen. 6 pp. Berlin, G. Reimer. Rept. from *Deutsche Klinik* 7, 1855.

1856

Über contractile Klappensäcke an den Venen der Menschen. *Deutsche Klinik.* **8**: 32, 1856.

Bemerkungen zu der von Herrn Duchenne de Boulogne im zweiten Heft der Schmidt'schen Jahrbücher der gesamten Medicin (Jahrg. 1856) gegebenen Beurtheilung meiner Schrift "Über methodische Elektrisierung gelähmter Muskeln." *Deutsche Klinik.* **8**: 125–127, 1856.

Second edition of Über methodische Electrisierung (1855).

Über die Enden der Nerven im electrischen Organ der Zitterrochen. *Müller's Arch.* 1856, 467–472.

Neue Beiträge zur physiologischen Therapie der Lähmungen und Contracturen. *Deutsche Klinik.* **8**: 257–258, 1856. Reprinted in 134: 209.

Über die Lösung paralytischer Contracturen mittelst constanter galvanischer Ströme. *Deutsche Klinik.* **8**: 289, 1856. Reprinted in 134: 213.

**Spenersche Zeitung, Berlin.* 19 August, 1856.

Über die Heilwirkung des constanten galvanischen Stromes bei Contracturen Lähmungen und Atrophien der Muskeln. *Deutsche Klinik.* **8**: 353–354, 1856. Reprinted in Galvanotherapie, 245 (1858). Also separately printed, 1856. Berlin, G. Reimer.

Sur l'action physiologique et thérapeutique du courant galvanique constant sur les nerfs et les muscles de l'homme. (Commissaires MM. Andral, Rayer, Velpeau.) (Sept. 22, 1856.) *C. R. Acad. Sci. Paris* **43**: 603–605, 1855. Reprinted in Galvanotherapie, 215 (1858).

Über die Anwendung galvanischer Ströme zur Heilung von Lähmungen und Contracturen. *S. B. d. Hufeland. Ges. Berlin,* **28**: III, 1856. Reprinted in Galvanotherapie, 207 (1858).

Note additionelle au Mémoire sur l'áction physiologique et thérapeutique du curant galvanique constant sur les nerfs et les muscles de l'homme. lu le 22 Septembre par m. Remak. (Commissaires Andral, Rayer, Velpeau.) *C. R. Acad. Sci. Paris* **43**: 655, 1856. (29 Sept. 1856.) Reprinted in Galvanotherapie, 217 (1858), and separately printed 1856. Paris, Mallet-Bachelier.

1857

Über die Verdickung der Muskeln durch constante galvanische Ströme. *Deutsche Klinik.* **9**: 435, 1857. Partly reprinted in Galvanotherapie, 222 (1858).

Elektrotherapeutische Mitteilungen. *Deutsche Klinik.* **9**: 489–490, 1857.

Über die Heilwirkung des constanten galvanischen Stromes bei Lähmungen Schmerzen und Krämpfen. (Aus dem Protokolle der Gesellschaft für wissenschafliche Medicine vom 19. Januar 1857.) *Allg. Med. Centralzeitung.* **12**. Stück No. 30, 1857. Reprinted in Galvanotherapie, 218 (1858).

Über die physiologischen Grundlagen der Anwendung galvanischer Ströme zur Heilung von Lähmungen. *B. d. Hufeland. Ges. Berlin.* 27. III. 1857. Reprinted in Galvanotherapie, 220 (1858).

1858

Über die Theilung der Blutzellen beim Embryo. *Müller's Arch.* 1858: 178–188.

Über peripherische Ganglien an den Nerven des Nahrungsrohrs. *Müller's Arch.* 1858: 189–192.

Über den antiparalytischen Wert inducierter electrischer Ströme. *Deutsche Klinik.* **10**: 17–19, 1858. Reprinted in 134: 230.

Eine Verspätete Erwiederung auf die in No. 47 des vorigen Jahrganges enthaltenen Bemerkung des Herrn Hugo Ziemssen über die Verdickung der Muskeln durch galvanische Ströme. *Deutsche Klinik.* **10**: 250, 1858.

Über die Behandlung der Tabes dorsalis mit constanten galvanischen Strömen. *S. B. d. Hufeland. Ges. Berlin.* 26. III. 1858. Reprinted in Galvanotherapie, 238 (1858).

On the therapeutical action of the constant galvanic current. *Medical Times and Gaz.* **16**: 479–480, 1858. Reprinted in Galvanotherapie, 241 (1858).

Constant galvanic current. *Medical Times and Gazette* **16**: 642, 1858.

Galvanotherapie der Nerven und Muskelkrankeiten. Berlin, A. Hirschwald. XV + 461 pp. 8°, 1858. To the 89th birthday of Alexander von Humboldt.

1860

Sur les ganglions péripheriques des nerfs. (July 2, 1860.) *C. R. Acad. Sci. Paris* **51**: 28–29, 1860.

Klinische Mitteilungen I, II. *Österr. Zsch. f. pract. Heilkunde* **6**: 721–726, 1860. I. Über centrale Übertragungen peripherer Anesthaesie. II. Über centrale Übertragungen von reflectorischen Krämpfen.

Galvanothérapie. Trad. de l'allemand par A. Morpain. Avec les additons de l'auteur: XX, 461 pp. 8°. (1860. Paris, J. B. Baillière & fils.)

Action centripète du courant galvanique constant sur les nerfs de l'homme. (August 27, 1860.) *C. R. Acad. Sci. Paris.* **51**: 327–331, 1860.
Klinische Mitteilungen III. Über Neuritis. *Österr. Zsch. f. pract. Heilk.* **6**: 769–776, 1860.
*Remarques sur l'action du courant galvanique continu. *Brown Séquards J. de Physiol.* **3**: 439–443, 1860.

1861

Über Anwendung elektrischer Ströme in der Praktischen Heilkunde. *Österr. Zsch. f. prakt. Heilk.* **7**: 717–721, 1861.
Über endogene Entstehung von Eiter und Schleimzellen. *Virchow's Arch.* **20**: 198–202, 1861.
Anatomische und physiologische Beobachtungen. I. Über den Bau und die Funktion der Nieren. II. Über den Bau und die Zusammenziehung der Muskelfasern. *S. B. Wiener Akad. d. W.* **44** (Abth 2): 413–423, 1861.

1862

Über das Epithel der Lungenbläschen. *Deutsche Klinik.* **14**: 197–198, 1862.
Über die Wiedererzeugung von Nervenfasern. *Virch. Arch.* **23**: 441–444, 1862.
Neurologische und elektrotherapeutische Ergebnisse. I. Über Tabes dorsalis. *Deutsche Klinik.* **14**: 479–483, 1862.
Über die embryologische Grundlage der Zellenlehre. *Reichert & Du Bois Archiv* 1862, 230–241. (English translation in: *Microscop. Soc. J.* **2**: 277–284, 1862.)
M. Depretz présente au nom de M. Remak profeseur de médécine à l'université de Berlin la note suivante concernant une pile galvanique portative dont il fait usage. (Nov. 5, 1862.) *C. R. Acad. Sci. Paris* **55**: 697, 1862.
Klinische Mittheilungen. IV. Über die Heilbarkeit der progressiven Muskelatrophie. *Österr. Zsch. f. prakt. Heilkunde.* **8**: 1–6, and 29–35, 1862.
Klinische Mitteilungen. V. Über Tabes dorsalis. (Nach einem am 31. Oktober 1862 in der Hufeland' schen Gesellschaft gehaltenen Vortrag.) *Österr. Zsch. f. prakt. Heilkunde.* **8**: 937–941 and 953–956, 1862.

1863

Neurologische und elektrotherapeutische Ergebnisse. Vorl. Mitt. II. Über den Einfluss der Centralorgane des Nervensystems auf Krankheiten der Knochen und der Gelenke. *Deutsche Klinik.* **15**: 107–108, 1863.
Klinische Mitteilungen. VI. Über haemorrhagische Hemiplegien. *Österr. Ztsch. f. prakt. Heilkde.* **9**: 177–181, 1863. VII. Über den Einfluss der Centralorgane des Nervensystems auf Krankheiten der Knochen und Gelenke. *Ibidem* **9**: 193–196, 1863. VIII. Über Torticollis und Chorea. *Ibidem* **9**: 224–225, 1863.

1864

Sur le traitement de quelques névroses ayant leur siège a la base du cerveau. *C. R. Acad. Sci. Paris* Sept. 12, 1864.
Über nervöses Contagium. *Berlin Klin. Wsch.* **1**: 458, 1864.
Discussion to a paper read by E. A. von Gräfe "über die Basedow'sche Krankheit." (Paper read in the Berl. Mediz. Gesellschaft March 6. 1864.) *Klin. Monatsbl. f. Augenheilkunde.* 1864, 185.
Vorstellung zweier Krankheitsfälle. *Berl. Klin. Wsch.* **1**: 167–168 and 175–176.
Über Gesichtsmuskelkrampf. *Berl. Klin. Wsch.* **1**: 209–212 and 221–223 and 229–232.
Über vitale Wirkungen des konstanten Stromes. *Berl. Klin. Wsch.* **1**: 269–270, 1864.
Über Tabes. *Berl. Klin. Wsch.* **1**: 321–323, 1864.
Neue Beiträge zur Lehre von der Tabes. *Berl. Klin. Wsch.* **1**: 393–398, 1864.
Sur le traitement de quelques nevroses ayant leur siége a la base du cerveau (5 Sept. 1864.) *C. R. Acad. Sci. Paris.* **59**: 482–484, 1864.
L'application thérapeutique du courant galvanique constant. *C. R. Acad. Sci. Paris* **59**: 856, 1864.
Mémoire déposé 5. Dec. 1864 (pp. 952 and 996). (Renvoi a l'examen des commissaires déja désignés M. M. Velpeau, Rayer, Bernard.)

1865

Über spasmus alternans transversus. *Berl. Klin. Wsch.* **2**: 94–95, 1865.
Zusatz zu dem vorigen Aufsatze. *Berl. Klin. Wsch.* **2**: 124, 1865.
Über dentale Neurosen des Herzens. *Berl. Klin. Wsch.* **2**: 257–259, 1865.
Über Gesichtmuskelkrampf. *Berl. Klin. Wsch.* **2**: 280–281, 1865.
Application du courant constant au traitement des névroses. Leçons faites a l'Hôpital de la Charité. 41 pp. 8° Paris, G. Baillière, 1865.

REFERENCES

1. Augustin, F. L. 1803. Versuch einer vollständigen Geschichte der galvanischen Electricität und ihrer medizinischen Anwendung. Berlin, Felisch.
2. Becher, W. 1891. Rudolf Virchow. Berlin, S. Karger.
3. Benedikt, M. 1865. Nachruf. *Wiener Med. Presse.* **37**: 915.
4. ——. 1906. Aus meinem Leben. Erinnerungen und Erörterungen. Wien, C. Konegen.
5. Bidder, F. H. 1847. Zur Lehre vom Verhältnis der Ganglien-Körper zu den Nervenfasern. Leipzig, Breitkopf & Härtel.
6. Bidder, F. H., and A. W. Volkmann. 1842. Die Selbständigkeit des sympathischen Nervensystems durch anatomische Untersuchungen nachgewiesen. Leipzig, Breitkopf & Härtel.
7. Braun, Gustav. 1926. Rudolf Virchow und der Lehrstuhl für pathologische Anatomie an der Universität Zürich. Zürich, O. Füssli.
8. Burdach, Karl. 1848. Rückblick auf mein Leben. Leipzig, L. Voss.
9. Callisen, A. C. P. 1830–1845. Medicinisches *Schriftstellerlexikon.* 33 v. Copenhagen and Altona.
10. Carus, Carl Gustav. 1866. Lebenserinnnerungen und Denkwürdigkeiten. Leipzig, F. A. Brockhaus.
11. Du Bois-Reymond, Emil. 1860. Gedächtnisrede auf Joh. Müller. *Abh. d. K. Akad. d. Wissensch. zu Berlin* 1859: 25–176.
12. Duchenne de Boulogne, G. 1856. Ueber methodische Elektrisierung gelähmter Muskeln. *Canstatt's Jahresber.* 1856: 250.
13. Ehrenberg, C. G. 1833. Nothwendigkeit einer feineren mechanischen Zerlegung des Gehirns und der Nerven vor der Chemischen, dargestellt aus Beobachtungen. *Poggendorfs Annalen der Physik und Chemie* **28**: 449–473.
14. Ehrlich, Ad. 1865. Nekrolog. *Allg. Ztg. d. Judentums.* **1865**: 619.
15. Eulenburg, A., and P. Guttmann. 1873. Die Pathologie des Sympathicus auf physiologischer Grundlage. Berlin, A. Hirschwald.
16. Fontana, F. 1787. Abhandlungen über das Viperngift. Berlin, C. F. Himburg.
17. Fulton, John F. 1929. Edward Selleck Hare (1812–1838) and the syndrome of paralysis of the cervical sympathetic. *Proc. Roy. Soc. Med.* **23**: 152–157.
18. ——. 1929. Horner and the syndrome of paralysis of the cervical sympathetic. *Arch. of Surg.* **18**: 2025–2039.

19. Geiger, Ludwig. 1908. Zum Andenken an Moritz Veit. *Monatsschrift f. Gesch. u. Wissensch. d. Judentums.* **52**: 513–539.
20. ——. 1915. Robert Remak. *Allgem. Ztg. des Judentums* **79**: 354–355.
21. ——. 1916. Briefe Alexander von Humboldt's an Dr. Remak 1839–1855. *Jahrb. f. jüdische Geschichte und Literatur.* **19**: 112–134.
22. Gluge, Gottlieb. 1850. Atlas der pathologischen Anatomie. 2 v. Jena, F. Mauke.
23. ——. 1853. Atlas of pathological histology. Translated by Joseph Leidy. Philadelphia, Blanchard & Lea.
24. Graefe, A. v. 1864. Note. *Klin. Monatsbl. f. Augenheilk.* **3**: 185.
25. ——. 1865. Sitzungsbericht, Berliner Medizinische Gesellschaft. *Berl. Klin. Wochenschr.* **2**: 479.
26. Haberling, Wilhelm. 1924. Johannes Müller. Das Leben des Rheinischen Naturforschers. Leipzig, Akad. Verlag.
27. Hannover, Adolph. 1840. Die Chromsäure ein vorzügliches Mittel bei mikroskopischen Untersuchungen. *Müller's Archiv* **1840**: 549–558.
28. ——. 1843. Mikroskopiske Undersögelser of Nervesystem. *Kgl. Danske Videnskabernes Selskabs Afhandl.* **10**: 1–113.
29. ——. 1844. Recherches microscopique sur le systeme nerveux. Copenhagen, Paris and Leipzig, Philipsen.
30. Helmholtz, Hermann. 1842. De Fabrica Systematis nervosi evertebratorum. Doctoral thesis, Berlin, Typis Nietackianis.
31. Henle, J. 1841. Allgemeine Anatomie. Leipzig, L. Voss.
32. ——. 1882. Theodor Schwann. *Arch. Mikr. Anat.* **21**: I–XLIX.
33. Hensel, S. 1882. Die Familie Mendelssohn. 2 v. 3rd ed. Berlin, B. Behr.
34. Horner, J. F. 1869. Ueber eine Form von Ptosis. *Klin. Monatsbl. f. Augenheilkunde* **7**: 193–198.
35. Humboldt, A. v. 1797. Versuche über die gereizte Muskel-und Nervenfaser. 2 v. Posen und Berlin, Decker & Co. (see vol. **1**: 324).
36. Johnstone, James. 1764. Essay on the use of the ganglions of the nerves. *Phil. Trans. Roy. Soc. London.* **54**: 177–184.
37. Johnston [*sic*], J. 1767. History of a foetus born with a very imperfect brain to which is subjoined a supplement of the essay on the use of ganglions. *Phil. Trans. Roy. Soc. London.* **57**: 118–131.
38. Johnstone, James. 1771. An essay on the use of the ganglions of nerves. Shrewsbury, J. Eddowes.
39. Johnstone, James. 1795. Medical essays and observations with disquisitions relating to the nervous system. Evesham, J. Agg.
40. Kalisch, M. 1860. Die Judenfrage in ihrer wahren Bedeutung für Preussen. Leipzig, Veith & Co.
41. Kisch, Bruno. 1951. Horner's syndrome an American discovery. *Bull. of Hist. of Med.* **25**: 284–288.
42. Koelliker, A. v. 1844. Die Selbstständigkeit und Abhängigkeit des sympathischen Nervensystems, durch anatomische Beobachtungen bewiesen. Zürich, Meyer & Zeller.
43. ——. 1899. Erinnerungen • aus meinem Leben. Leipzig, Engelmann.
44. Königsberger, Leo. 1902–3. Hermann von Helmholtz. 3 v. Braunschweig, F. Wieweg & Sohn.
45. Kronthal, Arthur. 1933. Die Beziehungen Robert Remak' zum Polentum. *Deutsche Wissensch. Zeitschr. f. Polen.* **1933**: 123.
46. Lazarus, M. 1913. Aus meiner Jugend. Frankfurt a.M., J. Kauffmann.
47. Leyden, Ernst. 1893. Zum hundertjährigen Geburtstage Johann Lucas Schönlein's. *Deutsche Med. Wochenschr.* **19**: 1249–1253.
48. Merkel, Fr. Jacob Henle. *Abh. d. Kgl. Ges. d. Wissensch. z. Göttingen.* Göttingen.
49. ——. 1891. Jacob Henle. Braunschweig.
50. Michaelis. E. 1877. Albrecht von Graefe, Berlin, Reimer.
51. Mitchell, S. Weir, G. R. Morehouse and W. W. Keen. 1864. Gunshot wounds and other injuries of nerves. Philadelphia, J. B. Lippincott & Co.
52. Müller, Joh. 1844. Handbuch der Physiologie des Menschen. v. I, 4th ed. Coblenz, J. Hölscher.
53. Naunin, B. 1908. Die Berliner Schule vor 50 Jahren. *Volkmann's Sammlung Klinischer Vorträge.* No. 478. Leipzig, Breitkopf u. Härtel.
54. Nothnagel, H. 1876. Ueber Neuritis in diagnostischer und pathologischer Beziehung. *Volkmann's Sammlung klinischer Vorträge.* No. 103. Leipzig, Breitkopf u. Härtel.
55. Oppeln-Bronikowski, Friedrich v. 1928. David Ferdinand Koreff, Berlin u. Leipzig, Gebrüder Paetel.
56. Pagel, J. 1897. Die Entwicklung der Medicin in Berlin. Wiesbaden, J. F. Bergmann.
57. ——. 1889. R. Remak. *Allg. Deutsche Biogr.* **28**: 191–192.
58. Pagel, W. 1945. The speculative basis of modern pathology. Jahn, Virchow and the philosophy of pathology. *Bull. Hist. of Med.* **18**: 1–43.
59. Purkinje, J. E. 1838. *Ber. über d. Vers. Deutscher Naturforscher u. Aerzte in Prag.* Prag.
60. Rabl, Marie. 1906. Rudolf Virchow. Briefe an seine Eltern 1839–1864. Leipzig, W. Engelmann.
61. Remak, Robert. 1836. Vorläufige Mitteilung microscopischer Beobachtungen über den innern Bau der Cerebrospinalnerven und über die Entwicklung ihrer Formelemente. *Müller's Archiv* **1836**: 145–161.
62. ——. 1837. Weitere microscopische Beobachtungen über die Primitivefasern des Nervensystems der Wirbeltiere. *Froriep's Notizen,* 2nd Ser. **3**: 36–40.
63. ——. 1837. Vermischte Anatomische Beobachtungen. *Froriep's Notizen* **3**: 150–154.
64. ——. 1838. Observationes anatomicae et microscopicae de systematis nervosi structura. Doctoral thesis. Berlin, Reimer.
65. ——. 1938. O budowie nerwów i zwojów nerwowych. *Pamietnik Towarzystwa Lekarskiègo.* **2**: 325–374.
66. ——. 1842. Bericht über die Leistungen im Gebiete der Physiologie im Jahre 1841. *Canstatt's Jahresber. d. ges. Med.* Erlangen.
67. ——. [Signed R.R.-K.] 1844. Sphygmologia. *Encyclop. Wörterbuch d. med. Wissensch.* **32**: 46–57.
68. ——. 1845. Diagnostische und pathogenetische Untersuchungen, in der Klinik des Herrn Geh. Raths Dr. Schönlein auf dessen Veranlassung angestellt und mit Benutzung anderweitiger Beobachtungen veröffentlicht. Berlin, A. Hirschwald.
69. ——. 1850–1855. Untersuchungen über die Entwicklung der Wirbeltiere. Berlin, G. Reimer.
70. ——. 1852. Ueber die Enstehung des Bindegewebes und des Knorpels. *Müller's Archiv* **1852**: 63–72.
71. ——. 1852. Ueber extracelluläre Entstehung thierischer Zellen und Vermehrung derselben durch Zellteilung. *Müller's Archiv* **1852**: 47–57.
72. ——. 1856. Ueber methodische Elektrisierung gelähmter Muskeln. 2nd ed. Berlin, A. Hirschwald.
73. ——. 1858. Galvanotherapie der Nerven und Muskelkrankheiten. Berlin, A. Hirschwald.
74. Retzius, G. 1900. Briefe von Johannes Müller and Anders Retzius. Stockholm, Aftenbladets Artieboligs Tryckeri.

75. RILLE, J. H. 1926. David Gruby. *Derm. Wochensch.* **82**: 512–526.

76. SACHERO, G. 1843. Delle functioni dei nervi spinali e cerebrali e del Nervo Sympathico. Libri quattro del professore G. Valentin. Torino.

77. SALOMONSON, CARL J. 1950. Reminiscences of the summer semester, 1877, at Breslau. Translated with notes and a biographical index by C. Lilian Temkin. *Bull. of Hist. of Med.* **24**: 333–351.

78. SMITH, HAMILTON. 1882. Memoir of Charles A Spencer. *Proc. of the Soc. of Microscopists* **1882**: 49–74.

79. STAHL, ERNST. 1904. Matthias Jacob Schleiden. Jena, G. Neuenhahn.

80. STIEDA, L. 1899. Geschichte der Entwicklung der Lehre von den Nervenzellen und Nervenfasern während des 19. Jahrhunderts. Festschrift zum 70. Geburtstag von Carl v. Kupffer. Jena, G. Fischer.

81. VIRCHOW, RUDOLF. 1847. Ueber die Reform der pathologischen und therapeutischen Anschauungen durch die mikroskopischen Untersuchungen. *Virchow's Arch.* **1**: 207–255.

82. ——. 1854. Handbuch der speciellen Pathologie und Therapie. v. 1. Erlangen und Stuttgart, F. Enke.

83. WALDEYER-HARTZ, WILHELM VON. 1920. Lebenserinnerungen. Bonn, F. Cohen.

84. WALTHER, PHILIPP F. v. 1803. Ueber die therapeutische Indikation und den Technicismus der Galvanischen Operation. Wien.

85. WRZOSEK, ADAM. 1925. Stosunek Roberta Remaka do nauki Polskiej i Spoteczenstwa Polskiego. *Arch. Hist. i. Filoz. Medicyny.* **3**: 173–187.

86. 1847. Der Orient. 5th of Nov.: 357.

87. 1855. Einfuhrbehandlung der sogenannten magnetischen Amulette. *Oesterr. Ztschr. f. prakt. Heilkunde* **1**: 207.

88. 1858. *Notizen. Oesterr. Zeitschr. f. prakt. Heilkunde* **4**: 755.

89. 1859. Anonymous review in *Med. Times and Gazette* **18**: 372–373.

90. 1860. Fünfzigjährige Jubelfeier der Berliner Universität. *Oesterr. Zeitschr. f. prakt. Heilkunde* **6**: 702.

91. 1864. Dr. Remak in Paris. *Oesterr. Zeitschr. f. prakt. Heilkunde* **10**: 965.

92. 1865. *Berlin. Klin. Wochensch.* **2**: 372.

93. 1865. *Allgem. Zeitg. d. Judentums.* **1865**: 602.

94. 1865. Eulogy. *Deutsche Klinik.* **1865**: 413.

95. 1905. Medicina in Nummis. A catalogue of the firm Robert Ball. Berlin, Ball.

96. 1898. 30 Jahre experimentelle Pathologie. Leipzig and Vienna, F. Deuticke (see p. 25).

97. 1945. Three American microscope builders. Buffalo, N. Y., American Optical Co.

IV. LEOPOLD AUERBACH

1828–1897

INTRODUCTION

In 1828, the same year in which G. G. Valentin entered the University of Breslau as a student of medicine and natural sciences, Leopold Auerbach was born in the same town in Silesia, the son of a Jewish merchant.

The course of Auerbach's life bears some similarities to that of his famous compatriot Valentin. Eagerness to study and enthusiasm for research in the field of natural science led him to enter the university despite the desire of his parents to make him an efficient merchant. As in the case of Valentin, this devotion lasted to the end of his life and led him to outstanding discoveries in the field of modern medicine.

Like Valentin, Auerbach, though he was not an orthodox Jew, retained his Jewish faith all his life and therefore never had a chance to secure a position in Germany commensurate with his knowledge and his achievements, nor was he given any encouragement there despite the recognition he received for his scientific work throughout the entire medical world. Less fortunate than Valentin, no opportunity was opened to him outside of Germany to be assigned his own laboratory; thus, he was compelled to limit his research work to such investigations as he was able to carry on in his private home, in two small rooms on the third floor of an apartment house in Breslau. And even that he could do only as far as his limited means permitted him, without neglecting the needs of the large family he raised. The main official recognition that Auerbach received for the purpose of furthering his work came toward the end of his life when, in 1889, the Berlin Academy of Sciences (Akademie der Wissenschaften in Berlin) loaned him a modern Zeiss microscope and a microtome at the suggestion of his old admirer and friend, Professor Waldeyer.

If we bear in mind that the man who had so little success in his personal career was the one who discovered the nervous *Plexus Myenthericus* in the intestinal tract, who proved that the endothelium in capillaries and lymphatic vessels consists of a layer of nucleated cells, who was the first to see the conjugation of two nuclei in the fertilized egg, and reported the figures later described in detail by Bütschli, Hertwig, and others, it is inconceivable that his name and his contributions should be practically forgotten today.

Two previous biographical sketches, eulogies written shortly after Auerbach's death, were sources for the writing of Auerbach's biography. One of these was by the embryologist Professor Born of Breslau, well acquainted with Auerbach and a friend and steady guest in his home for many years. This eulogy was published in the fourteenth volume of the *Anatomische Anzeiger* in 1898 (4).[1] There is also a small pamphlet printed in Breslau in 1898 (6) containing the text of the funeral oration delivered on October 3, 1897 by Auerbach's close friend, the famous botanist Ferdinand Cohn of Breslau, and a short biography of Auerbach (6). Ferdinand Cohn survived his friend by only a very short time. Graetzer's well known history of famous physicians of Silesia, which appeared in 1889, does not give any data on Auerbach except for the short statement that he became a member of the Leopoldinische Carolinische Academy of Science in February 1881. This valuable book concerns only already deceased physicians from Silesia, and Auerbach was still alive at the time of its publication. A few data on Auerbach's activities are obtainable from biographical sources like the *Allgemeine Deutsche Biographie* (11)

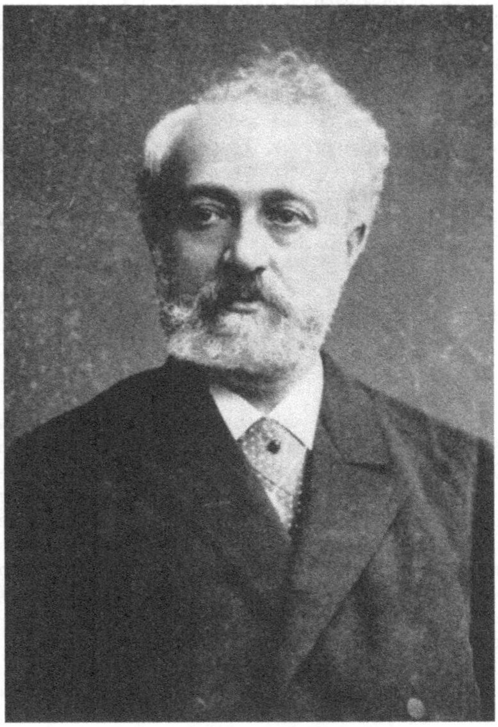

FIG. 57. Leopold Auerbach. Courtesy of the University of Wraclaw (Breslau), Poland.

[1] Numbers in parentheses indicate references at end of chapter, p. 313.

and other biographical dictionaries concerning famous physicians. But all these sources do not amount to much and are based largely on the two above-mentioned eulogies.

For the following biography all of Auerbach's publications had to be studied, including the short autobiography (Vita) in his doctoral thesis of 1849 (2). In addition, there exists an autobiographical sketch by Ferdinand Cohn (7), also instructive with regard to his friend Auerbach. A great deal of original material, including many interesting letters by Auerbach as well as those written to him by well known persons like Ferdinand Cohn, Waldeyer, Moritz Traube, Lothar Meyer, and Jacob Moleschott, and some letters addressed to his family on the occasion of his death, is still extant. All this material and Auerbach's complete work were carefully assembled and preserved by his oldest son, Dr. Felix Auerbach, Professor of Physics at the University of Jena (Germany), outstanding as a scientist, a fine artist, and a humanistically well educated person. He and his congenial wife were very fond of their niece Ruth Kisch-Arndt, and from them she and this writer inherited all the pertinent documents when Felix Auerbach and his wife after fifty years of happy companionship chose to leave this life together in 1933 when their beloved Germany fell prey to cruel barbarism.

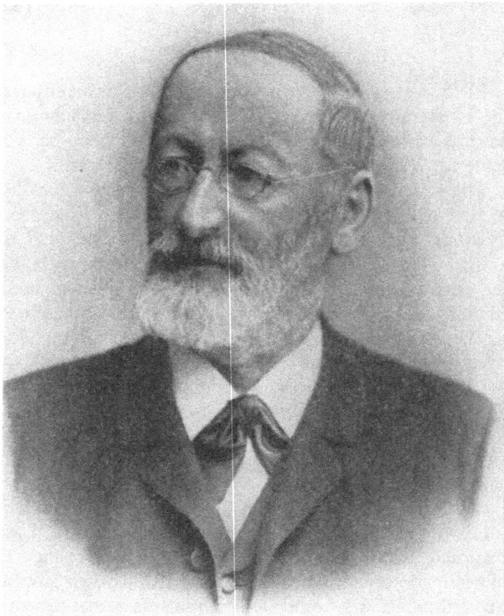

FIG. 58. Professor Ferdinand Cohn in Breslau. The famous botanist and lifelong friend of Auerbach. From heliogravure in the author's possession.

YOUTH

Leopold Auerbach was born of Jewish parents on April 28, 1828, in Breslau, the capital of German Silesia. His father was Salomon Auerbach and his mother Julia Danziger. Leopold Auerbach was three months the junior of his life long friend and colleague in the field of research, Ferdinand Cohn, who was born in the same city on January 24, 1828, and who was to become the leading botanist and plant physiologist of his time, the founder of the modern system of bacteriology, and full professor at the University of Breslau. Cohn gives in his autobiography a vivid picture of conditions in his home town at the time when Auerbach was born (7).

As far back as the early 1800's, Breslau had, by a decree of Napoloeon I, ceased to be a fortress. However, in 1828 the town had not yet spread beyond the limits of the old battled wall. There were still reminders of the Napoleonic wars; the bridges connecting the suburbs with Breslau that had been burned in 1808 were only poorly restored.

In the southwestern corner of the city, between the river Ohle and the town moat, was situated the Jewish Ghetto. There were no gates, as in other German towns, to lock in the Jewish quarter every night, but the Jewish inhabitants nevertheless crowded in the small streets of this part of the city, and only a few dared to live and have their places of business outside the Ghetto. The number of Jews permitted to settle in Breslau was still limited at the beginning of the century. Some were compelled to live under the designation of servants, even if they were independent persons, in order to obtain as Jews permission to stay in the city. But if one of these unfortunate pseudo-citizens died, the body could not be buried in Breslau; it had to be brought to one of the towns in the neighborhood where a Jewish cemetery existed. In the early years of the nineteenth century most of the Jewish families in Breslau were very poor; it was only when the political status of the Jews legally improved in 1812 and when, later, the railroad system made Breslau more important, and the natural resources of Silesia more useful, that the financial condition of its inhabitants, Jews and non-Jews alike, improved. However, there still remained some discrimination, and in 1847, for instance, Ferdinand Cohn had to go to Berlin in order to be able to graduate as a doctor from the philosophical faculty, for, as a Jew, he was not admitted to the essential examinations in Breslau (7). It was not until 1859 that a decree of the Prussian Minister declared that Jews should be awarded the doctor's degree under the same conditions as Christians and that they should be admitted to lecturing positions in the law faculty of Breslau University.

Among the Jewish business men of Breslau who lived in comfortable financial circumstances in the middle of the last century was Leopold Auerbach's father, Salomon Auerbach. There is a remark by Ferdinand Cohn, who knew him very well for many decades, characterizing his personality in a letter to his friend Leopold on August 3, 1870, a few days after the death of Salomon Auerbach on July 30, 1870. Cohn speaks of him as an "unpretentious, kind hearted, pious" man. Leopold Auerbach was his oldest son. He and three brothers are mentioned in the father's last will deposited with the Koenigliches Stadtgericht at Breslau on January 23, 1865. There the four children are mentioned in the following sequence, with their Jewish second names added: (1) Leopold (Gabriel, Loebel), practicing physician in Breslau; (2) Ludwig (Lipman), *medicinae doctor* in Berlin; (3) Hermann (Hirsch), merchant in Breslau; (4) Wilhelm (Wolf) merchant in Breslau. In this will also a brother of Salomon Auerbach who lived and died in Posen was left an annuity up to his death. That Salomon Auerbach was a rather well-to-do man can be also be assumed from the marriage contract of his son, Leopold, signed by the notary Carl Moritz Fraenkel, Justizrat and lawyer in Breslau. In this contract of January 18, 1855 Salomon Auerbach promised his son Leopold on the occasion of his wedding the sum of 10,000 Thaler, equal approximately to 10,000 American dollars at that time, a quite large sum of money. Leopold Auerbach was fortunate enough to grow up in a prosperous and, as we know from other indications, very cultured family.

He received his first instruction in reading and writing from private teachers and did not enter school until 1838, when he was admitted to the Elisabeth Gymnasium in Breslau. At that time it was customary for a Jewish boy, having reached the age of thirteen years, to turn to a profession or occupation in which he was expected to earn his livelihood later. That may have been the reason why, according to his report cards, Auerbach left the Elisabethanum in 1841. His last school report is dated July of that year. It is noteworthy that the grades he received in the various subjects during these three years were only average, without any special excellence. This is true especially for French, Latin, German, and history. In Hebrew his progress was satisfactory, but he came late to the classes. Only in science and physics were the marks better. Thus his parents may have been under the impression that their oldest son was neither a prodigy nor so outstanding a scholar that it would have been a crime not to allow him to continue his studies at the Gymnasium.

Auerbach followed the wish of his parents that he enter a business as an apprentice. But he was as little satisfied with the activities of a businessman as his contemporary famous colleague from Frankfurt, Moritz Schiff, who as a child was also supposed to become a merchant, but who later became physiologist and professor. Auerbach's parents did not wish to force their son to enter a career for which he had no desire, and so he picked up his studies again at the Royal Catholic Gymnasium (St. Matthias) in Breslau. Only fourteen and a half years old, he was admitted to the highest class (prima) in this institution. His school grades there were much better, showing improvement with progressing adolescence. In 1844, at the age of only sixteen years, he was able to graduate from this school. This graduation entitled him to enter the University of Breslau, where he immediately began to study medicine.

The report on his graduation from the Gymnasium has the following to say about him: "He was on good terms with his classmates, he was always respectful to his teachers and he always endeavored to show proper and decent behavior. Highly talented, he was diligent and careful and, thus, he was happily able to reach his goal at so young an age and with honors." The detailed account of Auerbach's achievements on his graduation certificate mentions that he was able to translate well and easily Latin and Greek texts, and that he had a good understanding of the meaning of the classics. He is also commended for his well grounded knowledge of German literature, and for his mastery of the German as well as the French language. It appears that he was not eager to continue with his Hebrew studies, for the report states that he did not attend these classes. His knowledge of the Bible was regarded as not satisfactory, but in mathematics, history, and geography, as well as in the natural sciences and philosophy, he did so well that he passed the examination (Maturitätsprüfung) before the Royal Commission, which decided on August 17, 1844 to permit him to enter the medical or any other faculty of a University.

MEDICAL STUDIES IN BRESLAU AND BERLIN

On October 14, 1844, Auerbach was admitted to the medical faculty of the University of Breslau. There he remained for two years; he left in 1846 with the intention of continuing his studies in Berlin. The certificate he received from the University of Breslau gives his birth date as April 25, 1828, and as the date of matriculation October 12, 1844. These first years of university work were devoted to very intensive study. In contrast to his report cards from the lower schools, the Breslau certificate of his first two years as medical student is full of praise for his diligence and application. It mentions all the classes he attended, the instructors, and, in the old fashion, also the grade for conduct given him by each, which was unanimously one of the highest praise. It is indicative of the times and of political conditions in Germany that the certificate also states that Auerbach was not suspected of having taken part in any of the illegal student fraternities at the University. It is signed on October 12, 1846, by Purkinje as Dean of the Medical Faculty.

Purkinje at that time was the outstanding personality on this faculty. Auerbach attended his classes repeatedly, for instance the physiology class of the summer term of 1845. During the winter term 1845–1846, he attended a class called Physiology of Sexual Life and one called Histology of Men, both given by Purkinje. His other instructors at Breslau, who are worth mentioning as outstanding scholars, were the botanist Nees von Esenbeck and the chemist Goeppert. Auerbach studied anatomy there with Otto and Barkow and, as required, he took botany, zoology, mineralogy, chemistry, and physics in addition to medical subjects. That he also took courses in mathematics, philosophy, and astronomy at that time may have been owing in part to the influence of Ferdinand Cohn. The friendship with the latter started in their childhood. Of course, each family in the Ghetto knew all the others well. The religious life, so beautifully described by Cohn in his autobiography (7), the common lot and the common problems of daily life, of the education of the children, and so forth brought families with similar background and ideals close together. In the text of his disputation, after his inauguration lecture as Privatdozent in 1863, Auerbach mentions that at that time their friendship was already of two decades' duration. An entry in Cohn's diary (7) in 1846 mentions Auerbach with whom in that year he climbed the Riesengebirge Mountains to the highest point, the Schneekoppe. Cohn characterizes his companion as "his very lovable friend." They hiked together to all the famous hills, valleys, and the little towns on the border of Silesia and Bohemia, where they experienced together "free and happy, wonderful, blissful moments in the mountains and in the valleys; moments which I never will forget."

This was the wonderful enthusiastic, though sentimental, atmosphere of romanticism that surrounded the German youth of the end of the eighteenth and the first half of the nineteenth centuries. This was a time of heroism, revolutionary street fighting, jubilant war spirit, but also a time of self pity and the weeping spirit of unhappy romance, as expressed by so many of Heine's love poems. Cohn's diaries mirror this sentiment as distinctly as a great deal of the German literature of that time. The high spirit of this epoch of German idealism embraced the two university students from Breslau's Ghetto, and their friendship is no less intense, though on a higher level, than that between two of their average Teutonic colleagues united in a color-bearing, politically active German fraternity.

Unfortunately, Auerbach's diaries are not preserved, and we find him only occasionally remembered in Cohn's. The spirit of their friendship and the nature of their activities can be seen in various remarks in Cohn's diaries. For instance, on January 27, 1846 Cohn describes his working day: "Up to 4 P.M.," he writes, "I was in college, up to 8 P.M. with Auerbach discussing different problems, then we went to the 'Ring' [a famous promenade in Breslau] and we admired the wonderful starry sky in spite of frost, wind and all the people." On February 2, 1846 he writes how he "together with Auerbach did not study," as intended, Pohl's electromagnetism, but many other things and "many good resolutions were made." What those things were is revealed in the February 2 entry: "with Auerbach we discussed much about the perfectness of the universe and about perfectionism." The friends visited the Bernardiner Church together, enjoying the music and the sermons of the popular preacher, Krause, and when Krause was replaced by another minister they preferred to walk and discuss their problems in the free air. The main problem for both of them was the continuation and completion of their university education in the best possible way, and they planned to do this at another university. Such a change to another institution was and still is customary with students in Germany. Auerbach must have been tempted by the growing fame of Berlin as an outstanding center for medical study in Germany; for his friend other considerations existed too. Under the law, Cohn, as a Jew, as mentioned before, could not receive his Ph.D. degree at Breslau. Thus it was that the two students decided to go together to Berlin. On October 17, 1846 Auerbach was admitted to the University of Berlin, as a student in the medical faculty, and there he remained for more than two years. Time and again we find his name in the interesting diaries of Ferdinand Cohn (7), and from these diaries we learn how they both experienced all the excitement of the days of the Revolution of 1848 and the fighting in the streets of Berlin.

During their stay in Berlin the close friendship between Auerbach and Cohn and their frequent meetings continued in spite of the fact that they were students of different faculties and lived in different quarters. Cohn's diary reports on January 10 that they discussed meteorological problems and apparatus: "We discussed that with Auerbach (Tierarzneischulplatz 3) whom I visited that evening and talked about our home town, homesickness, the register of the stove and atmospheric pressure." Two days later the diary records Auerbach's and Samoje's (a common, close friend) visit at Cohn's quarters, where they did *not* consume, as was usual for German students of their age in these days, beer in great quantities, but an "excellent home made chocolate." Once when the two friends did not meet for an entire week, in that pre-telephone time, Cohn's diary mentions this fact as something unusual.

When, finally, on November 13, 1847, the nineteen-year-old Ferdinand Cohn received his Ph.D. degree, his four best friends, Pohl, Friedländer, Samoje, and Auerbach, participated in the solemn festivities following the graduation. When Cohn, in accordance with historical custom, had to defend his doctor's thesis publicly (5), Leopold Auerbach figured as the first of his opponents, an honor that was usually bestowed upon the closest friends of the doctor-to-be. Sixteen years later, when Auerbach was in a similar position publicly defending his thesis for the diploma of a lecturer (Privatdozent) at the University of Breslau, we find Ferdinand Cohn as one of his three official opponents. After his graduation, Cohn received the permission of his parents to remain in Berlin and to continue with his research. Then it was that both friends lived together through the stirring times of 1848. It is typical that when the news of the French (February) Revolution reached Berlin and Cohn heard it first, in his ecstatic excitement he ran to bring the news to Auerbach. He found him at home, busy with his books and studying. Both hurried to the Zeitungshalle, a place where newspapers of various types and from different countries could be found. Here they witnessed together the arrival of the latest news reporting the proclamation of the French Republic and the dethronement of Louis Philippe. The youthful romanticists were deeply impressed. The diary reports: "It is impossible to describe our sentiments. The impression remains unforgettable. Tears, embracing, everyone is jubilant in the feeling of fraternity."

The French Revolution was the beginning. A few weeks later followed the revolution of the people in Berlin and all over Germany. That was an extremely exciting time for the two friends, as it was for everyone in Berlin and in the entire country, but after a short and brilliant success, the German revolution collapsed, and the reaction and the persecution of democrats by military and police forces started. "Gegen Demokraten helfen nur Soldaten"[2] was the slogan. The political hangover came and Cohn returned to his home town, Breslau. Auerbach remained in Berlin, using all the opportunities it offered to continue his studies and taking full advantage of the modern development of German medicine, which had started just a few decades before and soon made Berlin a world renowned center of medical progress.

At Breslau two of Auerbach's professors, Purkinje (1787–1869), already well advanced in years, and Goeppert, may be regarded as the outstanding and most inspiring members of the medical faculty at that time. It was different at Berlin. Many famous names were among the faculty members there, everyone of them known as a stimulating personality, leaving their permanent traces in the field of medical research. It must have been extremely impressive to each academic newcomer that the world renowned Johannes Müller, at that politically dangerous time of 1848 Rector of the University, or another of the luminaries of medicine or science, personally took his oath of allegiance to Berlin University. Johannes Müller, who in 1846 was Dean of the Medical Faculty, admitted Auerbach as a student and was his professor in pathological anatomy. Auerbach studied histology, embryology, and microscopical semiotics under Robert Remak. The latter was only thirty-two years of age but already famous for his

[2] "The only remedy against democrats is soldiers."

neuro-histological studies and in 1847 had just won his struggle to be admitted as a lecturer at Berlin's University without the usually demanded baptism. Christian Ehrenberg was Auerbach's instructor in physiology of living organisms of microscopical dimensions. In clinical medicine and pathology he had the privilege of working under Romberg, Schönlein, L. Traube, and the young Virchow, the rising star on the medical horizon, who also had just started lecturing at Berlin in 1846. In 1847 the first issue of a medical *Archiv* appeared, which was founded by the twenty-six-year-old Virchow in collaboration with his friend Reinhardt. Virchow was officially appointed Privatdozent at Berlin University in 1847. The lectures of the interesting young doctor, a vigorous revolutionary in medicine as well as in politics, were in Berlin's medical circles the sensation of the time. He was able to report in letters to his father (9) that since 1847 even old medical digni-

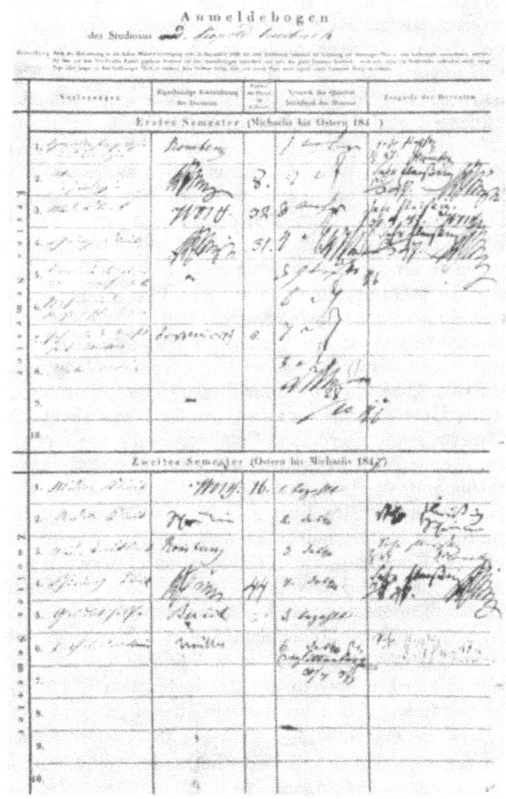

FIG. 59. Page from Auerbach's book of registered classes with teachers' signatures (among them Romberg, Poggendorff, Schoenlein, Joh. Müller), 1846–47. In the author's possession.

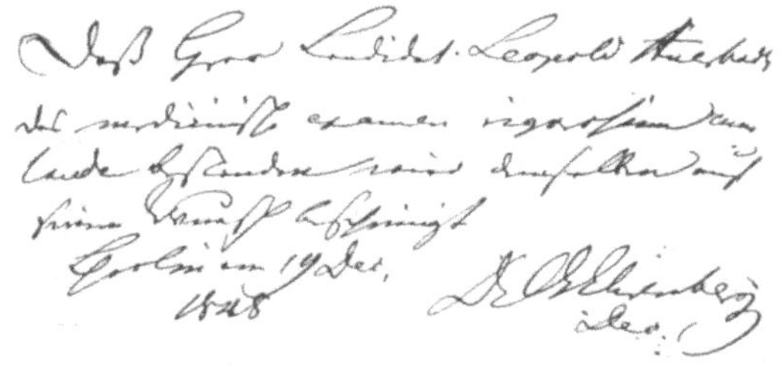

FIG. 60. Certificate signed by Ehrenberg as Dean of the Faculty, that L. Auerbach passed his examination *cum laude*. In the author's possession.

taries as well as young doctors and students were present in his audience (15).

This was a group of teachers of such extraordinary importance that every student of medicine at Berlin could consider himself extremely fortunate and was the envy of all his less privileged colleagues at other universities. Although we know that Auerbach had close personal contact with his teacher Remak (4), he must have been influenced by his other instructors as well, who imparted to the Berlin Medical Faculty the high lustre of its golden age (6). He was unquestionably influenced also by continuous contact with Ferdinand Cohn and other gifted young students. He was privileged in another way too, unusual for a student at that time, in that he became the owner of a good microscope. Some of the professors then permitted a favored pupil the use of their own microscope, but only the singularly fortunate among the students received from their parents the necessary funds to buy one (6). The cost of a good microscope during the first half of the nineteenth century was about 300 Thaler. That was a small fortune, considering that—as we know from the biography of Ernst Abbe (1)—the *annual* salary of a full professor at the University of Jena in those days was about 200 Thaler a year. Ferdinand Cohn received a fine modern microscope from his father while he was studying at Berlin, and Auerbach was given by his parents a similar microscope from the firm of Schieck (6). It was the same type of instrument as that used by Auerbach's teacher, Ehrenberg, for his studies on Infusoria (now called Ciliata) and by young Virchow (15). Although Auerbach unquestionably had some instruction from his teachers, such as Johannes Müller, Ehrenberg, and Remak, it was mainly by the autodidactic method that he had to learn how to use this instrument efficiently. As Ferdinand Cohn pointed out, it was at that time largely the eagerness and ability of the owner of such a microscope that determined whether he would become a good microscopist or not (4, 6, 7).

After all the commotion of the turbulent year of 1848 had subsided, Auerbach graduated as a medical doctor from the University of Berlin on January 18, 1849, with a thesis (2) dedicated to his parents, written in Latin and titled, "De Irritamentis Nervorum Studia Critica" (Critical Studies on Nervous Irritation). In this thesis Auerbach stressed the point that not heat itself, but change of temperature brought about by warming or cooling, was an irritating stimulus for nerves, just as a steady electric current did not produce action of the nerve, but changes in the intensity of the current or of the voltage. This thesis was undoubtedly written under the influence of the impressive work of Johannes Müller's pupil and assistant, Emil Du Bois-Reymond, whose investigations in animal electricity were just published in 1848. Auerbach also refers in his considerations to the fact of thermoelectricity. He emphasizes that in certain crystals (tourmaline) an increase or decrease in temperature produces the appearance of electric phe-

DE

IRRITAMENTIS NERVORUM

STUDIA CRITICA.

DISSERTATIO

INAUGURALIS NEUROPHYSIOLOGICA

QUAM

CONSENSU ET AUCTORITATE

GRATIOSI MEDICORUM ORDINIS

IN

ALMA LITTERARUM UNIVERSITATE

FRIDERICA GUILELMA

UT SUMMI

IN MEDICINA ET CHIRURGIA HONORES

RITE SIBI CONCEDANTUR

DIE XVIII. M. JANUARII A. MDCCCXLIX.

H. L. Q. S.

PUBLICE DEFENDET

AUCTOR

LEOPOLDUS AUERBACH

VRATISLAVIENSIS.

OPPONENTIBUS:

J. FRIEDLAENDER, Dr. phil.
H. HIRSCHFELD, Dr. med. et chir.
O. POHL, Cand. med.

BEROLINI,

TYPIS FRATRUM SCHLESINGER.

FIG. 61. Front page of Auerbach's Doctoral Thesis. Berlin, January 18, 1849. In the author's possession.

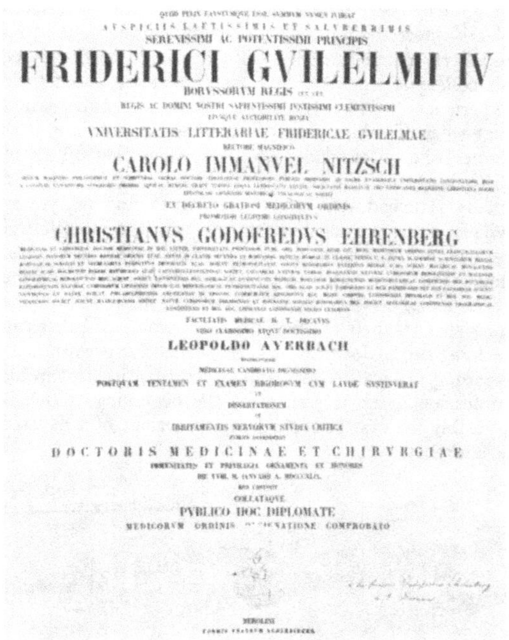

SERENISSIMI AC POTENTISSIMI PRINCIPIS

FRIDERICI GVILELMI IV

BORVSSORVM REGIS

VNIVERSITATIS LITTERARIAE FRIDERICAE GVILELMAE

CAROLO IMMANVEL NITZSCH

CHRISTIANVS GODOFREDVS EHRENBERG

LEOPOLDO AVERBACH

POSTQVAM TENTAMEN ET EXAMEN RIGOROSVM CVM LAVDE SVSTINVERAT

DOCTORIS MEDICINAE ET CHIRVRGIAE

PVBLICO HOC DIPLOMATE

FIG. 62. Doctoral diploma of Auerbach, with the seal of the Medical Faculty of the Berlin University and signature of the Dean, Ch. Ehrenberg. In the author's possession.

nomena, but as soon as the temperature is held steady, there is no more electricity traceable.

GENERAL PRACTITIONER IN BRESLAU

After his graduation, Auerbach returned to his home town, Breslau, and took up the life of a general practitioner. His practice, although it was never overwhelmingly large, kept him busy continually.

During the later years of his life Auerbach specialized increasingly in neurology. However, even when his practice claimed more and more of his time, he never allowed it to keep him entirely away from scientific research, which was really his vocation until the end of his life. Stimulating and inspiring during the early years of his scientific career was his steady contact and close friendship with other brilliant and enthusiastic young scholars. They were, next to Cohn, the physiologist Aubert, the gynecologist Wilhelm Alexander Freund, and others who were at that time active in Breslau and later gained fame and recognition.

"Intellectual friendship," as A. W. Freund called it, united Auerbach in his home town Breslau in a lifelong bond with other physicians who, like himself, were young and eager to do research and to contribute their share to the modern development of science and medicine (10). They created at that time a kind of "Academy," and in monthly meetings presented their new plans and ideas and the results of their research, and discussed and criticized them thoroughly. The members of this inner circle were Richard Forster, the ophthalmologist; Wilhelm Alexander Freund, the gynecologist; Herman Aubert, the physiologist; Heinrich Neumann, the psychiatrist; and a non-medical member, the famous chemist Moritz Traube, Ludwig Traube's brother. After the scientific part of each meeting they remained gayly together till the morning. For the most part they enjoyed themselves listening to music, Freund as violinist and Neumann as pianist entertaining the others with Mozart and Beethoven sonatas. More than half a century later Freund, in his published autobiographical sketch (1913), still reminisces about those happy days and nights (10).

During the first years of Auerbach's practice his research work was concentrated partly on neurological problems and partly on problems of muscle physiology, but the principal area of his interest throughout his life remained microscopical investigation.

Worth mentioning among the publications of his early period is a paper in 1853 on "The Psychic Functions of the Spinal Cord." It contains, on the basis of his own experiments on frogs, fish, lizards, snakes, and rabbits, many valuable experimental observations, and some valid objections to the various laws concerning reflexes set up by Pflüger. Auerbach, like Pflüger, was of the opinion that the spinal cord was able to perform certain independent psychic functions. In the introduction to the paper its author confesses his strict adherence to the materialistic point of view of his day. Psychic activity is a function of organs. In lower animals the "psychic energy" is distributed through the entire substance of the animal or at least through most of it. That is the point of view of the contemporary materialism of Molechott, Vogt, and others. The high spot of this attitude was reached in 1855 in Ludwig Büchner's often reprinted book, *Kraft und Stoff* (*Energy and Matter*).

EARLY RESEARCH

In 1855 Auerbach published his first really important contribution to science. It was an extensive paper that appeared in the seventh volume of von Siebold and Koelliker's *Zeitschrift für die wissenschaftliche Zoologie,* entitled "Über die Einzelligkeit der Amoeben" ("On the Unicellularity of Amoebas"). It was the first proof that this type of living organism is unicellular. But the paper was of higher importance than the title would indicate. It was valid support for the opinion expressed by Koelliker and von Siebold too, that all protozoa are unicellular animals. This view was by no means generally accepted at that time. It was the opinion of many outstanding experts that amoebas have no cell membrane and no nuclei. The excellent and thorough studies of Auerbach demonstrated the exist-

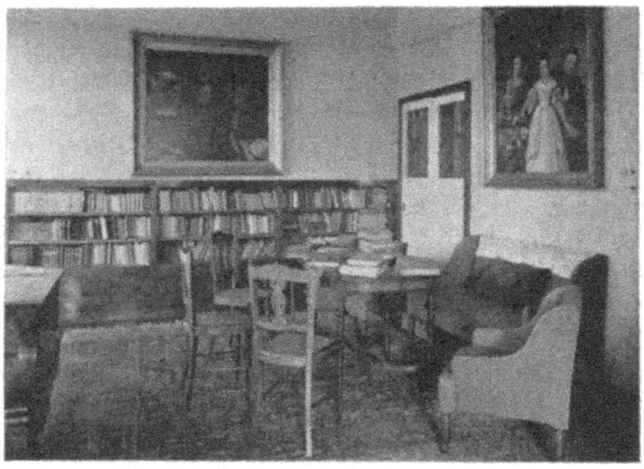

FIG. 63. Drawing room of the late Professor Felix Auerbach in Jena. On the wall is a portrait of his grandparents (parents of Arabella Hess) and their children.

ence of a distinct nucleus in each amoeba. Later the nuclei of cells continued to be a favorite subject of Auerbach's studies.

The year 1855 was noteworthy in Auerbach's private life, too. It was then that he found in Miss Arabella Hess the congenial partner of his future years. He set up a family and established a home that for decades remained a most enjoyable and harmonious center for the small circle of his friends. Professor Born at Breslau asserted in his eulogy (4) that the hours he was privileged to spend in Leopold Auerbach's house were among the happiest memories of his own youth. Arabella Hess, like her husband, loved music and played the piano very well. Later when the six lively children grew up, the house may have become somewhat crowded, but the spirit in it was always a happy one, especially as the children inherited the musical inclinations of their parents. Auerbach's eldest son, Professor Felix, the physicist, a pupil of Hermann Helmholtz, not only was a very gifted musician, but also wrote several interesting books on the physical aspects of music. Another son, Frederic, an outstanding chemist, played the cello very well, and their brother Max became a professional musician and a well known pianist in Breslau.

The young, newly married doctor was still extremely devoted to his medical research. There is an anecdote about his honeymoon which his children who read it in his diary, since lost, remembered. The young couple went to Würzburg, where Koelliker, the famous anatomist and histologist, Auerbach's colleague in this field, and editor of a scientific journal, had the chair of anatomy and physiology and where young Virchow, once Auerbach's teacher at Berlin, was professor of pathology. For Auerbach, such attractions made Würzburg the best honeymooning place to visit with his young wife. As soon as they arrived in this town he left her alone at the Hotel Schwan, promising to be back early enough to go with her to dinner in one of these nice small places where the food was as famous as the wine in its peculiarly shaped bottles. Meantime he went to see his colleague Koelliker and the two talked about their experiences. They were so engrossed in the discussion that when Koelliker invited Auerbach to continue it at dinner, the latter gladly accepted, forgetting all about his bride who was waiting for him in the hotel! He finally returned late in the evening to find his young wife in tears packing their valises with the intention of returning to her parents, disappointed in her neglectful young husband. But no real damage was done, and the relationship between this husband and his wife over the long span of their life was the most wonderful that can be imagined. However, it surely called for great understanding toward her husband's absorbing interest in his profession, later as well as in the beginning, which is probably the case in every happy marriage of a devoted scientist.

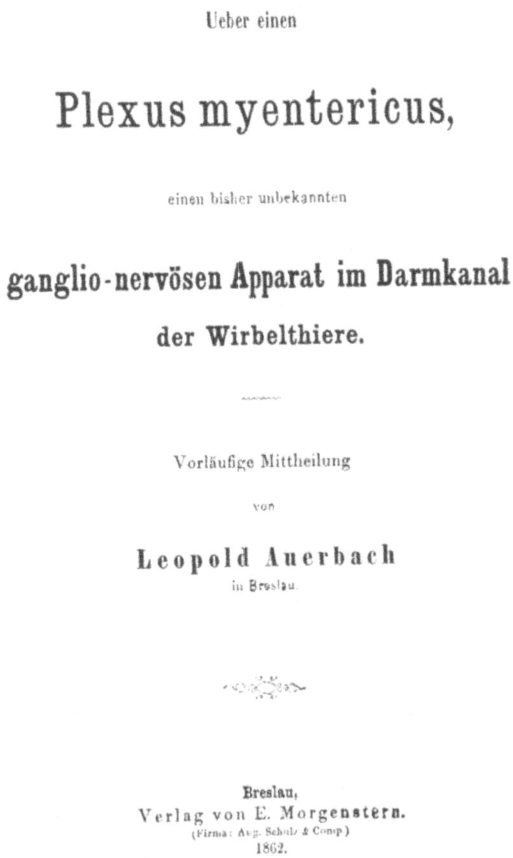

Ueber einen

Plexus myentericus,

einen bisher unbekannten

ganglio-nervösen Apparat im Darmkanal

der Wirbelthiere.

Vorläufige Mittheilung

von

Leopold Auerbach

in Breslau.

Breslau,

Verlag von E. Morgenstern.

(Firma: Aug. Schulz & Comp.)

1862.

FIG. 64. Title page of the pamphlet publishing the discovery of the Plexus Myentericus (Auerbach's Plexus). In the author's possession.

DISCOVERY OF AUERBACH'S PLEXUS

The next years of Auerbach's research were devoted to studies of muscle physiology and their application to clinical problems. But during all this time he did not neglect his studies in microscopy, and in 1862 he published one of the most outstanding discoveries which even today is connected with his name: the discovery of a ganglionic nervous plexus in the intestines of vertebrates located between the various intestinal muscle layers. Auerbach called it the plexus myentericus, usually known as Auerbach's plexus. We know that Auerbach's teacher Remak published a book on the intestinal nerves in 1847 at the time when Auerbach was attending his lectures as a student. Remak, however, overlooked this fundamental element in spite of the fact that he himself was the first to discover ganglionic cells in organs of the body like the heart, the lungs, and the stomach.

It is strange that the preliminary report of Auerbach's plexus was not published in any of the well known archives of these days. Auerbach may have been anxious to establish his priority by putting his findings into print as quickly as possible. So the account of the discovery of Auerbach's plexus was published as a pamphlet, printed in 1862 in Breslau (by E. Morgenstern), bearing the title, *Über einen Plexus Myentericus, einen bisher unbekannten ganglio nervoesen Apparat in Darmkanal der Wirbeltiere. Vorläufige Mitteilung von Leopold Auerbach in Breslau.* This little pamphlet, once for sale at the publishers for 5 Silbergroschen (about twenty-five cents), is today one of the rarest items sought by collectors of medical bibliophylica. It does not contain any pictures, only a description of the discovery. Soon followed several papers by Auerbach on the same subject. The preliminary report, for instance (1862), appeared in the *Proceedings* of the Schlesische Gesellschaft für vaterländische Kultur and in the reports of the Convention of German Physicians and Scientists at Carlsbad (also in 1862, p. 202).

The first publication of 1862 is a classical document of modern medicine in its concise, clear expression, its excellent observation, and the logical evaluation of the new discovery. This contribution is the more admirable when we consider that it was made before the time of modern tissue differentiation by dyes, with the most primitive methods of the modern microscopic era.

It was in 1857 that G. Meissner (1829–1903) discovered a layer of nerve fibers of ganglia and single nerve cells in the submucose tissue of the intestine. Even this fact—the existence of what is now called Meissner's plexus—originally met with skepticism and sharp criticism from the profession. In his pamphlet Auerbach announced that he had found, in addition to Meissner's plexus, "another very interesting ganglio-nervous stratum to be present in the wall of the intestines of birds and mammals," rich in nerve connections, ganglia, and single ganglionic cells. This plexus is present all over the intestinal canal, from the pylorus to the rectum, in a continuous layer. Its position in the muscles of the intestines is precisely between the circular muscles and the longitudinal muscles. Wherever the colon lacks longitudinal muscles, the nerve plexus is on the outside of the ring muscles, just beneath the peritoneal cover.

When Auerbach's pamphlet was issued, he had already investigated the following species of animals: pigeon, chicken, sparrow, rabbit (where for the first time he also confirmed the existence of Meissner's plexus), and man. He gives an exact and detailed histological description of this stratum, calling it plexus myentericus.

Auerbach was also aware of the physiological importance of his discovery. He emphasized, on page 12 of his first publication, that the nerve fibers of the plexus terminate in the muscle layer of the intestines and have as their purpose to initiate their contractions. It sounds very modern, when he states:

> Because unbiased physiological observation has for a long time already hinted that the peculiar form of peristaltic movement of the intestines is caused by intrinsic, so to say automatically working, sources of excitation, which are in a certain sense independent of the cerebro-spinal center, the successive and slow transmission of excitation is conducted from each point of the intestines in both directions. Therefore nothing is more obvious than to ascribe this function to the ganglia which I have discovered in the musculature.

He is of the opinion that Meissner's plexus rules the contractibility of muscular fibers in the mucose membrane and serves trophic and vegetative functions.

Auerbach's discovery was made at a time when the masters of anatomy and histology had already investigated with their pupils, so to say, every square millimeter of the human body. It made Auerbach the equal, in histological skill, of his teacher Remak, of Koelliker, Virchow, and others. Through his discoveries it was shown for the first time that the major portion of the intestines is connected by and probably is under the functional control of what we call today the autonomic nervous system.

Already on September 19, 1862, at the thirty-seventh meeting of German scientists and physicians in Carlsbad, Auerbach was able to add to his previous findings the new fact that a similar plexus myentericus can also be found in the stomach. His discovery was soon confirmed by Koelliker, by H. Frey, and others.

PRIVATDOZENT IN BRESLAU

The reputation Auerbach had gained mainly through his discovery of the myenteric nerve plexus brought him one of the rare recognitions he received during his lifetime. In 1863 he was admitted as lecturer (Privatdozent) to the medical faculty of the University of Breslau. At that time his more fortunate friend,

Ferdinand Cohn, was already assistant professor (*extraordinarius*) on the philosophical faculty at the same University. No salary was connected with the position of Privatdozent, nor did a laboratory go with it nor a right to receive help for scientific work. All that it brought was the right to announce lectures on a subject, agreed upon by the head of the department and by the faculty, and a slight expectancy of promotion in an academic career. For an unbaptized Jew this expectation was extremely slight indeed, regardless of his scientific achievements and teaching ability. In order to be admitted as Privatdozent Auerbach had to submit a special thesis and defend it in public against any objections that might be made. This he did on May 5, 1863. The subject of this thesis was "the muscular stomach of birds." This thesis contains an exact anatomy and comparative anatomy of the stomach of birds, with special reference to the nervous plexus in it.

DE VENTRICULO CARNOSO AVIUM.

SCRIPSIT

ET

IN ALMA LITERARUM UNIVERSITATE VIADRINA

GRATIOSI MEDICORUM ORDINIS

AUCRORITATE

AD

IMPETRANDAM DOCENDI VENIAM

DIE V. MENSIS MAJI MDCCCLXIII

H. L. Q. C.

PUBLICE DEFENDET

LEOPOLDUS AUERBACH

MED. ET CHIR. DR.

ASSUMTO SOCIO:

PHIL. STEUER, DR. MED.

OPPONENTIBUS:

HERM. COHN, DR. PHIL. ET MED.

GUIL. AL. FREUND, DR. MED PR. DOC.

FERD. COHN, DR. PHIL. PROF. P. E.

VRATISLAVIAE,

TYPIS GRASSII, BARTHII ET SOCII (W. FRIEDRICH).

FIG. 65. Title page of the Thesis of L. Auerbach to become lecturer at the University of Breslau.

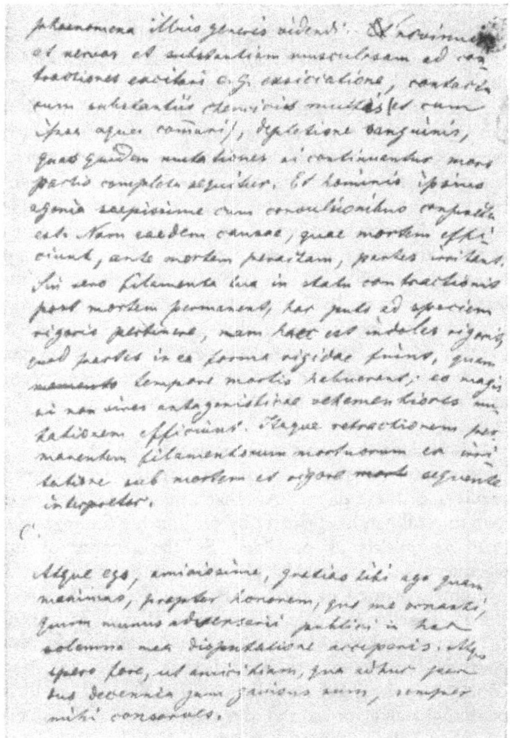

FIG. 66. Outline of the disputation remarks, written by Auerbach in Latin on the last pages of his personal copy of the thesis. Last paragraph presents his answer to the opponent Ferdinand Cohn (C.). In the author's possession.

Auerbach submitted a request to the Minister of Education for permission to write this thesis and discuss it in the German language, but this unusual request was refused on February 2, 1863 by the Prussian Minister of Instruction and Medicine (Minister der Geistlichen, Unterrichts-und Medizinal Angelegenheiten). Consequently, the thesis had to be printed and the discussion held in Latin. Auerbach's three official opponents were his friends Herman Cohn, Ph.D. and M.D., William A. Freund, M.D. and Privatdozent, and Ferdinand Cohn, Ph.D. and Professor Extraordinarius.

Auerbach's own copy of the thesis contains eight pages in his own handwriting with the main points to be defended in Latin. The last passage is the Latin acknowledgment directed to Ferdinand Cohn, which conveys something of the relationship between the two friends. It reads in translation:

I am extremely grateful to you, my best friend, for the honor that you have agreed to bear the burden of being officially appointed in this solemn disputation. I hope that

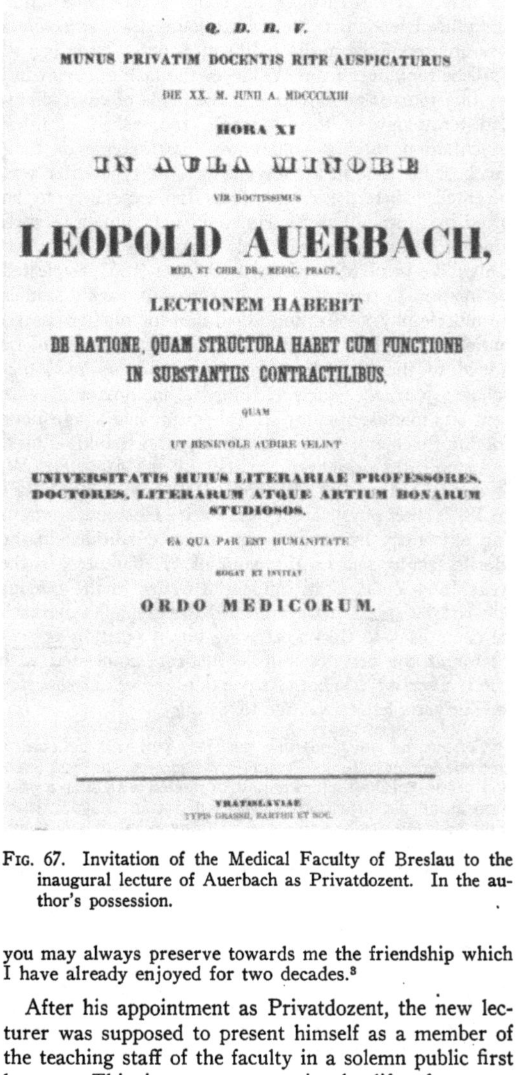

Q. D. B. V.

MUNUS PRIVATIM DOCENTIS RITE AUSPICATURUS

DIE XX. M. JUNII A. MDCCCLXIII

HORA XI

IN AULA MINORE

VIR DOCTISSIMUS

LEOPOLD AUERBACH,

MED. ET CHIR. DR., MEDIC. PRACT.,

LECTIONEM HABEBIT

DE RATIONE, QUAM STRUCTURA HABET CUM FUNCTIONE
IN SUBSTANTIIS CONTRACTILIBUS,

QUAM

UT BENEVOLE AUDIRE VELINT

UNIVERSITATIS HUIUS LITERARIAE PROFESSORES,
DOCTORES, LITERARUM ATQUE ARTIUM BONARUM
STUDIOSOS,

EA QUA PAR EST HUMANITATE

ROGAT ET INVITAT

ORDO MEDICORUM.

VRATISLAVIAE
TYPIS GRASSII, BARTHII ET SOC.

FIG. 67. Invitation of the Medical Faculty of Breslau to the inaugural lecture of Auerbach as Privatdozent. In the author's possession.

you may always preserve towards me the friendship which I have already enjoyed for two decades.[8]

After his appointment as Privatdozent, the new lecturer was supposed to present himself as a member of the teaching staff of the faculty in a solemn public first lecture: This important event in the life of an academic instructor in Germany took place for Auerbach at 11 o'clock on June 20, 1863. The subject of his lecture was: "De ratione quam structura habet cum functione in substantiis contractilibus" ("The Relationship between Structure and Function in Contractile Substances").

Once more Auerbach returned to his famous discovery of the myenteric plexus when he published a short summarizing survey in 1864 in Virchow's *Archiv*[4] and reported on this subject to the medical section of the *Schlesische Gesellschaft für vaterländische Cultur* (July 1, 1864). There he announced certain further findings, such as the discovery of connections between the plexus and the nerves of the mesenterium and some additional histological details. The report on the paper which he read on July 1, 1864 before the *Schlesische Gesellschaft* mentions that an illustrated monograph on the entire subject was under preparation at that time. However, it seems that this project was never finished. Nothing of this sort appears in the Bibliography of Auerbach prepared by his son Felix and published by Born, nor could this author trace such a publication in the literature. The responsibility of a growing family consisting of wife and six children, the problems of a busy practitioner, who as Privatdozent automatically was regarded as a consultant, the lack of laboratory facilities and of any kind of technical assistance and secretarial help, together with the burden of other duties, may have prevented this endeavor. Finally, new discoveries of importance apparently claimed Auerbach's mind more urgently than the literary task of summarizing old and—in the main—already published work.

DISCOVERY OF THE ENDOTHELIAL CELLS

It was in 1864 and 1865 that Auerbach's indefatigable eagerness for research was blessed with two further discoveries of high importance. Again it was microscopical research that yielded to the master a treasure not yet found by other outstanding experts in microscopy.

At that time the microscopical technique was already enriched by a method of silver impregnation devised by Recklinghausen, who discovered in the lymph vessels cell-like boundaries. He did not, however, see nuclei, nor did he find real cell structures. It was Auerbach who established that the blood capillaries, as well as the smallest lymph vessels, consist of flat epithelium-like cells, each having a nucleus. But while Auerbach was the first to make and to publish this discovery, the existence of endothelial cells of the capillaries had been postulated more than twenty years before by Auerbach's teacher Remak. In 1842 Remak had reviewed in Canstatt's *Jahresberichte* the progress of physiology in the year 1841. He says in a footnote on page 19 of his report: "Therefore the capillaries cannot be metamorphosed cells, but their walls must consist of cells."

The actual discovery of the existence of these cells was Auerbach's contribution. The same discovery was made independently and simultaneously and was published shortly afterwards by Eberth in Würzburg and by Aeby in Bern. Auerbach published only a short note on the blood capillaries, but an excellent and extensively illustrated paper by him devoted principally to the

[8] "Atque ego amicissime gratias tibi ago quam maximas, propter honorem, quo me ornasti, quam munus advertatione publici in hac solemna mea disputatione acceperis, atque spero fore, ut amicitiam, qua adhuc per duo decennia jam gavisus sum semper mihi conserves."

[4] 30: 457, 1864.

lymph vessels, appeared in Virchow's *Archiv*.[5] A report on the structure of the blood capillaries of the lungs in the *Proceedings* of the Schlesische Gesellschaft followed in 1865, and in the same year he presented his discovery at the meeting of the German Physicians and Scientists in Hannover.

About that time the progress of Auerbach's research work was again interrupted by his duties as a practicing physician and the lack of adequate help and working facilities.

In Germany, during the period of 1859 to 1871, politics, war, and the struggle for national unity and power affected each person's life. Auerbach, too, was involved, for instance, in the war of 1866, as lazaret-physician in Breslau. He was never permitted to concentrate on his research work exclusively. The opportunity to do so was only vaguely offered to him at that time if he could decide to move from Breslau to Berlin.

INVITATION TO GO TO BERLIN

To evaluate fairly Auerbach's achievements up to that time and to compare them with the achievements of other famous contemporary research workers, we must always bear in mind that Auerbach was left without any material encouragement or help in his work. The only encouragement he enjoyed was contact with his scientifically minded friends, including Waldeyer, the well-known anatomist. Waldeyer remained faithful in his friendship and admiration even when later he became professor of pathology at Breslau, and still later, when he obtained a leading position at Berlin University. In his research work, Auerbach was compelled to do everything himself. He had to clean his instruments, each beaker and each test tube that he used. Whatever literature he required he had to borrow from the libraries, in Breslau and outside, because the amount he was able to spend for his research was limited. He had to pay out of his own funds for material, instruments, chemicals, and books. His worst handicap, of course, may have been that his time had to be devoted mostly to his patients and, in order to be a scientist, he had to snatch at whatever opportunities presented themselves to escape temporarily from his duties as a physician. Furthermore, there were lectures to be prepared carefully, because, in Born's opinion, he was not a naturally good or compelling speaker as was his friend Ferdinand Cohn.

Other duties had to be discharged too; reviews had to be written for journals. He had been asked to take on the responsibility of this work by L. Rosenthal in Berlin for his *Centralblatt,* as well as by others. Especially after the outbreak of the Franco-Prussian War, when many of the contributors to the *Centralblatt* were called to military service, Rosenthal was in despair. He seriously considered discontinuing the publication of the journal and wrote despondent letters to Auerbach for help. It was through the cooperation of the latter and other friends that the publication of the *Centralblatt* was uninterrupted in those difficult years. Even before 1870 he took over from Waldeyer the task of reviewing for this journal publications in the fields of embryology and teratology. Other journals, too, asked him for contributions and a voluminous correspondence took much of his time in the days before the typewriter was invented, when a secretary was too expensive to be hired by a practitioner. He could not indulge in such kind of luxury. It was surely gratifying to him when a man like Jacob Moleschott, in October, 1863, requested permission to reprint in his journal Auerbach's studies on muscle physiology, and asked him for further contributions as well as Auerbach's consent to have his name added to those of the regular contributors to Moleschott's journal. Zuelzer, from Berlin, time and again sent him manuscripts for critical editing and suggestions for improvement, a time consuming and thankless task.

Letters are preserved, written by the same Dr. W. Zuelzer, Professor of Hygiene at Berlin and, from 1871 to 1877, chief physician at the Charité Hospital, containing extremely interesting reports on conditions in the Berlin faculty and on the work of W. Kühne. In the year 1864 Zuelzer, an influential figure in the famous Charité Hospital in Berlin, tried to persuade Auerbach to come back to Berlin, offering him a position as prosector at the new anatomical institute connected with the University. What this position offered, as reported in Zuelzer's letter, was the following:

> Concerning your possible position, you will be able to get one immediately as Prosector, as soon as the first opening occurs. Like Lieberkühn, who started with such a position as an old practitioner, you will retain all your spare time and will not be hampered. In any event, if you would like to come here now, you can be sure of lecturing a profitable course in mycology for *Cursenten* [that means for graduate and post-graduate participants in courses in microscopy, especially those to be soon examined to receive their degree], and a *repetitorium* for students. It is impossible to promise more for the time being. However, I hope you will keep in mind the aim here, as I do. It will surely be of advantage for you to move to Berlin as soon as possible. Couldn't you come here for your own orientation? The competition here is heated, but here laurels also grow and life here has one advantage: one is strongly stimulated.

Expectations of this kind seem not to have been promising or reliable enough either for Auerbach or for his friend Lothar Meyer, whom Auerbach was supposed to persuade to make the decision also to leave Breslau for Berlin.

EVENTS AND HANDICAPS IN HIS CAREER

At the same time, Auerbach's good services were employed to influence Lothar Meyer, the famous chemist—who, with Mendeléev, is to be regarded as the founder of the modern system of elements in chemistry—to accept a paid position at Berlin.[6] In 1864 Meyer had just published his work on modern theories in chemistry, a

[5] 33: 340, 1865.

landmark in modern chemistry, and in 1869 followed his epochmaking paper on the *Nature of Chemical Elements* as the function of their atomic weights. After having studied physics and chemistry in Zürich (Switzerland), Würzburg, Heidelberg, and Königsberg, he graduated from Breslau in 1858 and became a lecturer there at the University. At Breslau he became a friend of Auerbach, who was only two years his senior.

Zuelzer at Berlin was very eager for both of them to come to the capital. Meyer, well aware of his own worth, hesitated very much, as his letters to Auerbach show,[6] to take a step in this direction without the assurance of a satisfactory offer, and so did Auerbach. The atmosphere of "heated competition," mentioned in Zuelzer's letter, is mirrored in his several letters [6] soliciting Auerbach's and L. Meyer's criticism and critical reexamination of the work of W. Kühne, apparently much decried at that time in Berlin. Such an atmosphere, without a definite offer of an independent position in the Berlin faculty, was not too enticing to a man like Auerbach who, like most of the Silesians, was a great local patriot.

This factor, too, may have kept Auerbach from accepting the invitation to move to Berlin, even though at Breslau conditions were far from ideal for him. A letter from the above-mentioned Lothar Meyer to Auerbach, dated November 8, 1865,[6] shows how unpleasant was the position of a Privatdozent at Breslau University. Meyer wrote on November 8 that one student registered for his classes on Monday and Thursday, and that he expected more to register, and therefore he requested Auerbach to reserve for him the auditorium in the physiological laboratory, which was used up to that time by Auerbach for his lectures. These were not pleasant working conditions. It was still less pleasant to read in a letter from Waldeyer, written in 1870 when some important discoveries by Auerbach were already well known and recognized, that he, Waldeyer, then Professor at Breslau University and chief of its new Laboratory of Pathological Anatomy, was extremely sorry to notify him that the suggestion of the faculty, submitted to the Minister, to make Auerbach, after seven years of lectureship, a Professor Extraordinarius, in other words, to award him the title of Professor, was not agreed to by the ministry in Berlin.

Despite the friendship of Waldeyer, dating back to the time in 1864 when Waldeyer was assistant and Privatdozent in Heidenhein's physiological laboratory in Breslau, and the support of the faculty, it took two more years before Auerbach acquired the prestige necessary for a Jew to be nominated professor in accordance with the ruling of the Minister, a long since forgotten man. The title of professor was bestowed on Auerbach on May 31, 1872. In the same year he was elected to succeed Waldeyer, as secretary of the Schlesische Gesellschaft für vaterländische Kultur. No salary or any special prerogatives were attached to the title of professor, but it was the highest rank ever bestowed upon Auerbach by the government, disregarding the very unimportant fact that he received the Rote Adler Orden (Fourth Class) from the Emperor, a medal of no great significance. On February 25, 1881, Auerbach was elected a member of the Academy Leopoldino-Carolina of natural scientists. While the Prussian Minister was still hesitating to bestow the title of professor on Auerbach, because as a rule a Jew had to offer more in the way of outstanding achievements than his non-Jewish colleagues before he could obtain half the credit from the Prussian Government, Auerbach was already well advanced in new research work, and a new fundamental discovery had already been made, fully evaluated by his friend Waldeyer, but up to the present not adequately recognized in the history of embryology.

[6] The letters are in this author's possession.

INVESTIGATIONS ON THE FERTILIZED EGG

The new discovery Auerbach made during those years concerned the problem of what happens anatomically in the fertilized egg with reference to the conjugation of the two nuclei, the typical changes of the position of the nuclei and the discovery of central radiation (see figure). In a letter of 1897 Waldeyer still mentioned how much he was impressed by the paper dealing with these matters, which Auerbach read in 1874 at a meeting of scientists in Breslau. Not until 1874 were the details of many years of research published in two little volumes. Like his first preliminary report on the myenteric plexus, these volumes were published by Morgenstern in Breslau. Auerbach calls them *Organologische Studien,* and here, finally, he presents more details on nuclei and on capillary vessels. These studies dated back many years. Especially in the second part, his findings on fertilized eggs and on the early stages of cleavage were accompanied by impressively exact drawings. The illustration giving the first stages of the development of the fertilized egg leaves no doubt that what the embryologist Born (4) says about the importance of this work is justified. "Auerbach laid the first lasting basis for the modern knowledge of fertilization, and it should never be forgotten that this credit goes entirely to Auerbach." The influence which this publication of Auerbach's, together with his detailed studies on the nuclei, had on his contemporaries and on the development of our knowledge in biology and medicine may be judged by a few quotations from outstanding experts of his time. First to be mentioned is Oscar Hertwig, who, in the following year (1875), published his fundamental first paper on the behavior of the nucleus during the cleavage of the fertilized egg (13). In 1873, shortly before Auerbach's papers had appeared, an expert like J. Heitzmann (12) had emphasized that nuclei, nucleoli, the network, and the granula in the cell

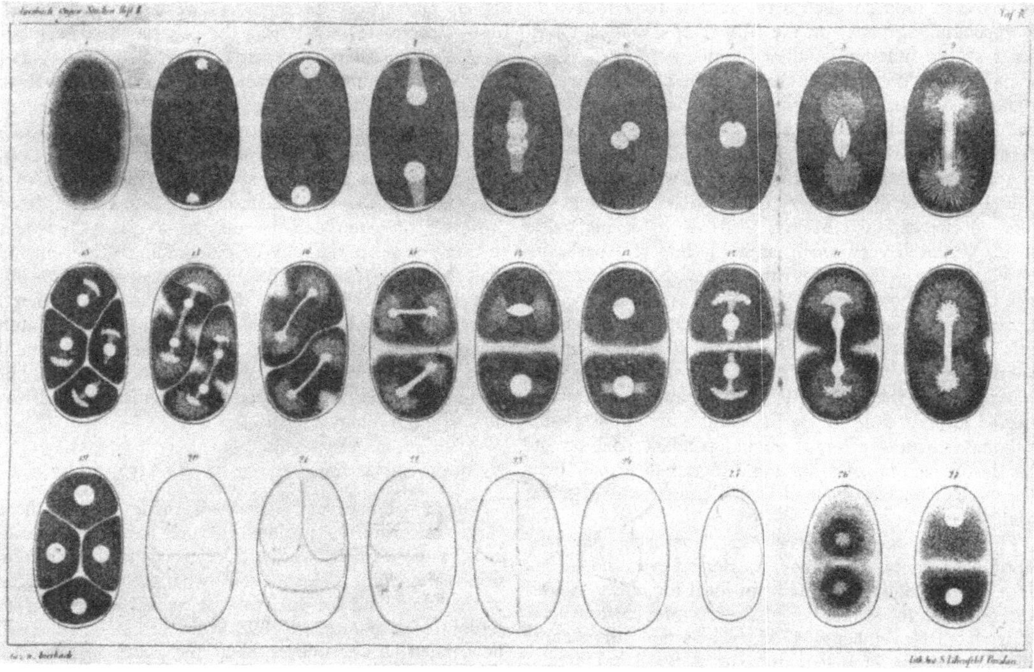

FIG. 68. Table with pictures of the progressive changes of the nuclei in the fertilized egg. Published by Auerbach in his *Organologische Studien*, in 1874. These were the first published observations of this kind.

were all one and the same substance, viz. the protoplasma of the living contractible matter.

Hertwig (13) characterizes Auerbach's work by saying in the introduction to his history-making paper:

> Auerbach has to be credited with the fact that he, through a number of systematically performed investigations, called attention to the cell nuclei and again aroused the interest of the investigators in this problem. In his "Organologische Studien," extensive material to solve the problem of the nuclei was for the first time collected and arranged under general viewpoints. Observations of former investigators were checked, remaining gaps were filled with systematically performed investigations. In this way Auerbach created a good basis for further studies and at the same time showed how much still remained to be done in this field, how many unsolved riddles waited for a solution.

It is to the everlasting credit of Oscar Hertwig's sincere character and noble personality that he begins the presentation of his most important discoveries with the confession that (p. 348)

> Auerbach's investigations also provided the stimulus for the herein presented research. The recently printed second issue [i.e., of Auerbach's *Organologische Studien*], especially, induced me to devote a stay of several months duration by the sea to further studies of the nuclei and the process of the division of the eggs of the animals.

On page 388 Hertwig makes the statement: "Comparing the results of my observations on sea urchins with those of Auerbach on nematodes, there is no doubt concerning the exact correspondence of both." Hertwig also confirmed—against the opposing opinion of Strasburger—Auerbach's observation that the nuclei of the daughter cells in cell division do not originate within the centrosomes but appear more centrally in the protoplasm.

A few years later (1882), Walter Flemming, another outstanding authority on cytology and a sincere historian of the development of our knowledge in this field, wrote his well known book, *Zellsubstanz, Kern und Zellteilung*. In the following statement Fleming, who himself played a leading role in the early development of modern cytology, pays his respects to Auerbach. "In his *Organologische Studien* (1874), he studied the influence of acetic acid on the nuclei, and he and (8) Th. Eimer were the first to see definite structures in the nucleus." On page 139 Flemming observes that modern knowledge of the nucleus starts with the work of Frommann, Eimer, Auerbach, Flemming, and Hertwig. "Auerbach discovered the existence of nuclei without nucleoli, and that in many cells the number of nucleoli changes periodically under certain physiological conditions. He saw the division of the nucleus." Flemming, too, gives Auerbach credit for having been the first one to devote a systematic, monographic study to the nucleus (1874). He regards as a long step forward Auerbach's objectively sound statement that formations ("geformte Dinge") are present within the nucleus. "Eimer and Auerbach," says Flemming, "were the rediscoverers of those structures, seen by Frommann, who was not aware of the importance of his findings."

But no less important was Auerbach's discovery of details concerning the radiating figures in the dividing cells. Auerbach observed the fusion of two nuclei in the fertilized egg (see fig. 68), though not realizing their true nature as the nuclei of the egg and the spermatozoön. He thought that both nuclei disappear (Auerbach's Karyolyse), and that the appearance of a stretched figure is only their residue (karyolytische Figur). On both ends of this dumb-bell-like figure he noticed radiating figures. According to Auerbach the daughter nuclei appear centrally and not within the radiating figures, as was later corroborated by Hertwig. This type of cell propagation Auerbach called palingenetic (palingenetische Zellvermehrung). Besides, as he emphasized, there also exists a direct division of nuclei as already found by his teacher Remak. Without any doubt Auerbach deserves credit for having first recognized the central role the nucleus plays in cell division and cleavage and for having called attention to this matter with his monograph.

That the fame of Auerbach's work soon extended far beyond the boundaries of his native country, can be seen from a review by the famous zoologist E. L. Mark, published (14) in 1881 in the *Bulletin of the Museum of Comparative Zoology* of Harvard University, in Cambridge, Massachusetts. Mark says in his review (p. 259): "Probably no single work in the past few years has furnished a greater impetus to the investigations of the structure of nuclei than the extensive and systematic observations published by Auerbach in 1874." Mark emphasizes especially Auerbach's statement that in the egg of vertebrates, articulates, and worms, the nuclei of the young cells are destitute of nucleoli in a certain early stage of embryonic development.

Knowing how inspiring Auerbach's work was to his entire generation and how highly esteemed it was by the most outstanding research workers of his time, it is sad to read the preface to the first volume of Auerbach's *Organologische Studien,* in which (1874) the meek but indefatigable scholar apologizes for the delay in completing and publishing his work, which was three-quarters finished before the year of the war, 1870. This delay was due mainly to the fact that Auerbach was never privileged to devote all his time to research and to enjoy all the assistance and facilities, the means and the personnel, of the laboratories that already existed at all the universities, where soon other scientists were able to spend all their time exploiting the results and harvesting the fruit of Auerbach's pioneer work in a virgin field of science.

DISCOURAGEMENT AND NEW RESEARCH

With profound bitterness Auerbach realized that a general practitioner, compelled to be at the disposal of his patients all day and night, cannot buy with his limited income modern instruments like those that now were already in every university laboratory. It became clear to him that in these conditions a free lance biologist or anatomist was necessarily unable to play a leading role in the rapid progress that medicine was making during the second half of the nineteenth century. At the same time the activities of his young, growing children filled Auerbach's house with gayety and excitement. All of this accounts for the fact that there was a lull in his research and a period of literary inactivity of more than ten years.

Not that Auerbach was idle or neglected research entirely in the period between 1874 and 1890, but his craving interest and research activities were devoted now to certain clinical problems. As early as 1870 and 1871 he published some papers on muscle physiology and reported a case of true muscular hypertrophy. In the succeeding years his attention turned repeatedly to this field, and in 1888 he published an extensive study on the mechanics of suction and of inspiration.

It was in 1889 that Auerbach received belated but nevertheless inspiring assistance in his research endeavors. His old friend Waldeyer in 1872 had become head of the anatomical department of the University of Strassburg and later Professor of Anatomy on the medical faculty of Berlin, and also a member of the Berlin Akademie der Wissenschaften. Now he was instrumental in providing Auerbach with an important loan from this Academy: a modern Zeiss microscope with all the latest accessories as well as a modern microtome. At the time Auerbach was already sixty-one years old and microscopic methods had changed fundamentally since the early days when he discovered the plexus myenthericus and the endothelium of the capillaries. However, with new enthusiasm and youthful eagerness he studied the new methods of using a microtome, of embedding specimens in paraffin, and of staining slices.

A new epoch of microscopical research began for Auerbach. First he studied the blood cells of the batrachians. A great deal of work was then devoted to the differentiation of various cells, especially their nuclei, by using various kinds of stains and, through Waldeyer's kind offices, the results were published in the *Proceedings* of the Berlin Academy of Sciences. The various sex cells (spermatozoa and eggs), in particular, showed typical staining differences. The data reported by him were differently interpreted later by different research workers, especially in botany, and urgently need evaluation from a modern point of view. Auerbach himself was led by these observations to his last extensive and excellent histological studies on spermatogenesis.

Here he discovered and correctly evaluated the conjugation of spermatozoa in an insect *Ditiscus marginalis.* Only one other scholar, Ballowitz, had ever before seen similar microscopic pictures and he had mentioned his observations in a few words without paying any special attention to the fact. This paper had escaped the attention of Auerbach, as well as of most other biologists. Auerbach saw in this conjunction of spermatozoa an implication important from the point of view of heredity. It restricted too great variations, thus safeguarding the constance of a species. A very modern idea.

This study, followed by various other excellent investigations along the same lines, was concluded with a monograph of 150 pages (1896) on the *Spermatogenesis of Paludina Vivipara.* This was Auerbach's last original publication. After it there was only one extensive discussion of a lecture by Professor Volz on the evaluation of remains of *Pithecanthropus erectus,* Dub., given on March 18, 1897.

In 1896 Auerbach lost his beloved wife. His only consolation, aside from his attachment to his children, was concentration on his research work. But not for very long did he have to carry on a lonely existence, after more than forty years of happy and blessed companionship with Arabella Hess. In July 1897 he fell sick. The real nature of his illness was never determined. After several attacks of a kind of septic fever, he died on September 30 of that same year. Even during the fever delirium of his last days, his mind was continually occupied with new problems arising from his last experiments on spermatogenesis (6).

FAMILY LIFE

It was gratifying to Auerbach and to his wife in their advanced years to witness the brilliant achievements of their highly gifted children and the beginnings of their careers. Two of his three sons were highly talented scientists, one a good professional musician. He lived to see his eldest son Felix receive his Ph.D. under Helmholtz at Berlin at the age of nineteen and his appointment as a Privatdozent in Physics at the University of Breslau; he was present at Felix's marriage to the charming and brilliant Anna Silbergleit; took great pride in his call to a professorship at the University of Jena and in his award of a prize by the Academy of Sciences in Venice. Auerbach was fortunate enough also to attend the graduation of his much younger son Frederic, a physical chemist who, in 1893, received his Ph.D. degree *summa cum laude* at the University of Breslau. To some extent, the father's fate befell this son: Extrinsic factors, appearing a year after his graduation, kept him for nine years far from any research work. From 1904 until his death in 1925, however, he worked as an outstanding member and imperial Regierungsrat of the Reichsgesundheitsamt in Berlin.

This biographical sketch of Leopold Auerbach should be concluded with an appreciation of his work and his personality, as given in a letter of sympathy written by his friend Professor Waldeyer in Berlin and addressed to Professor Felix Auerbach, on October 3, 1897. In literal translation it reads:

> I admired his unselfish love of research and work, which he demonstrated so splendidly by never getting tired and by starting very fruitful laborious research work at an age so advanced that any expectation of a material reward was entirely excluded. How many would have, in such conditions, decided indignantly to remain idle? Your dear father accomplished much more than many of those who have reached the goal of a full professorship. I remember his many investigations of primitive animals, of the structure of muscle fibers, of the endothelium of vessels, of the plexus myentericus—a discovery of high importance—of the fertilization process, where he, one of the first, observed the copulation of the nuclei, their position, and the radiation. I remember vividly his lecture on this subject at the convention of natural scientists in Breslau in 1874. I remember his *Organologische Studien,* and his studies on spermatozoa. His name will retain an honored place in the history of science . . Everyone of us could consider himself fortunate if posterity would only remember us in the way that it will unquestionably remember your father.

BIBLIOGRAPHY OF LEOPOLD AUERBACH'S PUBLICATIONS

De irritamentis nervorum studia critica. Doctoral Thesis, Berlin, Schlesinger Bros. 1849.

Über psychische Tätigkeiten des Rückenmarks. *Günsburg's Zeitsch. f. Med.* **4**: 452–496, 1853.

Über Encystirung von Oxytricha Pellionella. *Z. f. wiss. Zool.* **5**: 430–433, 1854.

Über die Einzelligkeit der Amoeben. *Z. f. wiss. Zool.* **7**: 365–430, 1855.

Über den Muskeltonus. *Jahresber. d. Schles. Ges.,* 1854: 7–10.

Über die Natur des Muskeltonus, Historisches und Experimentelles. *Jahresber. d. Schles. Ges.,* 1854: 32–34 and 127–130.

Über Muskelcontractionen durch mechanische Reizung am lebenden Menschen. *Jahresber. d. Schles. Ges.,* 1860: 134–140.

Über die Wirkungen topischer Muskelreizung. *Abhandl. d. Schles. Ges.* 1861: 291–326.

Über Percussion der Muskeln. *Zeitschr. f. ration. Med.* **14**: 215–231, 1862.

Über einen Plexus myentericus, einen bisher unbekannten ganglio-nervösen Apparat im Darmkanal der Wirbeltiere. Vorläufige Mitteilung, Breslau, E. Morgenstern, 1862.

Über einen Plexus gangliosus myogastricus. *Abhandl. d. Schles. Ges.,* 1862, and *Amtl. Ber. d. Naturf.-Vers. zu Carlsbad,* 1862: 202.

De ventriculo carnoso avium. Ad impetrandam docendi veniam. Breslau, Grassius, Barthius et Socii, 1863.

Fernere vorlaeufige Mitteilung über den Nervenapparat des Darmes. *Virchow's Arch.* **30**: 457–460, 1864; also *Jahresber. d. Schles. Ges.,* 1864.

Neue Beobachtungen über den Bau der Lymphadern. *Jahresber. d. Schles. Ges.,* 1864: 167–168.

Über den Bau der Lymph- und Blut-Capillaren. Vorläufige Mitteilung, *Centralb. f. d. med. Wiss.,* 1865, No. 12; also separately printed. Berlin, H. S. Hermann, 1865.

Untersuchungen über Lymph und Blutgefässe. *Virchow's Archiv.* **33**: 340–395, 1865.

Über den Bau der Lungen-Capillaren. *Amtl. Ber. d. Naturf.-Vers, zu Hannover,* 1865; u. *Jahresber. d. Schles. Ges.,* 1865: 157–158.

Über die Einwirkung des Lichtes auf befruchtete Froscheier. *Centralbl. f. d. med. Wiss.*, No. 23, 1870.

Schreibkrampf und Schreiblaehmung. *Jahresber. d. Schles. Ges.*, 1870: 172–173.

Ein Fall von wahrer Muskelhypertrophie. *Virchow's Archiv.* **53**: 234–266 and 397–417.

Organologische Studien, Heft 1, Breslau, E. Morgenstern, 1874.

Organologische Studien, Heft 2, Breslau, E. Morgenstern, 1874.

Zur allgemeinen Muskelphysiology. *Tageblatt. d. Naturf.-Vers. zu Gratz* 1875: 106.

Über erweiternde Wirkung der Längsmuskeln der Gefässe. *Nachtrag z. Jahresber. d. Schles. Ges. f. 1875,* vom Nov. 1877.

Zur Lehre von der Vermehrung der Zellkerne. *Centralb. f. d. med. Wiss.* 1876, No. 1.

Zelle und Zellkerne. *Beitraege zur Biologie d. Pflanzen* **2**: 1–26, 1876.

Über die streifige Spindelfigur der Zellkerne. *Vortrag, geh. in d. 50, Naturf.-Vers. zu München,* 1877; *Allg. Wien med. Ztg.*, 1–3, 1877.

Zur Mechanik des Saugens und der Inspiration. *Du Bois-Reymond's Archiv f.* [Anat. u.] *Physiol.*, 1888: 59–128.

"Saugen" in Eulenburg Realencyklopädie der ges. Heilk., Wien & Leipzig, Urban & Schwarzenberg: 2. Aufl, 1–8.

Zur Frage der wirklichen oder scheinbaren Muskelhypertrophie. *Centralb. f. med. Wiss.* **27**: 802–803, 1889.

Über die Blutkörperchen der Batrachier. *Anat. Anz.* **5**: 570–578, 1890.

Die Blutkoerperchen der Batrachier. *Verhandl. d. X. internat. med. Congress in Berlin* **2**: 72–76, 1890.

Zur Kenntnis der tierischen Zelle. *S. B. d. Preuss. Akad. d. Wiss.* 1890: 735–749.

Ueber einen sexuellen Gegensatz in der Chromatophilie der Keimsubstanzeh. nebst Bemerkungen zum Bau der Eier und Ovarien niederer Wirbeltiere. *S. B. d. Preuss. Akad. d. Wiss.* 1891: 713–750.

Über einen sexuellen Gegensatz in der Chromatophilie der männlichen und weiblichen Geschlechtsproducte. *Verh. physiol. ges. Berlin* **17**: 1–4, 1890–1891.

Zur Charakteristik von Ei und Samen. *Berl. klin. Wochnschr.* **28**: 908–910, 1891.

Über einen Gegensatz in der Chromatophilie der männlichen und weiblichen Geschlechtsproducte. *Du Bois-Reymond's Archiv f.* [Anat. u.] *Physiol.*, 1891.

Über merkwürdige Vorgänge am Sperma von Dytiscus marginalis. *S. B. Preuss. Akad. Wiss.* 1893: pp. 185–203.

Zu den Bemerkungen des Herrn Dr. Ballowitz. betreffend das Sperma von Dytiscus marginalis. *Anat. Anz.* **8**: 627–630, 1893.

Zur Theorie des Doppelfärbungen. *Jahresber. d. Schles. Ges.* 1894.

Spermatologische Mitteilungen. *Jahresber. d. Schles. Ges.* 1894: 11–38.

Zur Entstehungsgeschichte der zweierlei Samenfaeden von Paludina vivipara. *Jahresber. d. Schles. Ges.* 1896: 1–8.

Untersuchungen über die Spermatogenese von Paludina vivipara. *Jenaische Zeitschr. f. Naturw.* **30**, N. F. **23**: 405–554, 1896.

Discussion on Wilhelm Volz Pithecanthropus erectus Dub. *Jahresber. Schles. Ges.* 1897.

REFERENCES

1. Auerbach, Felix. 1918. Ernst Abbe. Leipzig, Academische Verlagsgesellschaft.
2. Auerbach, Leopold. 1849. De irritamentis nervorum studia critica. Doctoral Thesis. Berlin, Schlesinger.
3. ——. 1863. De ventriculo carnoso avium. Vratislaviae, W. Friedrich.
4. Born, G. 1898. Leopold Auerbach. *Anatom. Anz.* **14**: 257–267.
5. Cohn, Ferdinand Julius. 1847. Symbola ad Seminis Physiologiam. Doctoral Thesis, Berolini.
6. ——. 1898. Leopold Auerbach. Ein Nachruf. Breslau, Grass, Barth & Co.
7. Cohn, Pauline. 1901. Ferdinand Cohn. Blätter der Erinnerung. Breslau, J. K. Kern.
8. Eimer, Th. 1872. Zur Kenntnis vom Baue des Zellkernes. *Arch. f. Mikr. Anat.* **8**: 141–144.
9. Flemming, Walter. 1882. Zellsubstanz, Kern und Zellteilung. Leipzig, F. C. W. Vogel.
10. Freund, A. W. 1913. Leben und Arbeit. Gedanken und Erfahrungen über Schaffen in der Medizin. Berlin, J. Springer.
11. Grützner, P. 1902. Leopold Auerbach. *Allg. Deutsche Biogr.* **46**: 85.
12. Heitzmann, J. 1873. Untersuchungen über das Protoplasma. II. *S. B. Kais. Acad. Wissensch. Wien. Math.-Nat. Kl.* Abt. 3, **67**: 141–160.
13. Hertwig, Oscar. 1875. Beiträge zur Kenntnis der Bildung, Befruchtung und Teilung des Tierischen Eies. *Morphol. Jahrb.* **1**: 347–434.
14. Mark, E. L. 1881. Maturation, fecundation and segmentation of Limas campestris, Binney. *Bull. of the Museum of Comp. Zool. Harvard Coll.* **6**: 173–625 (see p. 259).
15. Rabl, Marie. 1906. Rudolf Virchow. Briefe an seine Eltern. Leipzig, W. Engelmann.
16. Retzius, G. 1900. Briefe von Johannes Müller an Anders Retzius von den Jahren 1830–1857. Stockholm, Aftenbladets Aktieboligs Tryckeri.

INDEX OF NAMES

www.ingramcontent.com/pod-product-compliance
Lightning Source LLC
LaVergne TN
LVHW081937200926
848484LV00009B/2449